Managing a Canadian Healthcare Strategy

Edited by

A. Scott Carson and Kim Richard Nossal

Queen's Policy Studies Series
School of Policy Studies, Queen's University
McGill-Queen's University Press
Montreal & Kingston • London • Ithaca

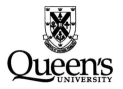

Queen's | Policy Studies

Publications Unit
Robert Sutherland Hall
138 Union St
Kingston, ON, Canada
K7N 3N6
www.queensu.ca/sps

R A
3 9 5
, C 3
M 3 6
2 0 1 6

Library and Archives Canada Cataloguing in Publication

Managing a Canadian healthcare strategy / edited by A. Scott Carson and Kim Richard Nossal.

(Queen's policy studies series)
Includes bibliographical references.
Issued in print and electronic formats.
ISBN 978-1-55339-502-7 (paperback).--ISBN 978-1-55339-503-4 (pdf).--
ISBN 978-1-55339-504-1 (epub)

1. Medical policy--Canada. 2. Health services administration--Canada. 3. Medical care--Canada. I. Carson, A. Scott, editor II. Nossal, Kim Richard, editor III. Queen's University (Kingston, Ont.). School of Policy Studies, issuing body IV. Series: Queen's policy studies series

RA395.C3M34437 2016   362.10971   C2016-902835-6
                                                 C2016-902836-4

TABLE OF CONTENTS

ACKNOWLEDGEMENTS

This volume is the product of a multiyear collaboration of Queen's University's Faculty of Health Sciences, the Queen's School of Policy Studies, and the Smith School of Business, in parallel with the Queen's Health Policy Change Conference Series. It would not have been possible without the support of Dr. Richard Reznick, Dean, Faculty of Health Sciences, and Dr. David Saunders, Dean, Smith School of Business at Queen's. The support of the University, particularly that of Principal Daniel Woolf and Chancellor Emeritus David Dodge, has been invaluable. Funding for the publication of this volume has been made possible by the generous support of the Joseph S. Stauffer Foundation. Administrative support was provided by Peter Aitken of the Queen's School of Policy Studies. Our thanks to our copy editor, Anne Holley-Hime, and to Mark Howes of the Publications Unit of the Queen's School of Policy Studies, for coordinating the publication of this collection.

CONTRIBUTORS

Owen Adams is chief policy advisor at the Canadian Medical Association (CMA), based in Ottawa, Ontario. Since joining the CMA in 1990 he has contributed to the association's research and policy development in areas such as physician human resources, health system financing and health reform. Prior to joining the CMA he spent 12 years in the Health Division of Statistics Canada. He holds a BA and MA in Sociology from Western University and a PhD in Population Health from the University of Ottawa.

Lisa Ashley is senior nurse advisor at the Canadian Nurses Association and current chair of the Chronic Disease Prevention Alliance of Canada. A registered nurse, Ashley has worked in leadership positions in acute care, home health, and public health. She has extensive experience in healthy public policy, program development, organizational planning, financial and information management, education, and stakeholder engagement. Ashley is an academic consultant for the School of Nursing at the University of Ottawa. She has published on a variety of topics in national and international peer-reviewed and other journals. In addition to a BScN in community health from Ryerson University and a Master in Education from the University of Ottawa, Lisa has certification in Multiple Intervention Programming, Health Management, and is proud to be CNA Certified in Community Health Nursing.

Talitha Calder is a policy analyst at the Government of Ontario's Ministry of Children and Youth Services. Prior to entering the public service, Talitha was a legislative intern at the Legislative Assembly of Manitoba, and worked as a research assistant and project manager with nonprofit organizations in Canada and abroad. Talitha recently graduated from Queen's University's School of Policy Studies with a Master in Public Administration and also holds a Bachelor of Arts (Honours) in Political Science and International Development Studies from McGill University where she was a Loran Scholar.

Dr. A. Scott Carson is the Stauffer-Dunning chair of Policy Studies and executive director of the School of Policy Studies, Queen's University. Previously, he was professor of Strategy and Organization, and director of The Monieson Centre for Business Research in Healthcare at Smith School of Business at Queen's. Professor Carson's career has combined academe with both government and business. He has been a dean at two Canadian university business schools and the CEO of an Ontario government secretariat. In business he was a vice-president of corporate finance at a major Canadian bank. He is chair of the Board of Kingston General Hospital and has been a director of many other public and private sector organizations. He is a graduate of Mount Allison University (B.Comm.) and Dalhousie University (B.Ed., MA), and received his PhD from the University of London (UK).

Adam Cresswell is a former Australian national health journalist who served as director of Communications for Australia's National Health Performance Authority from 2012 to 2016. He was the health editor of the national broadsheet newspaper *The Australian* from 2004 to 2012, where he became a well-known commentator on health policy issues and won a number of national awards for his reportage. Before that he worked at *The Australian Financial Review*, and was deputy editor of the medical newspaper *Australian Doctor*.

Keith Denny is a director with CIHI's Research & Analysis Division. Previously, he was director of Research & Policy at the Canadian Healthcare Association, overseeing all aspects of policy development, research projects and advocacy-related initiatives, and a manager with CIHI's Population Health Initiative (CPHI), where he led the development of analytical reports and mixed methods approaches to policy analysis, and oversaw the development and delivery of education products. Keith has also worked at Toronto's University Health Network, where he led the planning, implementation and evaluation of community-based health education programs, and developed and managed interdisciplinary education programs. Keith has graduate degrees in library science and adult education and a PhD from the University of Toronto's School of Public Health. He is an adjunct research professor in the Department of Sociology and Anthropology at Carleton University.

Don Drummond is the Stauffer-Dunning Fellow in Global Public Policy and adjunct professor at the School of Policy Studies at Queen's University. In 2011–2012, he served as chair for the Commission on the Reform of Ontario's Public Services. Its final report, released in February 2012, contained nearly four hundred recommendations to provide Ontarians with excellent and affordable public services. Mr. Drummond previously held a series of progressively more senior positions over 23 years in Finance Canada with the final being associate deputy minister. He subsequently was senior vice president and chief economist for the TD Bank (2000–2010), where he took the lead with TD Economics' work in analyzing and forecasting economic performance in Canada and abroad. He has honorary doctorates from Queen's and the University of Victoria and is a member of the Order of Ontario.

Jay Handelman is associate dean, Research and the Commerce '77 Fellow in Marketing at Smith School of Business. He was the founding director of Smith School of Business Centre for Corporate Social Responsibility (now called the Centre for Social Impact). His research and teaching interests centre on ways in which marketers integrate emotional, social, and cultural dimensions into their product/service and branding strategies. This has led to areas of investigation that include the ways in which marketers interact with not only consumers, but also a broader range of societal constituents such as consumer activists and NGOs.

Réjean Hébert is now professor in the Department of Health Administration at the School of Public Health of the Université de Montréal. He spent 30 years as professor at the Faculty of Medicine and Health Sciences at the Université de Sherbrooke and was dean of that faculty from 2004 to 2010. He was the founding scientific director of the Research Centre on Aging in Sherbrooke and of the Institute of Aging of the Canadian Institutes of Health Research. From September 2012 to April 2014, he was minister of Health and Social Sciences of the province of Québec, Canada.

Niek Klazinga, MD, PhD, has been professor of Social Medicine at the University of Amsterdam since 1999, and has been coordinating OECD's Health Care Quality Indicator program since 2007. His research focus is on health system performance and the measurement and improvement of quality of care. In addition to more than 200 articles published in peer-reviewed journals, he has supervised 32 PhD students to date. Present engagements include board of trustees membership of a teaching hospital and mental healthcare institute in the Netherlands and a visiting professorship at the Institute for Health Management, Policy and Evaluation at the University of Toronto.

Monica C. LaBarge is an assistant professor of Marketing at the Smith School of Business, Queen's University. Dr. LaBarge's research interests centre around public policy issues in marketing and how marketing can positively affect consumer well-being, particularly in the domain of health. Previous and ongoing research projects centre around health promotion, charitable giving and non-profit marketing, as well as how vulnerable consumer populations cope with and overcome vulnerability in the marketplace.

Dr. Julia M. Langton is a health services researcher with experience evaluating the quality of healthcare in both the Canadian and Australian settings. In her current role as a research associate at the Centre for Health Services and Policy Research (UBC) she is involved in research measuring the functioning of primary care. Specifically, she coordinates research across 12 pan-Canadian teams of community-based primary healthcare research and is involved in developing primary care performance portraits as part of one of these teams (Transformation team). She also involved in a program of work using health administrative data to examine end-of-life care in Australia through her affiliation with the Centre for Big Data Research in Health (UNSW Australia).

Harvey Lazar studied at McGill University, the University of British Columbia and the London School of Economics from which he received a PhD in 1975. He joined the federal public service in the 1960s and held policy advisory positions in various government departments, with his last assignments as deputy chair of the Economic Council of Canada from 1986 to 1992 and senior assistant deputy minister Strategic Policy, Human Resources Development Canada from 1992 to 1996. He was the director of the Institute of Intergovernmental Relations and adjunct professor in the School of Policy Studies at Queen's University from 1998 to 2006. His research interests included fiscal federalism, social policy and, more recently, health policy. His most recent book, *Paradigm Freeze*, an analysis of why it is so hard to reform healthcare policy in Canada, was published by McGill-Queen's University Press in 2013. He is currently adjunct professor, School of Public Administration, University of Victoria.

Alex Mitchell is a doctoral candidate in marketing at the Smith School of Business at Queen's University. His research focuses on understanding social and technological changes in markets, and the ways in which consumers, marketers, and other stakeholders influence these changes. He has examined these phenomena in healthcare and social enterprises settings, and more recently in the emerging markets for 3D printing.

Kim Richard Nossal is a professor in the Department of Political Studies, Queen's University. He was the director of the Queen's School of Policy Studies from 2013 to 2015, and co-editor, with A. Scott Carson and Jeffrey Dixon, of *Toward a Healthcare Strategy for Canadians* (2015).

Dr. Chris Simpson is professor and head of Cardiology at Queen's University, medical director of the Cardiac Programs at Kingston General and Hotel Dieu Hospitals, and the past-president of the Canadian Medical Association as well as current chair of the Canadian Wait Time Alliance. He received his MD from Dalhousie in 1992 and did post-graduate training at Queen's and Western. His health policy interests include medical fitness to drive, patient flow, wait times and seniors' care.

Neale Smith is a study coordinator with the Centre for Clinical Epidemiology and Evaluation, part of the Vancouver Coastal Health Research Institute; and an adjunct assistant professor in the University of Alberta School of Public Health. He is a qualitative researcher with more than 15 years experience in public health and healthcare policy, and author or co-author of more than 40 peer reviewed papers. Neale holds an MA in Political Science and a Masters in Environmental Design (Urban and Regional Planning).

Peter C. Smith is emeritus professor of Health Policy at Imperial College Business School, London, UK. Most of his research and teaching has been in the economics of health and the broader public services, with a particular interest in the link between research evidence and policy. He has advised many overseas governments and international agencies, including the World Health Organization, the International Monetary Fund, the World Bank, the European Commission and the Organisation for Economic Co-operation and Development.

Brenda Tipper is a senior program consultant, Health System Performance, at the Canadian Institute for Health Information, Toronto. She has worked on health system performance assessments as a consultant to the World Health Organization. Previous consulting work with the Ontario Ministry of Health and Long-Term Care included development of a primary healthcare scorecard for Ontario.

Jeremy Veillard, PhD, is an executive at the Canadian Institute for Health Information, currently on leave with the World Bank, where he works as a strategic policy adviser for the health global practice. He is also an assistant professor (status only) at the University of Toronto's Institute of Health Policy, Management and Evaluation, and the past-president of the Canadian Association for Health Services and Policy Research. An expert in health policy development and health system reforms, he has extensive professional experience in Europe and in Canada. He was the vice-president, Research and Analysis at the Canadian Institute for Health Information (2010–2015), and the regional adviser for Health Policy and Equity at the WHO Regional Office for Europe (2007–2010). Jeremy has a PhD in health systems research from the faculty of medicine of the University of Amsterdam (Netherlands) and Masters' degrees in healthcare management and history.

Dr. Karima Velji is the vice-president for patient care and quality at St. Joseph's Health Care. Most recently, Velji was the chief operating officer and chief nursing executive at Baycrest, a global leader in innovations on aging and brain health, and was vice-president of patient care and chief nursing executive at the Toronto Rehabilitation Institute, now a program in the University Health Network. Along with her position as president and chair of CNA's board of directors, she is board vice-chair with Accreditation Canada. Cross-appointed to the University of Toronto and McMaster University, Velji is also a consultant to global sites, including in East Africa, the Middle East and Asia, for the development of quality care and academic plans.

Dr. Diane Watson became interim chief executive officer of Australia's National Health Performance Authority in February 2012, shortly after the agency was set up, and was appointed to the position permanently in June 2012. Dr. Watson is a prominent international expert in the field of health performance reporting, with previous roles including that of inaugural chief executive officer of the New South Wales Bureau of Health Information as well as management and senior scientist positions in Canada. In 2005, Dr. Watson was a Harkness Fellow in the International Health Policy Program with the Commonwealth Fund. She has a PhD in Health Policy, Management and Evaluation and Master of Business Administration.

Dr. Sabrina T. Wong, PhD, RN, is a professor in the School of Nursing at the University of British Columbia. She is the director of the Centre for Health Services and Policy Research, co-director of the BC node for the Canadian Primary Care Sentinel Surveillance Network, and the research lead, Strategy for Patient Oriented Research BC node of Primary and Integrated Health Care Innovation Network. Her research examines the organization and delivery of healthcare services within the context of primary healthcare. She is a recognized leader in research involving patient-reported quality of care. Her work contributes to informing practice and system level interventions that seek to decrease health inequalities among Canadian residents, including people who face multiple disadvantages in accessing and using the healthcare system such as those who have language barriers and live in poverty.

LIST OF ABBREVIATIONS

ABF	activity-based funding
ACO	Accountable Care Organizations
AIDS	acquired immune deficiency syndrome
ALP	Australian Labor Party
AMI	acute myocardial infarction
BSC	balanced scorecard
CAHO	Council of Academic Hospitals of Ontario
CCF	Co-operative Commonwealth Federation
CEO	chief executive officer
CFHI	Canadian Foundation for Healthcare Improvement
CHA	Canada Health Act
CHBOI	core hospital-based outcome indicator
CHST	Canada Health and Social Transfer
CIHI	Canadian Institute for Health Information
CLHIA	Canadian Life and Health Insurance Association
CMA	Canadian Medical Association
CMWF	Commonwealth Fund
CNA	Canadian Nurses Association
COAG	Council of Australian Governments
CPA	chartered public accountant
CPAC	Canadian Partnership Against Cancer
CPCSSN	Canadian Primary Care Sentinel Surveillance Network
DHCPR	Dutch Health Care Performance Report

ECHI	European Core Health Indicators
ED	emergency department
EICP	Enhancing Interdisciplinary Collaboration in Primary Healthcare
EPF	Established Programs Financing
ER	emergency room
EU	European Union
FFS	fee-for-service
FPT	federal/provincial/territorial
GP	general practitioner
HCC	Health Council of Canada
HCIWG	Health Care Innovation Working Group
HCT	Health Care Transformation
HEAL	Health Action Lobby
HIDSA	Hospital Insurance and Diagnostic Services Act
HiT	Health Systems in Transition (EU)
HIT	Health Information Technology
HSMR	hospital standardized mortality ratio
HSPA	health system performance assessment
ICES	Institute for Clinical Evaluative Sciences (Ontario)
IHI	Institute for Healthcare Improvement
LHIN	Local Health Integration Networks (Ontario)
MBA	master of business administration
MCA	Medical Care Act, 1966
MIS	management information systems
MRI	magnetic resonance imaging
NDP	New Democratic Party
NEC	National Expert Commission (CNA)
NFP	not-for-profit
NHHRC	National Health and Hospitals Reform Commission (Australia)
NHPA	National Health Performance Authority (Australia)
NHS	National Health Service (UK)
NICE	National Institute of Health and Care Excellence (UK)
NPM	New Public Management
NSW	New South Wales
NWAU	national weighted activity unit (Australia)
OECD	Organisation for Economic Co-operation and Development
P3	public private partnership
P4P	pay-for-performance
PAF	Performance and Accountability Framework
pCPA	pan-Canadian Pharmaceutical Alliance
PHAC	Public Health Agency of Canada

PHC	primary healthcare
PHCTF	Primary Health Care Transition Fund
PPP	purchasing power parity
PQ	Parti Québécois
PREMs	patient-reported experience measures
PROMs	patient-reported outcome measures
RHA	regional health authority
SARS	severe acute respiratory syndrome
SHA	System of Health Accounts (OECD)
SPOR	Strategy for Patient-Oriented Research
TFSA	Tax-Free Savings Account
UK	United Kingdom
US	United States
WTO	World Health Organization

Introduction

MANAGING A CANADIAN HEALTHCARE STRATEGY

A. Scott Carson

Managing a Canadian Healthcare Strategy is a companion volume to *Toward a Healthcare Strategy for Canadians* (Montreal & Kingston: McGill-Queen's University Press, 2015). Both collections of essays by distinguished Canadian and international scholars and healthcare leaders resulted from a three-part conference series organized by Queen's University entitled the Queen's Health Policy Change Conference Series that was held in Toronto between 2013 and 2015. There are two major differences between our approach and other contributions to the healthcare reform discussion in Canada.

First, these volumes draw on a particular blend of contributors: our contributors come not only from government, academia and the healthcare sector, but also from business. Management academics who specialize in strategy, economics, data-analytics, and marketing, can give fresh perspectives to the health system debate. Analyses of industry, as well as institutional levels of strategy, are central to their discipline, so we can gain insights into our healthcare system by looking at it in terms of the models and frameworks drawn from management thinking. Further, international participants have brought to us valuable lessons-learned from their own reform processes. It is not turnkey solutions they provide, but rather insights that can lead us to see potential alternatives, effective processes, and unexpected outcomes.

Second, our approach is pan-Canadian in scope. Canadians are typically sty-

Managing a Canadian Healthcare Strategy, edited by A. Scott Carson and Kim Richard Nossal. Montreal and Kingston: McGill-Queen's University Press, Queen's Policy Studies Series. © 2016 The School of Policy Studies, Queen's University at Kingston. All rights reserved.

mied by the politics of reform. Because healthcare governance, administration and delivery come under provincial/territorial authority, it is an unquestioned assumption that there can be no overarching Canadian strategy. As a consequence, few observers take seriously the idea that we could, or even should, have a system-wide strategy that brings together the many jurisdictional and crosscutting foundational strategies (e.g., electronic health records and health human resources) into a comprehensive and coherent framework has been not taken seriously. Cynics think that ideological commitments to jurisdictional rights will foreclose any legitimate discussion about a Canadian strategy; skeptics presume that a lack of political will among the federal, provincial and territorial government leaders would make a common strategic framework impossible to achieve. So the debate about a Canadian system-wide strategy never gets started.

Canadians should not allow themselves to be put off by the naysayers. A system-wide strategy means neither that provincial/territorial rights are denied, nor that provinces/territories cannot pursue individual strategies that meet the needs of their own populations. Rather, it posits that we could be more sustainable, efficient and effective if we aligned the provincial/territorial strategies with each other, focused them on common problems and knit them together into a comprehensive and coherent whole. Indeed, throughout world history independent political bodies have formed federations, confederations, alliances, and constellations to pursue common objectives. Is it so unthinkable that Canadian provinces and territories, in conjunction with the federal government, could establish a unified strategy that they collectively would oversee but individually administer and deliver?

Our primary rationale for unity in Canadian healthcare should be performance-based. At present, our healthcare system—the aggregation of the federal/provincial/territorial systems—is one of the most expensive among developed countries. In fact, the cost of Canada's healthcare system is about 30 percent higher than the Organisation for Economic Co-operation and Development (OECD) average, yet its performance across the standard measures of health system performance—efficiency, effectiveness, access, and equity—is mediocre at best. Even this is a generous assessment by some accounts. For instance, a Commonwealth Fund study (2014), places Canada second to last in an eleven-country comparison.

Influential stakeholders such as the Canadian Medical Association (CMA) and Canadian Nurses Association (CNA) have been advocating for national strategies in wait times, pharmacare, and seniors' care. And even cynics should agree that pan-Canadian strategies and administrative structures can work; certainly benefits but not harms have been created by, for example, the Canadian Blood Services and Canadian Institute for Health Information (CIHI). As for the skeptics, we could point to the Australian experience, namely that of a country with a similar political structure to ours, which established unified national primary care and performance reporting strategies. Perhaps a hopeful sign at the time of writing (January 2016) is that the *Report of the Advisory*

Panel on Healthcare Innovation (Naylor Report, 2015) which called for a national innovation fund and a national agency to promote innovation (known as the "zombie report" for the lack of attention to it given by the previous federal government) is now being discussed at a meeting between the federal minister of health, Jane Philpott, and her provincial/territorial counterparts. And the Queen's Health Policy Change Conference, scheduled for June 2016 on Canadian healthcare innovation, will begin with Dr. David Naylor as its opening speaker. These are positive early steps.

It must be kept in mind that just having any strategy is not enough to improve the performance of Canadian healthcare. We need an *effective* strategy. The test of such a strategy would be both the extent to which it leads to improvements in our own system's performance as measured by internationally accepted standards of quality, and how over time we improve our performance-ranking in comparison with our OECD peer countries. Of course we do have strategies in Canada today. The problem is that we have federal, provincial and territorial governments, each with its own strategy. This fragmentation inhibits the achievement of system-wide cost efficiencies, performance effectiveness through shared innovations and the collection of standardized management data to assess performance and manage progress.

Part of what stymies the debate about Canadian strategy is confusion about what such a strategy means, or could mean. To be fair, there are many different terms being used without much clarity as to what they entail and how they differ from one another. For instance, does a Canadian strategy mean a "federal strategy," "national strategy," "pan-Canadian strategy," "system-wide strategy," "strategy-of-strategies," or what? As a result of this ambiguity, outright dismissal of a made-in-Canada strategy is often based on meaning: it means different things to different people. The first volume, *Toward a Healthcare Strategy for Canadians*, sought to address this issue head-on by sketching in detail a possible form, governance, and content of a Canadian healthcare strategy.

Managing a Canadian Healthcare Strategy builds on this framework. It is organized in four sections. Part I, "From Performance Measurement to Management," starts where the preceding book left off. If a Canadian balanced scorecard, or something like it, is needed in order to translate the goals and objectives of a pan-Canadian, system-wide strategy into concrete plans with measurable targeted outputs, then how could we use this scorecard to manage the system? The answer is that system-management requires reliable information. But it is not enough just to have data: it must actually be used to manage— to make decisions. So the first section of the book contains three chapters that start with CIHI's framework and rationale for a balanced scorecard, a robust program of system data gathering and analysis and system management. An extensive account of how Australia's reforms dealt with these issues is next. This is followed by an international comparison of four countries with each other, and then those four with Canada. Part II, "Patients as Active Participants," extends the discussion of data and analysis to make the case for the importance of patient input in performance management. Further, the management of the healthcare system must now adjust to the new dynamic of patient-centred care and the active role of the patient in it. Part III, "Stakeholders as Agents of Change," addresses the expanded role of stakeholders in the process of reform within our system. The business community is usually viewed as being only in a contractual relationship with providers; however, greater opportunity for health system innovation exists in partnership and strategic alliance relationships. Part IV, "Moving Healthcare Reform Forward" goes beyond the usual statement of barriers to change by pointing out possible future scenarios for Canadian healthcare reform. As well, it details the enabling conditions and necessary steps for change.

FROM PERFORMANCE MEASUREMENT TO MANAGEMENT

In Chapter 1, Jeremy Veillard, Keith Denny, Brenda Tipper, and Niek Klazinga bring the important perspective of the Canadian Institute for Health Information (CIHI), Canada's premier source for population health data and analysis. They point out that in the health sector there has been dramatic growth over the past 25 years in the use of performance measurement and reporting. Contributing to this has been pressure to contain costs, public demand of access to medical information, public accountability imperatives, and advances in information technology. The internationalization of reporting data has led to comparisons and rankings of countries with the consequence that "Linking performance measurement with strategic goals on the performance of the healthcare system as a whole, or the services of which it consists, is increasingly seen as a key driver towards better results." In Canada, the good news is that each of the provinces has defined its own strategic priorities and related performance indicators; the bad news is that there is no common set of indicators for the whole country, even after 15 years of trying to develop them.

The problem is not an absence of participants in the data-gathering landscape. Contributors include federal and provincial governments, government agencies, a myriad of pan-Canadian organizations, and international organizations, such as the OECD, the World Health Organization (WHO), and Commonwealth Fund. And as Veillard et al. note, "A growing body of research indicates that the use of strategy-based performance management tools in the public sector can result in substantial improvements in both health outcomes and cost-effectiveness." What is missing in Canada is an environment conducive to system-level performance management and a desire on the part of provincial health ministries to align health system design with strategic goals, resource allocation and incentives. The overall challenge is to reduce system fragmentation, duplication, and inefficiency.

The strategic integration tool that Veillard et al. promote is the balanced scorecard approach (BSC). Created by Kaplan and Norton (2005), the BSC approach links strategic objectives with measurable goals; targets are set and outputs assessed. The BSC approach recognizes the important causal relationship among the strategic objectives. And from these objectives is created a strategy map as a framework that guides implementation. Veillard et al. note that the BSC is conventionally used at an organizational level, but it can be adapted to an entire health system as was done by the Ontario Ministry of Health and Long Term Care in 2006. Indeed, as Carson discusses in detail in "If Canada Had a Healthcare Strategy, What Form Could It Take?" (Carson, 2015), the reforms of the NHS, England in 2013 were presented as a balanced scorecard. Like Carson, Veillard et al. believe that the BSC approach provides a useful tool for identifying and managing a system-wide strategic implementation.

Veillard et al. conclude that making performance management effective in Canada requires that we establish "shared strategic goals and objectives through the alignment of federal and provincial frameworks centred on the elaboration of shared health system priorities." As well, they propose a cascading set of metrics to provide policymakers with a system-wide view of performance that cuts across the sectors of care, and provide system managers and support staff with the tools to drill down into performance measures, such as hospital readmission rates, mortality from major surgery, or wait times for emergency rooms. In addition, it is this data that promotes cross-provincial learning. Finally, in order for Canada's fragmented health system to transition to a harmonized, high performing population health system, we need the engagement of Canadians: governments, provider organizations, policymakers, professionals and managers.

Chapter 2, by Adam Cresswell and Diane Watson of the Australian National Health Performance Authority (NHPA), an organization similar to CIHI, chronicles the Australian reform experience and the emergent use of data for system management. Cresswell and Watson describe the policy context and political processes by which performance reporting has increasingly become a driver of health system reform in Australia. Because of the similarities between the Canadian and Australian political systems, and state/provincial jurisdictional governance of healthcare, there are important parallels and lessons for Canada. As the authors note, over the past 30 years in both Australia and Canada, there has been an increasing demand for performance information and the publication of health statistics. While Canadians have focused more on data published by national agencies dealing with provincial-level performance, the Australians have moved toward creating a narrative about the relative performance of local health systems and the organizations that comprise them. With the objective of putting smart data in the hands of consumers, patients, and health professionals to understand better the health system and where action should be taken, NHPA reports on the performance of more than 1,000 public and private hospitals, primary care organizations, and local health systems. Cresswell and Watson outline many of the Australian reforms using this data for support.

The Australian path toward performance-based system management provides a useful case study for Canadians. The establishment of the NHPA as a small agency with independent leadership has been important to ensuring editorial independence, which has been valuable to building confidence in the integrity of the data and analyses. And the importance attached to the communications function of NHPA has led to a different mix of staff than in an organization whose primary role is health statistics analysis. Further, the task of data collection, analysis, and publication from thousands of health organizations has required significant automation. Finally, the NHPA has recognized that many of those wanting to improve healthcare sometimes value the narrative more than the health statistics alone. Indeed, the power of narrative has shown itself to increase the number and size of the audiences for performance information.

Perhaps the most valuable lesson for Canadians is contained in the tortuous political path of Australian healthcare reform. Jump-starting their process required the alignment of political will, public awareness, and a case for change. Canada needs all three. Dealing with the cynics requires the first of these; skeptics, the other two. In their detailed explanation of the path to reform, Cresswell and Watson show how all three conditions were met in Australia, even if imperfectly.

In Chapter 3, Peter Smith provides a valuable international context into which we can place the Canadian and Australian country system management discussions. Smith reinforces what we learn from the previous chapters: health system performance assessment (HSPA) is becoming a very important tool for system governance. Indeed, he says: "Since the *World Health Report 2000* there have been been several international efforts to promote the principles of HSPA, primarily in the form of internationally comparable report cards," (World Health Organization, 2000). A fundamental purpose of HSPA is using quantitative and qualitative indicators to make international comparisons between countries or regions, and even comparisons of a single system or subsystem over time. But HSPA has not been without challenges because there is not always consensus on how to incorporate health system functions such as service delivery, workforce planning, information resources, medical products, vaccines, technologies, and financing. Indeed, he is careful to point out the difference between analyses that can be used for health system guidance, and HSPA which is focused on accountability to populations, identifying priorities, developing strategy and tracking progress. The most commonly used categories with respect to the latter by agencies such as the OECD and The Commonwealth Fund are health status of the population, underlying health risk factors, access to care, quality of care, and healthcare resources. An important use to be made of these comparisons for countries such as Canada and Australia is that they can be a powerful instrument for reform by gaining both media attention and the interest of policymakers.

Smith provides a comparative analysis of Belgium, Estonia, the Netherlands, and the United States in which he summarizes the contrasting endeavours of each system in terms of their objectives, analytic frameworks and modes of presentation. He notes, for instance, that the focus in the Netherlands is on helping (or holding to account) the health ministry, while the other countries have the broader objectives of promoting transparency and accountability to citizens. The Netherlands, Sweden, and US reports focus strongly on health services, whereas the Belgians concentrate more on broader population health and equity. While there are commonalities among the reports, they reflect different target audiences and priorities. So the challenge is to ensure that when making comparisons between health systems, the performance indicators are genuinely comparable.

Smith makes this point again when referring to the chapter by Veillard et al. He notes the complexities that arise in a federal system such as Canada's where unitary provincial systems are compared. As he notes: "One of the strengths of a federal system should be that it facilitates experimentation in how services are organized, delivered, and governed." However, he goes on to say that in Canada "increased decentralization leads to a heightened need for standard information resources ... Such standardization can be achieved only at a national level, either through federal actions, or through collaboration between provinces." While not referring specifically to Canada, he makes a point that is applicable to us, namely that HSPA implicitly passes judgment on governments, which can lead to uncomfortable responses and controversial findings. Skeptics in Canada know this; but it is the price to be paid at the political level for reform.

Smith poses important and fundamental questions when he asks about accountability: "But who is to be accountable, and to whom? And how? Is it the accountability of governments to parliaments? Or of governments to citizens? Or of healthcare providers to patients?" The answers to these questions are central to the success of HSPA. This provides a useful transition to Part II.

PATIENTS AS ACTIVE PARTICIPANTS

An older tradition in healthcare system management, New Public Management (NPM), holds that system leaders—governments and provider executives—should manage stakeholders as being in a transactional relationship of providers and purchasers of services. Competing with this today is the patient-centred and citizen engagement approaches, which are characterized by engagement of patents and citizens in all aspects of improving system performance and quality of care.

In Chapter 4, Sabrina Wong and Julia Langton bridge the discussion of system performance assessment in the previous chapters to the role of patient contributions to both better system performance and individual quality of care. They argue that the transformative role of performance measurement and reporting should start with an understanding that patients define their own primary care needs and what they report from their experiences provides important information about the quality of healthcare delivery in the system. This contrasts with a provider centric transactional approach. They go on to claim that, at a system-level, strong community-based primary care (PHC), which includes patients' voices (including caregivers and family) leads to a more equitable system of care, with better population health outcomes at a lower cost. PHC provides not only system-level benefits, but also individual advantages because patients can affect their own quality of care by participating in treatment decisions. Doing so leads to a better understanding of their condition and increases their adherence to the recommended treatment. It also leads to fewer complaints, grievances and malpractice claims.

However, Wong and Langdon point out that while hospital-level performance reporting is growing, PHC reporting lags. Granted, there has been some provincial reporting, but the only significant national effort to date was a joint CIHI/Health Council of Canada population survey report in 2008. Wong and Langton go on to argue that system-level performance assessment requires creating a comprehensive performance measurement system by combining data sources that include the views of patients, providers, and payers. Unfortunately, the majority of indicators used currently in PHC are focused on the technical quality of care rather than on the outcome measures found by capturing patient experiences. While the method used to capture experience depends upon the goal to be achieved, Wong and Langton say: "Patients can be agents of change in the area of performance measurement and reporting by sharing their experiences through qualitative (e.g., stories, deliberative methods) and quantitative (e.g., surveys) methods that are used to collect information in a rigorous and systematic way."

Wong and Langton remind us that performance assessment is caught between two paradigms. The New Public Management approach, which emerged in the 1970s, depicts the healthcare system in terms of service providers and consumers in a competitive and transactional marketplace. Contrasting with this is the PHC, which emphasizes the importance of trust-based, long-term relationships between patients and clinicians. Stakeholders, they argue, need to be aware of the two paradigms in determining the purpose for which performance measures are used. Both promote different goals.

Chapter 5, by Monica LaBarge, Jay Handelman, and Alex Mitchell, starts where the preceding chapter ends, with the new paradigm of patient-centred care. LaBarge et al. explain that patient-centredness is a model in which healthcare providers partner with patients and families to address patient preferences. They note also that this has a moral grounding in respect for the patient as a unique person entitled to care on their own terms. They view the paradigm somewhat differently than Wong and Langton because they see the patient as a "consumer." Since patient dissatisfaction is prominent in the relationship between providers and patients, they look to the research literature on "complaining" behaviour to explain the new relationship dynamic and to propose ways for dealing productively with it.

Broadly speaking, complaining is a behavioural expression of dissatisfaction which functions as direct communication to a service provider by way of calls, letters, and word-of-mouth conversations with family, friends, and others. Complaining may simply be a way of venting frustrations or making small talk, but it can also influence the perceptions and behaviours of others. It can promote different ends such as warning others, obtaining redress, or gaining sympathy. This is important to healthcare providers because typically complaining takes place behind their backs, so they do not hear, or learn about, patient concerns. As patients reach out to broader audiences, especially through social media, this can further damage a provider's relationship with patients. Patient-centred care, however, can lead to better channels of communication between patients and providers. With this can come better patient outcomes: higher levels of patient satisfaction, interpersonal continuity of care, and greater patient compliance with treatment plans.

The result of patient complaining has relevance not just to individual patient advocacy, but collective advocacy as well. Enabled by digital technology, communication has been democratized: any patient is able to access not only information from everywhere in the world, but also to reach audiences and forums previously available only to an elite few. As LaBarge et al. comment: "The Internet and social media have given rise to a form of communication that empowers individual patients to connect to a network of social actors made up of individuals, small groups, and formal organizations, all of which present various narratives surrounding the nature of healthcare provision." In this new world of patient interests, perspectives, and experiences, the line is blurred between experts and the average person since they both share the same communication tools. The influence of social actors is less differentiated by health discipline-based expertise than social media competency. Importantly, "these social actors may not necessarily be driven by well-defined instrumental objectives, but rather by self-identity building projects, such as the pursuit of recognition for one's own points of view, and the corresponding social status that recognition affords within a given field."

What this means for healthcare providers is that they are not being confronted by a unified and organized activist group promoting a common end. Rather, in the democratized world of communications technology, the providers have become simply individual social actors having to navigate the diffused and complex social terrain comprised of many widely ranging social actors. Patients conduct and discuss their own research, which when combined with their personal experiences, creates a "local knowledge" that competes for legitimacy with "expert knowledge." Actions by providers to supplant or refute local knowledge by correcting it or educating patients will only further entrench the patient's dissatisfaction and further exacerbate the provider-patient relationship problems.

What LaBarge et al. argue is that providers need to understand and accept the new patient-provider dynamic and respond strategically to this. Traditionally, the healthcare system's "insiders" were the focus of organizational strategies. The patients, families and caregivers were "outsiders" whose expected behaviour was deference to insiders, namely to hospital authority figures—doctors, nurses, administrators, etc. This paternalism led to "inside-out" strategies. What is needed in the patient-centred environment is an "outside-in" approach to strategy in which a provider's leadership looks outside the institution to the interests and values of the stakeholders. Using a hospital case study, LaBarge et al. identify certain structural considerations for an outside-in strategy that is patient-centred: organizational culture that embraces the core principle of patient perspectives, integrated care across professional boundaries and, integration of patient voices into all aspects of organizational decision making.

In Chapter 6, Réjean Hébert complements the preceding chapters with a discussion of patient and citizen engagement, a coincident but broader concept than patient-centred care. Hébert takes patient engagement to mean the relationship between patients and healthcare providers working together to make both individual and collective healthcare decisions. He points out patient engagement is rooted in support groups such as Alcoholics Anonymous, AIDS awareness, and mental health activism, which have been effective in influencing health professionals and organizations to be more responsive to patient needs and to involving patients in the care process. Further, patient-engagement has application across the entire spectrum of healthcare: direct care, organizational design and governance, public policy making, professional training, and health research. In addition, he discusses three levels of engagement across each of the domains of care: consultation, involvement, and partnership.

In direct care, the patient can be engaged at the cognitive, emotional and behavioural levels: thinking, feeling and acting, respectively. The cognitive level is mainly in the form of consultation at which patients receive information. The patient becomes involved emotionally at the consultation level when he or she is asked about preferences in the treatment plan. However, a true partnership occurs only when consultation and involvement are extended to decision making between the patient and healthcare professionals. This can range from therapy groups that are co-led, to self-care using technology for the monitoring of patient information and communication with primary care providers.

Patient and citizen engagement can be achieved in the broader realms of governance and public policy through consultation using surveys and focus groups. A higher level of engagement is involvement and direct participation in which patients and citizens go beyond merely expressing opinions, just to express opinions, to making decisions about new programs or strategic orientations. As Hébert argues, "This type of health democracy is rapidly expanding in health organizations." Hébert also points out that public policy engagement can be understood as taking place at different levels in the system: macro (or governmental) level with respect, say, to program funding decisions; meso- (or health services and programs) level, such as in a provincial ministry; and micro (or local organizational) level in deciding about the rationalization of patient services.

An important component of Hébert's analysis goes beyond primary care to patient engagement in medical training and research. In his view, education is critical to changing the culture of medical professionals toward greater patient involvement and away from the hidden curriculum that perpetuates the paternalistic clinician and passive patient. Further, in research, the aim is not only to gain patient perspective in data gathering, but also to integrate patients better into the research process. They need to learn to be competent participants.

Hébert is careful to point out some of the limitations and pitfalls of patient and public engagement. While engagement is compelling in an era of personal autonomy, it must be sound from a scientific standpoint. He points to studies showing evidence of improved health literacy, clinical decision making, self-management and patient safety. But the main criticism is patient self-selection. As he puts it, "Patients involved in those programs are often more wealthy, better educated and highly motivated to be involved in the care process." It leaves out many of a society's marginalized citizens with the potential result that it affects the external validity of the studies and could lead to inequalities in healthcare.

Hébert concludes saying that despite these and other limitations, citizen engagement should be promoted. He points to its contribution to democratic processes and the positive contribution it could make to healthcare reform.

STAKEHOLDERS AS AGENTS OF CHANGE

Collaboration is the theme that underpins the three chapters linking system performance with patient-centredness and citizen engagement. The emphasis on collaboration continues in the two chapters to follow, the first dealing with healthcare partnerships and strategic alliances between business and government, and the second describing collaboration among the healthcare professions in their advocacy for healthcare improvement.

In Chapter 7, Scott Carson links health-system performance and innovation to achieving the ideals of a public system through collaboration between business and government. That is, the goals of social justice in Canada's public health system could be enhanced by the involvement of the business sector in healthcare, especially in the form of public private partnerships and strategic alliances with government.

Carson reminds those who have an ideological aversion to business participation in healthcare that the system is already 30 percent privately funded and that business concepts and management processes are already deeply imbedded in the system. Further, he distinguishes between the care of patients and the operation of hospitals, clinics, and other provider institutions. The operational side (e.g., finance, information technology, and human resources) is in many cases managed by many individuals with business credentials and experience, and that with respect to governance, 70 percent of the external directors on Ontario's academic hospital boards of directors have either business degrees or experience, or both.

Many Canadians believe that the self-interested underpinning of a corporate profit motive is at odds with the principle of fairness embodied in discourse regarding healthcare in Canada. However, Carson demonstrates that fairness, expressed in terms of access and equity, can best be achieved in a system that is functioning effectively, efficiently, and sustainably. Various forms of public private partnership—most especially, strategic alliances—bring business and government partners together in relationships. Important from the democratic perspective, is that in such partnerships the healthcare policy aspects are controlled by the government partner.

In order to promote the social goals of access and equity, Carson establishes a framework that is based on two primary operational pillars: resource allocation and growth. On those pillars there are six drivers of beneficial outcomes. Derived from resources are: (1) financing, (2) resource capacity and (3) expertise. And from growth are generated: (4) innovation, (5) learning, and (6) reputation enhancement. Acting in concert, these drivers can contribute to improved performance in the healthcare system that in turn can promote the social objectives of a public system. In terms of organizational structures to generate these beneficial results, what Carson demonstrates is that while government has a long history of establishing working relationships with business through various forms of regulation and contracting-out for services, the greatest potential lies in public private partnerships and strategic alliances.

Strategic alliances can be structured not only as a partnership among organizations, but also as constellations of multiple strategic alliances, partnerships, and individual organizations. In these more complex structures, democratic control could be achieved with a collaborative form of governance. Carson develops a model that he terms "bicameral governance." In this structure, separate but connected entities are created, one to oversee operational matters and the other a government entity to provide policy level oversight. To be effective, the operational entity needs to be independent from the government policy body, but it must operate within the policy framework determined by government. This structure can meet the tests of democratic fairness and of operational efficiency, effectiveness, and sustainability.

In Chapter 8, Christopher Simpson, Karima Velji, Lisa Ashley and Owen Adams show us that among the key agents of change in reshaping the national health policy agenda are the healthcare professionals themselves, and in particular their national organizations, such as the Canadian Nurses Association (CNA) and the Canadian Medical Association (CMA). In this chapter, Simpson, Velji, Ashley and Adams—all executives of key peak organizations—provide an extensive account of health policy initiatives which these professional organizations have undertaken through commissioned research, policy discussion papers, conferences, workshops, and meetings with government. Each organization has endeavoured to promote the triple aim approach of improving the patient experience of care, improving population health, and reducing the per-capita cost of care.

While each has independently advocated for policy change since its founding (CMA in 1867, and CNA in 1908), it is important to note that it was not until 1991, when they became two of the seven charter members of the action group of professions called the Health Action Lobby (HEAL), that they started working together. Since then, they have collaborated on many policy matters, including reduction in wait-times, creation of an integrated person and family-centred health system to enable better access for patients along the continuum of care, improvements to the social and environmental determinants of health, and pan-Canadian health human resource planning.

Simpson et al. describe what the CNA and CMA have done in concert and with other professional organizations, in terms of the substantive content of their policy recommendations. But it is not only their proposals for specific changes that have value. Value also derives from setting the groundwork for continuing policy research, analysis, discussion, debate, and advocacy. This is made clear when they talk about "creating an environment for change that results from building networks and relationships. ..." In part, what they think this requires is "collapsing power differentials" and "showcasing diversities." And the end toward which this is directed is "creating collaborative visions" and "building shared agreement." So, again in this chapter, as in the others, we see the important theme of "collaboration": not just what we should do, but how we should do it.

MOVING HEALTHCARE FORWARD

The final part of the book addresses both the process of change and what a changed Canadian healthcare system could look like. In Chapter 9, Neale Smith and Harvey Lazar examine the factors and conditions that could either help the process of pan-Canadian healthcare reform to advance, or could form barriers to system change. Specifically, they consider the tools available to the federal and provincial governments to enhance publicly funded healthcare and in doing so advance several scenarios in which certain types of change could occur.

Smith and Lazar provide a historical perspective by analyzing Canadian reform in two periods—pre- and post-1984. Pre-1984 was a period of innovation in which the policy agenda from 1945 onward helped to form the basis for the modern Canadian welfare state in which the symbolic capstone, Canada Health Act (CHA), was established. The agenda was impacted by political promises and election factors, but in the intergovernmental arena, provincial grants were the main tool for centrally directed change. However, in the post-1984 period, change has been incremental at best. Essentially, there has been consolidation and continuity with the reforms of the earlier period, and on-going public and political commitment to the CHA and the public funding of hospitals and physicians that are guaranteed in the Act. As Smith and Lazar argue, "governments have largely exhausted structural change such as re- or de-regionalization. There appear to be few prominent advocates of privatization or alternative payment plans, and there are vocal advocates for national pharmacare, but apparently little obvious governmental leadership, willingness, or commitment."

Smith and Lazar sketch five possible scenarios for pan-Canadian policy structure. The first possibility is the status quo, which presumes that change is slow and evolutionary. What they call the "Medicare plus" scenario involves incremental, but significant, change to the Medicare package in primary care, mental health, and catastrophic drug costs. This would require a more activist federal government and could entail greater federal transfers and new financial policy instruments such as refundable income tax credits. Collaboration and a willingness to navigate the complex terrain of competing political and professional interests would be needed. The third scenario is an enhanced egalitarian approach to promote the fairness agenda that would involve amending the CHA or creating new legislation to include the components of the Medicare plus scenario, and perhaps also to transfer funding and control of healthcare programs to indigenous peoples. This would be greater than any other policy change since the pre-1984 years. Scenario four is "technology-driven reform" that would see the policy agenda responding to the rapid developments in medical science and technology, especially in the areas of personalized medicine and bundled services. This is likely to result in expanded private financing of care reflecting some change toward private rights taking precedence over the social rights of citizenship. The fifth is public health emergency, which offers governments the opportunity to plan for future health challenges that cross national and international boarders, such as infections and multi-drug resistant "superbugs," such as Zika, Ebola, and others yet unknown.

Smith and Lazar maintain, in conclusion, that funding is the federal government's most effective tool for change. Commentators differ on the importance of federal leadership to effective change. Either way, perhaps the window for change is now open, whether through the leadership of a new Liberal government or new partnerships between those who wish to influence healthcare policy change. What this chapter gives us are some possible destinations that the process of change might reach.

In the concluding chapter, Don Drummond and Talitha Calder set out a strategy for government action to reform Canadian healthcare. Their basic premise is that consensus exists in Canada about the substance of meaningful reform, but political will to deliver is lacking. What is needed, therefore, is to create the environment for reform. Drummond and Calder suggest that a "national focus on health policy reform has some attractive features, such as supporting portability of care across provinces and territories, lowering costs through economies, and creating comparable standards for all Canadians." Moreover, they think that a national or pan-Canadian perspective is applicable in four areas: pharmacare, care for the elderly, healthcare innovation, and health information. However, they also maintain that in the current conditions the best prospects for change likely will come at the provincial/territorial level. That is, rather than a top-down approach, in which the federal and provincial/territorial governments agree and act on common standards, a bottom-up approach, in which best practices are emulated by others, has the greater prospects for success.

Central to the enabling conditions for change is communication with the public. This should start with a better definition of the problem, by which they mean that the fiscal argument about the unsustainability of the system needs to be broadened to provide an account of Canada's mediocre health outcomes and low level of efficiency. In addition, Canadians are conditioned to believe that because we have a public system, it is affordable for patients and their families. What needs to be better communicated is that the public nature of the system applies only to primary care and hospitals.

With respect to the process for reform, Drummond and Calder state that divided roles must be created between government and an independent body appointed by government "to provide an assessment of the provision of healthcare along with recommendations, informed by extensive consultations with stakeholders."

There are two aspects of healthcare that would have the greatest impact on the public. The first is a new pharmaceutical drug program in conjunction with the federal government and the provinces. The efficiency and effectiveness of pharmaceutical use could be improved by better data and analysis of the effectiveness of medications, and the sharing of that information with physicians and pharmacists. Second is seniors' care, which suffers the pressures of inefficiency, access, and poor levels of satisfaction by the elderly. In addition, there is the cost of long-term care services that will roughly triple in constant dollars over the next 40 years. A good starting point would be moving the focal point of strategy from the emergency departments of hospitals to community care settings. More broadly, a national seniors' care strategy could be moved forward if governments across Canada were prepared to state their goals, even if they were to be reached in different ways.

An important theme of this chapter is data and the use to which it can be put. Drummond and Calder argue that "Public policy often sets out lofty objectives but does not track their realization." Health data focuses on input and outputs, but not on the desired outcomes. If outcomes were more effectively tracked, and involved the perspective of patients and families, there could be better evaluations, hence more effective interventions. At the macro level, Drummond and Calder note that the Canadian Institute for Health Information (CIHI, 2008) is now making more cross-jurisdictional comparisons and that this should be combined with best practices from across the country which the Canadian Foundation for Healthcare Improvement (CFHI) is generating.

In conclusion, Drummond and Calder are optimistic: "It just takes a few more steps to create the winning conditions to get the public and stakeholders onside and then a comprehensive strategic plan." While they think a national approach is wise in some areas, a gradual approach with programs such as a national pharmaceutical plan and national seniors' care should be evolutionary rather than perceived as starting points.

CONCLUDING NOTE

Managing a Canadian Healthcare Strategy is based on the presumption that a made-in-Canada system-wide healthcare strategy is possible and desirable. Running through the book's chapters supporting this are recurring themes: need for system-wide performance enhancement, importance of data-driven management, legitimacy of patient-centredness, impact of multi-stakeholder change agency, and need for collaboration at all levels. Taken together, they create a picture of Canadian healthcare that is far removed from the provider-centric and unconnected structure with which Canadians are familiar. Change is inevitable, though. It is pushed by communications technology that has democratized patient information, and pulled by a growing public disquiet with the weak performance of our costly system. So we must ask ourselves whether we want to have a healthcare system whose direction is determined by the forces of change, or a system whose direction we determine by using those forces. The chapters of this book make a strong contribution to the latter.

REFERENCES

Canada Health Act, (R.S.C., 1985, c. C-6).

Carson, A. S. 2015. "If Canada Had a Healthcare Strategy, What Form Could It Take?" In *Toward a Healthcare Strategy for Canadians*, edited by A. Scott Carson, Jeffrey Dixon, and Kim Richard Nossal. Montreal and Kingston: McGill-Queen's University Press.

Carson, A. S., J. Dixon, and K. R. Nossal, eds. 2015. *Toward a Healthcare Strategy for Canadians*. Montreal and Kingston: McGill-Queen's University Press.

Canadian Institute for Health Information (CIHI). 2008. *Results from the Canadian Survey of Experiences with Primary Health Care (CSE-PHC)*. https://www.cihi.ca/en/phc_survey_cahspr2010_en.pdf

Commonwealth Fund. 2014. "Mirror, Mirror on the Wall: How the Performance of the U.S. Health Care System Compares Internationally." http://www.commonwealthfund.org/~/media/files/publications/fund-report/2014/jun/1755_davis_mirror_mirror_2014.pdf

Kaplan, R. S., and D. P. Norton. 2005. "Using the Balanced Scorecard as a Strategic Management System." In *Harvard Business Press Reprint* R0707M.

Report of the Advisory Panel on Healthcare Innovation (Naylor Report). 2015. *Unleashing Innovation: Excellent Healthcare for Canada*. Ottawa, ON: Health Canada, Her Majesty in Right of Canada.

World Health Organization. 2000. *The World Health Report 2000: Health Systems: Improving Performance*. Geneva, Switzerland: World Health Organization. http://www.who.int/whr/2000/en/whr00_en.pdf?ua=1

Part 1

MEASURING AND MONITORING A
HEALTHCARE STRATEGY

Chapter 1

FROM PERFORMANCE MEASUREMENT TO PERFORMANCE MANAGEMENT

JEREMY VEILLARD, KEITH DENNY, BRENDA TIPPER AND
NIEK KLAZINGA

There has been a dramatic growth in the use of performance measurement and reporting in the health sector in the last 25 years. In England, provisions for public reporting include Annual Quality Accounts for all healthcare organizations and an Outcomes Framework for the National Health Service (UK Department of Health 2011). In federal systems, the Patient Protection and Affordable Care Act in the United States (US Congress, 2010) mandates quarterly public reporting of performance information by institutions caring for Medicare patients, while in Australia quarterly and annual reports on health system performance are mandated (Council of Australian Governments 2011). The Netherlands has been reporting on a national healthcare performance framework since 2006 (van den Berg, Kringos, Marks, and Klazinga 2014).

Several factors have contributed to this growth in performance public reporting in the health sector, including pressure to contain healthcare costs, patients' and citizens' expectations of access to information, growing accountability imperatives, and advances in information technology (Smith, Mossialos, and Papanicolas 2008). International comparisons have added to this emphasis on performance reporting, especially in countries where international rankings have shown poor or uneven performance across a range of comparable indicators for Organisation for Economic Co-operation and Development (OECD) countries

Managing a Canadian Healthcare Strategy, edited by A. Scott Carson and Kim Richard Nossal. Montreal and Kingston: McGill-Queen's University Press, Queen's Policy Studies Series. © 2016 The School of Policy Studies, Queen's University at Kingston. All rights reserved.

(Commonwealth Fund 2011; OECD 2015; CIHI 2014a). Linking performance measurement with strategic goals on the performance of the healthcare system as a whole, or the services of which it consists, is increasingly seen as a key driver towards better results.

In Canada, most provinces have now defined clear strategic priorities and related performance indicators for their systems and/or services. For example, in Alberta, strategic priorities for government are supported by a small core set of 12 performance indicators covering the domains of health status, health system outcomes and health system performance (Alberta Health 2014). Yet there is no common set of performance expectations or performance indicators for the health sector that would apply to the entire country despite repeated efforts to do so since 2000 (Fierlbeck 2012; Fafard 2013). A recent effort of the Council of the Federation and its Innovation Working Group included releasing a common framework specifying key domains of quality of care (Health Care Innovation Working Group 2012).

One notable but limited exception is the joint effort undertaken in 2004 by Canadian provinces to reduce wait times for a small number of priority procedures through which provinces agreed to establish common, medically acceptable benchmarks and performance indicators for wait times in five areas: radiation therapy for cancer, hip and knee replacement surgery, cataract surgery, cardiac bypass surgery and diagnostic imaging. A third party organization (the Canadian Institute for Health Information) was mandated to monitor the provinces' progress. Interestingly, the addition of financial resources combined with independent public reporting, investments in information systems, innovation in payment systems, and initiatives to redesign care delivery processes and share best practices among provinces resulted in notable reductions in wait times and led Canada to become a better performer than many other OECD countries for cataracts surgeries and joint replacement surgeries (OECD 2015).

This focus on performance measurement and reporting as a key policy instrument is tightly connected to the emergence of performance management as the dominating paradigm in the delivery and management of public services. This movement is rooted in the influence and expansion of different waves of new public management and management by results since the 1970s (Groot and Budding 2008). Importantly, the concept of performance management is pivotal to different waves of new public management. It has been influenced by a variety of theoretical contributions from different disciplines, which can be grouped into three broad categories: neoclassical public administration and public management, management sciences, and new institutional economics (Groot and Budding 2008). These perspectives share the common objective of transforming public services through a greater focus on managing performance and service improvement (Osborne and Gaebler 1992). In the health sector, the emergence of greater demand for accountability and transparency since Codman's work a century ago (Donabedian 1989) has been an additional driver for a focus on performance measurement and reporting.

Still, although health system performance management has become an area of interest for policymakers, health system managers, and researchers, it remains poorly defined. We can build a working definition from the component parts of the term "health system performance management." The World Health Organization (WHO) defines *health systems* as all actors, institutions, and resources that undertake health actions—where the primary intent of a health action is to improve health (World Health Organization 2000). Although they vary throughout the world in their design and organization, health systems generally share the same core goals of good health, responsiveness to people's expectations, social and financial protection, efficiency, and equity (Smith, Mossialos, Papanicolas, and Leatherman 2009; World Health Organization 2000).

Performance can be defined as the maintenance of a state of functioning that corresponds to societal, patient, and professional norms (Veillard et al. 2005). Daniels defines performance *management* as a technology for managing behaviour and results, two critical elements of what is known as performance (Daniels and Daniels 2004) while for Smith it is a set of managerial instruments designed to secure optimal performance of the healthcare system in line with policy objectives (Smith 2002). In this chapter, our definition of *health system performance management* includes both the instruments and processes to improve health system performance (Veillard et al. 2010).

In this chapter, we review the state of affairs of performance measurement and reporting in Canada and how performance measurement and reporting could be better positioned to support the emergence of performance management as the paradigm for performance improvement in Canada's healthcare system.

PERFORMANCE MEASUREMENT AND REPORTING IN CANADA: THE INSTITUTIONAL LANDSCAPE

The healthcare performance measurement and reporting landscape in Canada includes multiple players, including provincial governments, their agents and other provincial entities, the federal government, non-governmental pan-Canadian organizations of different stripes, and international organizations whose performance reporting activities include Canada. Since 2004, the provinces have worked towards the development of benchmarks and indicators for wait times and all provinces now report wait time information publicly. Beyond wait times, progress across provinces in performance measurement and public reporting in general has been uneven. Most provinces report on health system performance to varying degrees through their ministries of health. In addition, provinces with specialized agencies responsible for performance reporting and/ or quality improvement (such as New Brunswick, Ontario, Quebec, and Saskatchewan) tend to have a well-established performance reporting function in place. These agencies produce regular reports on health system performance and health status at the provincial and, in some cases, the health region level. Health Quality Ontario, for example, was created in 2011 with a mandate to monitor and report on progress on health system performance following the introduction of the Excellent Care for All Act.

In addition to the reporting of provincial ministries and quality councils, there are additional health information and research organizations—such as the Newfoundland and Labrador Centre for Health Information, Ontario's Institute for Clinical Evaluative Sciences (ICES), the Manitoba Centre for Health Policy, and the University of British Columbia Centre for Health Services and Policy Research—that carry out research, analyze, and report on healthcare system data for their jurisdictions. The Manitoba Centre for Health Policy, for example, has produced the province's Indicators Atlas for Regional Health Authorities, which measures the health of Manitobans and their use of healthcare services. Cancer Care Ontario's Cancer Quality Council of Ontario monitors and publicly reports on the performance of the provincial cancer system.

The federal government is also a player in health system performance measurement, most notably through Statistics Canada, but also through Health Canada, the Public Health Agency of Canada, and Employment and Social Development Canada. Statistics Canada conducts the Canadian Community Health Survey and the Canadian Health Measures Survey, which are widely used across the country to inform the generation of performance indicators for the health sector. As the country's statistical agency, Statistics Canada has access to a wide range of data and draws on the census and other sources of Canadian socioeconomic data to report on health and healthcare.

The Public Health Agency of Canada (PHAC) Chronic Disease Infobase includes the Chronic Disease and Injury Indicator Framework, which consists of a set of indicators grouped within six domains, and the Canadian Chronic Disease Surveillance System, a network of provincial and territorial surveillance systems. Perhaps less known, Employment and Social Development Canada publishes the *Indicators of Well-Being in Canada*, which includes a section specifically on health reporting indicators on health status, mortality and influences on health such as health behaviours, access to primary care and patient satisfaction. Other sections include indicators on employment, education, housing, and social networks.

In addition to these major contributors to pan-Canadian health performance reporting, there are other national organizations that report publicly on health system performance. Most obvious among these is the Canadian Institute for Health Information (CIHI), created in 1994 to address what was then deemed the "deplorable" state of the country's health information infrastructure. With a mandate to collect and disseminate standardized, comparable pan-Canadian data and analyses, CIHI has since become Canada's lead agency for health system information and reports on health system performance at national, provincial, territorial, regional and hospital levels through its website http://www.yourhealthsystem.ca. In June 2015, CIHI publicly released a core set of quality indicators for 1,200 long-term care homes across the country.

Other organizations reporting on performance in specific diseases or sectors of health system performance include the Canadian Partnership Against Cancer (CPAC), specific disease-based associations, and private organizations such as the Conference Board of Canada and the Fraser Institute, both of which produce performance reports on the healthcare sector.

Finally, several prominent international organizations have health system performance reporting projects that include Canada. Most notably, these include the OECD's Health Care Quality Indicators Project, initiated in 2002, the World Health Organization and the Commonwealth Fund's International Health Policy Surveys.

A Proliferation of Indicators in Canada

Clearly, the performance measurement and indicator agenda has been adopted enthusiastically in recent years, producing a great deal of activity in the area. Strikingly, besides the general objective of greater transparency and accountability, the objectives and incentives related to public reporting initiatives in the health sector are often unclear or unspecified. The crowded field of performance measurement, marked by multiple players and a proliferation of indicators has led to a situation that has been described as "indicator chaos" (Saskatchewan Health Quality Council 2011). In practice, while a focus on measurement has taken hold and indicators have multiplied, from a big picture perspective, there has been an inadequate focus on developing an overarching logic for this activity to give it consistent purpose, common standards (in indicator development), coordination, and coherence, and to put indicators to use to stimulate performance improvement. A number of organizations including CIHI are now reviewing indicators published and retiring the indicators that show the least value for health system performance improvement (CIHI, 2015a).

Attempts to frame and strategically align health system performance indicators in Canada

Over the last 20 years, CIHI has worked in collaboration with Statistics Canada to develop measurement standards that enable pan-Canadian reporting of health indicators. In 1999, CIHI and Statistics Canada initiated a joint health indicators project that has since become internationally recognized. The indicators were identified through extensive consultation and developed primarily to support regional health authorities in monitoring progress in improving and maintaining the health of their populations and the functioning of the health system, as well as enabling reporting to governing bodies, the public, and health professional groups.

In 2012, CIHI launched a new initiative focusing its public performance reporting efforts on a small number of cascading indicators determined by a clarified health system performance framework and aligned with the strategic priorities of Canadian provinces. This initiative aimed to: stimulate performance improvement by reporting publicly on a small number of indicators aligned with priorities of the general public and of Canadian jurisdictions; focus public reporting instruments on the information needs of well-segmented audiences defined through various engagement mechanisms; and implement complementary analytical, research and capacity-building initiatives supporting the performance improvement efforts of jurisdictions.

A health system performance framework aligned with the main strategic objectives of Canadian provinces and territories (Figure 1.1) was designed to address questions about the quality of healthcare services, the health system's contributions to the overall health of the population and the extent to which our healthcare systems are optimizing resources.

This health system performance measurement framework incorporates Donabedian's (1966) framework for evaluating health services and the quality of care—the triad of structure (inputs and characteristics), process (outputs), and outcomes. It also adopts the three categories of the Triple Aim (Berwick, Nolan, and Whittington 2008) specifically for the measurement of health system outcomes: improve the health status of Canadians (in terms of health conditions, functioning, and well-being), improve health system responsiveness (the extent to which healthcare "meets the needs and expectations of the people it serves"), and improve value for money (the health outcomes produced for a given level of investment in health).

Taken together, the elements of the framework comprise a more holistic orientation to performance measurement and improvement and incorporate an inherent logic that was lacking in earlier indicator frameworks. The framework was used to derive a small set of 15 performance indicators aiming to meet the information needs of the general public and high level policymakers, then expanded to a set of 37 indicators designed for health system managers and covering more detailed performance information at the level of regional health authorities and hospitals. An additional set of nine indicators focused on the quality of long-term care homes were scheduled to be released in June 2015 (CIHI 2014b). Table 1.1, and the two quadrants which follow, provides a summary of the strengths and weaknesses of the Canadian health system based on an analysis of the core set of 15 performance indicators selected for the general public and policymakers, and presents complementary information on performance comparisons with other OECD countries and within Canadian provinces.

FIGURE 1.1
Canada's Health System Performance Framework, 2013

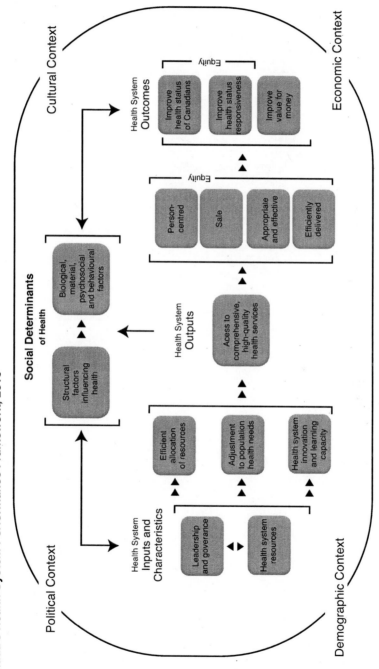

TABLE 1.1
Strengths and Weaknesses of the Canadian Health System

Dimension of Health System Performance	Canada Compared to Other Countries	Provincial and Territorial Variation Within Canada	Identified Indicator Development Priorities
Access to comprehensive, high-quality health services	HAVE A REGULAR DOCTOR 85% of all Canadians and 95% of Canadians over 55 have a regular doctor. These results are similar to higher performing countries in CMWF and OECD. However, having a regular doctor does not imply access when needed, with only 22% of Canadians reporting they could get an appointment the same or next day. Rates for Commonwealth Fund (CMWF) and OECD countries are much higher.	There is significant variation among provinces and territories in Canada, with many provinces having rates around 80% while others are well over 90%. Also, rates are extremely low (under 50%) in some sparsely populated regions of the country.	• Wait times for community health and social services, in particular mental health services for children and youth. • social services to support health of individuals with multi-morbidities and complex needs • home care and long-term care • Access to, and use of, palliative care and appropriate settings for end-of-life care

…continued

TABLE 1.1, continued

Dimension of Health System Performance	Canada Compared to Other Countries	Provincial and Territorial Variation Within Canada	Identified Indicator Development Priorities
	SPECIALIST WAIT TIMES In the 2013 CMWF survey, 29% of Canadians reported waiting longer than two months for a visit with a specialist, compared to the next highest rate of 18% for Australia and France. Some countries had rates of less than 10%.	In the Statistics Canada 2013 survey, 23.8% of patients in the province with the highest rate reported waiting more than three months for a specialist visit, nearly double the 12.3% in the province with the lowest rate. However, due to small sample sizes in this survey, there are wide margins of error in the results.	
	RADIATION TREATMENT WAIT TIMES No international comparisons available	Performance is high across the board and there is little variation within Canada on this measure. With two exceptions, 95% of patients in the 10 provinces began their radiation therapy treatment within four weeks. The two exceptions had rates of 88% and 90%. Wait times are not reported by the three Territorial governments.	

…continued

TABLE 1.1, continued

Dimension of Health System Performance	Canada Compared to Other Countries	Provincial and Territorial Variation Within Canada	Identified Indicator Development Priorities
	JOINT REPLACE-MENT WAIT TIMES Median wait times in Canada for hip replacement compare favourably with other peer OECD countries. Canada's median wait time for both procedures was fourth among OECD countries in 2014.	There is variation across provinces in wait times for joint replacements. The percentage of patients receiving a hip or knee replacement within six months ranged from close to 90% in three provinces to results in the 60s for four others. One small province had a result of 48%.	
Person-centred	POTENTIALLY INAPPROPRIATE USE OF ANTI-PSYCHOTICS IN LONG-TERM CARE In an international comparison of results for five countries Canada's rate of roughly 26% was similar to that of the US and lower than rates of 34% and 38% reported in Switzerland and Finland.	Of the eight provinces where some or all facilities report continuing care data, results vary from highs of roughly 35% of long-term care residents on anti-psychotic drugs without a diagnosis of psychosis for two provinces to lows of 20–25% for two other provinces.	• Patient and caregiver perspectives on continuity of care across sectors. This is also related to examining alignment of patients' treatment goals across various healthcare providers and organizations, particularly for individuals with multi-morbidities. • Engagement of patients in managing their own health and health care

...continued

TABLE 1.1, continued

Dimension of Health System Performance	Canada Compared to Other Countries	Provincial and Territorial Variation Within Canada	Identified Indicator Development Priorities
	REPEAT HOSPITAL STAYS FOR MENTAL ILLNESS In the 2011 report, Canada's results were above the OECD average but under the top 25%.	Results across provinces ranged from a high of 13.3% of mental health patients with at least three hospitalizations in a year to results under 10%. A small province and territory had rates under 10%, but these were not statistically significantly different from the national average.	
Appropriate and Effective	HOSPITAL DEATHS (HSMR) International comparisons of HSMR are not appropriate without a standardized measure of expected hospital deaths. However, on two measures of in-hospital deaths (within 30 days following AMI and stroke), Canada's results are mixed. On in-hospital deaths following admission for AMI, Canada's result is in the top third of OECD countries; however for deaths following admission for stroke, the result for Canada is only slightly better than the OECD average.	The two best performing provinces had HSMR results in the low 80s. Three smaller provinces had results just above 100 (actual hospital deaths in 2013 greater than expected deaths based on 2009 results).	• Medication reviews in community-based care, including flagging for inappropriate medications or combinations • Appropriateness of care settings, for example, patients cared for in hospitals who could be cared for in residential or home-care settings, as well as inappropriate use of emergency departments for non-urgent problems.

...continued

TABLE 1.1, continued

Dimension of Health System Performance	Canada Compared to Other Countries	Provincial and Territorial Variation Within Canada	Identified Indicator Development Priorities
		8.8% of hospital patients in Canada were readmitted within 30 days following discharge. There were two small jurisdictions with results close to 11%. However, all other results were less than 10%, with some provinces having results just over 8%.	
Safe	There is no high level measure of patient safety available in the core set of performance indicators reported yet.	There is no high level measure of patient safety available in the core set of performance indicators reported yet.	• Measures of in-hospital infection and hospital harm to become part of pan-Canadian reporting on performance in 2015

...continued

TABLE 1.1, continued

Dimension of Health System Performance	Canada Compared to Other Countries	Provincial and Territorial Variation Within Canada	Identified Indicator Development Priorities
Efficiently delivered	AGE-ADJUSTED PUBLIC SPENDING PER PERSON In 2013, Canada's total health expenditure per person was 10th highest among 34 OECD countries. The proportion of spending from private sources, however, tends to be higher than many countries at close to over 30%. Of the countries with higher total levels of per-person spending, only the US and Switzerland have a greater proportion of private spending.	Age-adjusted public spending per person varies significantly across jurisdictions in Canada. Spending is generally lower in larger provinces— Quebec is the lowest at $3,360, followed by BC and Ontario, while all three territories have the highest per person spending at close to or over $10,000.	• Extra spending related to (in) appropriate care settings. This would include, for example, patients cared for in hospitals, who could be cared for in residential or home-care settings, as well as inappropriate use of emergency departments for non-urgent problems. • Explore "waste" in healthcare— spending on inappropriate diagnostic and treatment interventions.

...continued

TABLE 1.1, continued

Dimension of Health System Performance	Canada Compared to Other Countries	Provincial and Territorial Variation Within Canada	Identified Indicator Development Priorities
	COST OF A STANDARD HOSPITAL STAY	The average cost in Canada for a typical hospital stay is just over $5,500. As with spending per person, costs of hospital stays tend to be lower in larger provinces, with Quebec and Ontario having the lowest costs at $4,900 and $5,300 respectively. A number of jurisdictions had average costs over $6,000, including Alberta at $7,300 and Saskatchewan at $6,500.	

QUADRANT 1.1

Dimension of Health System Performance	Canada Compared to Other Countries	Provincial and Territorial Variation Within Canada	Identified Indicator Development Priorities
Improve health status of Canadians	LIFE EXPECTANCY AT BIRTH Canada's life expectancy at birth was close to the OECD 34-country average and was 13th highest at 81.5 years. This is a significant drop from its position as the 3rd highest in 1990 and 8th highest in 2000.	The three largest provinces have life expectancies above the Canadian average of 81 years, with BC having the highest rate at 81.7 years. There are three provinces with results below 80 years. The territories have life expectancy results in the mid- to low-70s.	Mental health status of children and youth. Patient-reported outcome measures including population-based functional health status, and outcomes for specific interventions (e.g., joint replacement). Improvement in the health status of the elderly. Overall health and well-being.
	AVOIDABLE DEATHS In a comparison of 31 OECD countries published in 2011[1] Canada ranked 11 of 31 countries on amenable mortality (avoidable due to treatment).	Canada's rate per 100,000 for avoidable mortality (includes avoidable due to treatment and prevention) was 171. In a pattern similar to that for life expectancy, the results for the territories were significantly higher at over 230. The best results were for BC and Ontario at 158 and 163 per 100,000 respectively.	
Improve health system responsiveness			Measures of burden on informal caregivers of caring for relatives and friends. The burden of treatment and illness for patients.

[1] OECD (2011).

…continued

QUADRANT 1.1

Dimension of Health System Performance	Canada Compared to Other Countries	Provincial and Territorial Variation Within Canada	Identified Indicator Development Priorities
Improve value for money			Costs for "bundles of care" that could be related to outcomes; for example, costs of joint replacements across all sectors of care related to long-term patient-reported outcomes and economic benefit.

QUADRANT 1.2

Dimension of Health System Performance	Canada Compared to Other Countries	Provincial and Territorial Variation Within Canada	Identified Indicator Development Priorities
Structural factors influencing health			• Measures of structural and contextual factors to better understand the impact on the health system and on population health. • Expansion of capacity to disaggregate health status outcomes to focus on results for marginalized and vulnerable population groups (e.g., aboriginal peoples, refugees, people with disabilities). • Summary measure of the impact of income inequality on health status.
Biological, material, psychosocial and behavioural factors	SMOKING Canada had the 10th lowest rate of smoking among 34 OECD countries at 15% of adults compared to the OECD average of 20%.	The provincial rates of smoking among adults varied from highs of over 20% in a number of provinces to the lowest rate of 16.2% in BC.	

...continued

QUADRANT 1.2, continued

Dimension of Health System Performance	Canada Compared to Other Countries	Provincial and Territorial Variation Within Canada	Identified Indicator Development Priorities
	OBESITY Canada had the 7th highest rate of obesity among the 34 OECD countries, with a *measured* rate of 25.8% compared to the OECD average of 19%. While Canada's rate was lower than measured rates of five other countries, it was still higher than measured rates in many other countries including the UK. Obesity in Canada increased from 22% to 25.8% *between 2000 and 2013.*	The average rate of obesity in Canada, based on self-reported height and weight, was 18.8%. There is a significant spread among provinces and territories, with six provinces and territories having rates of 25% or higher, including some that were nearly 30%. The lowest provincial rate was almost half this at 15%.	
	CHILDREN VULNERABLE IN AREAS OF EARLY DEVELOPMENT	Just over one in four children at age five were identified as being vulnerable in one or more areas of early development. For the eight provinces and territories with reported results, the rates ranged from over 30% for four of these to a low of 17.2% with other results in the low 20% range.	

Putting the framework to work: Canadian health system performance management beyond wait times

The extent to which this initiative will have an impact on performance improvement will depend, in part, on institutional accountability cultures and strategic commitment to service improvement through performance management. Canada's recent experience with wait times provides a useful case study in this regard. The 2004 Health Accord focused on a narrow set of wait times with the expectation to provide care within wait times that were clinically acceptable. Provinces worked together to define what were clinically acceptable benchmarks, the federal government provided financial support to the initiative and CIHI was designated as the third party organization responsible for working with data suppliers (i.e., the provinces) to ensure the quality and comparability of the data provided, and to report on progress on an annual basis. Ten years after signing the accord, not only are provincial governments reporting on an annual basis through CIHI on wait times for key procedures and interventions, but much progress has been made despite a substantial increase in the volume of services delivered for these procedures (CIHI 2015b).

On the other hand, wait-times reporting also provides a useful example of what can occur in the area of performance reporting in the absence of the coordination and commitment described above—a situation that for the most part characterizes health system reporting beyond wait times. Table 1.2 illustrates that there is a great deal of consistency in reporting those areas identified as priorities. As noted above, this is at least partially due to the role of the federal government in providing financial support, and organizations such as CIHI and the Wait Times Alliance in reporting the data. Sustainable performance improvement through the use of standardized performance measurement, available evidence, and policy and political commitment is possible in Canada given the appropriate support. However, Table 1.1 also shows that for wait-times reporting for non-priority areas, we see much less consistency across jurisdictions and a considerably less coherent picture. In some cases, indicators are reported by jurisdictions but with non-comparable methodologies.

TABLE 1.2
Comparison of the Provincial Reporting of Access to Care Measures, 2014

		BC	AB	SK	MB	ON	QC	NB	NS	PE	NL
FEDERALLY FUNDED INDICATORS†											
Priority Areas	Joint replacement (hip and knee)	√	√	√	√	√	√	√	√	√	√
	Radiation Therapy	√	√	√	√	√	√	√	√	√	√
	Cataract Surgery	√	√	√	√	√	√	√	√	√	√
	MRI Scans		√	√	√	√			√	√	
	CT Scans		√	√	√	√			√	√	
	CABG	√	√	√	√	√	-	√	√	*	√
OTHER WAIT TIME INDICATORS‡											
Cancer Care	Wait time from referral to consult (all body sites combined)	√	-			√			√	√	
	Wait time from decision to treat to start of treatment (all body sites combined)	√	√	√	√	√	-	√	√	√	√
Cardiac Care (Scheduled Cases)	Electrophysiology						-		-	*	
	Cardiac Rehabilitation								-		
	Cardiac nuclear imaging				-				-		
Plastic Surgery	Breast reconstruction	-	-	-		√			√		
Pediatric Surgery	Advanced dental caries: carious lesions/pain					-			-	-	
	Strabismus						-		√	√	

†Source: Canadian Institute for Health Information, Wait Times for Priority Procedures in Canada, 2014

‡Source: Wait Time Alliance, Report Card on Wait Times in Canada, 2014

- Provinces report wait times for this specific procedure, but in a matter that could not be compared to the others

*PEI does not offer cardiac services; patients receive care out of province

CABG: coronary artery bypass graft; MRI: magnetic resonance imaging; CT: computerized tomography

TOWARDS A LEARNING HEALTHCARE SYSTEM: FROM PERFORMANCE MEASUREMENT TO PERFORMANCE MANAGEMENT

A growing body of research indicates that the use of strategy-based performance management tools in the public sector can result in substantial improvements in both health outcomes and cost-effectiveness. Specifically, the literature on balanced scorecards (Kaplan and Norton 1992) and strategy mapping (Kaplan and Norton 2001) illustrates the importance of linking strategy, performance measurement, and performance expectations (Veillard et al. 2010) into a coherent path towards a specified and shared goal. While the balanced scorecard provides a means for organizing strategic objectives and embodies the cause and effect relationships between them, the strategy map forms a framework—a common point of reference—to guide the implementation of strategy. It is the scorecard and map, used in tandem, that move an organization beyond performance measurement to strategic system management (Kaplan and Norton, 2001). If measurement involves reporting on the past, it also identifies areas for emphasis in the future, enabling organizations "to accomplish comprehensive and integrated transformations" (Kaplan and Norton 2001, 102).

Conventionally, the unit of application of the balanced scorecard and strategy maps is the organization. Adaptation is required if the approach is to be mobilized for the entire health system (see Carson 2015). In Ontario, for example, the Ontario Ministry of Health and Long Term Care developed a health system performance management framework in 2006 that adapted the seminal work of Kaplan and Norton to a system level and used this approach for the development of its new accountability policy for newly created Local Health Integration Networks (Veillard et al. 2010). This process is graphically depicted as a performance management cycle in Figure 1.2, in which a jurisdiction (a) sets its strategic priorities, (b) selects key performance indicators to monitor progress of the strategy, (c) uses these indicators to support resource allocation, (d) holds those receiving resources accountable for results, and (e) assesses whether performance improvements have the desired impact on the performance of the health system in order to adjust strategies accordingly.

To create an environment conducive to this form of system-level performance management requires forms of stewardship and governance that ensure a proper alignment between health system design, resource allocation and incentives, and health system goals and performance expectations (Veillard et al. 2011). It also requires that health ministries ensure a fit between strategy and institutional and organizational structure, and that there are efforts in place to reduce system duplication and fragmentation. It also implies that the health system has the capacity to adapt its strategies and policies to take into account changing priorities (Porter 1996).

Besides legislative and regulatory instruments, there are various policy tools that can be mobilized by provincial governments and system managers in Canada to manage the performance of the healthcare system. Table 1.3 presents a menu of possible instruments that can be used to manage health system perfor-

FIGURE 1.2
A strategy-based performance management cycle

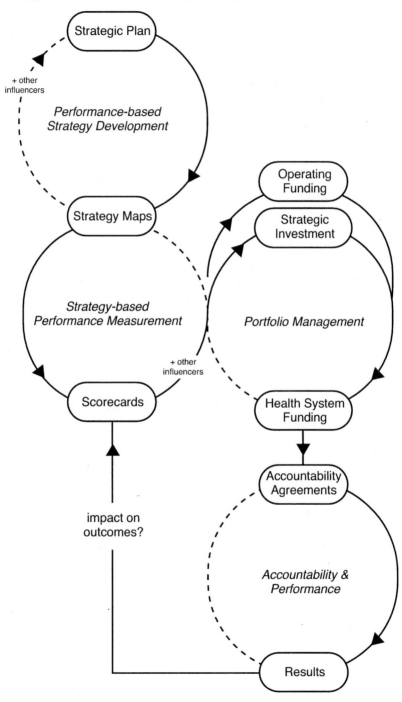

mance. Depending on goals pursued and context, a different combination of these policy instruments will be required to achieve performance objectives. Importantly, these policy instruments all rely heavily on the strategic use of performance information and evidence.

Wait times in Canada are an excellent example of the strategic use of performance information for management purposes. The combination of additional financial resources obtained through the 2004 Health Accord, of political attention, comparative performance reporting, and of specific interventions such as innovative financing mechanisms, introduction of financial and organizational incentives, process redesign, and spreading and scaling of best practices, delivered better results for Canadians despite the pressures of demographics, ageing, and changes in expectations from the population. In 2014, about eight Canadians out of 10 received these services within the clinical benchmarks. International comparisons also showed that for cataracts and joint replacements, Canada made enough progress in the last 10 years to become one of the OECD countries with the best access for these specific procedures (OECD 2015). Similar progress has been seen in Canada and several other OECD countries for cancer and cardiovascular care, where the combination of public reporting and transparency, innovation in planning and payment systems, clinical leadership and medical innovation have been combined to drive significant improvements. Interestingly, for other domains of performance with little monitoring and reporting, such as access to primary healthcare and specialists, little progress has been made and Canada still lags behind significantly in these domains when compared to other OECD countries (OECD 2015).

Criticisms of the Performance Management Paradigm

It should also be noted that a number of potential drawbacks and undesirable consequences have been identified with regard to the use of performance measurement to manage the performance of health systems (Exworthy 2011). These criticisms pertain to a number of issues, with gaming of financial incentives at the forefront (Bevan and Hood 2006). Other observers have raised a range of concerns, including: the fact that improperly mobilized performance indicators can result in sub-optimal service delivery, or a focus on meeting the target rather than substantively improving performance (Klazinga 2011; Mannion and Braithewaite 2012); the difficulty of improving performance in targeted areas while ensuring that other non-reported aspects of care or health system performance are not adversely affected (Mannion and Braithwaite 2012); the challenge of balancing formal (quantifiable) and informal (non-quantifiable) aspects of performance when measurement imperatives are predominant (Mannion and Braithewaite 2012); the difficulty of improving performance when interrelations and trade-offs between the different dimensions of health system performance are complex and poorly understood (Plsek and Greenhalgh 2001); and the need to act simultaneously on primary, secondary, and tertiary factors influencing health to achieve better outcomes (Mannion and Braithewaite 2012; Commission on Social Determinants of Health 2008).

TABLE 1.3
A possible menu of policy instruments for health system performance management

Instrument	Definition	Examples
Public reporting	Data, publicly available or available to a broad audience free of charge or at a nominal cost, about a healthcare structure, process, or outcome at any provider level (Totten et al. 2012).	Provincial quality councils Canadian Institute for Health Information
Target setting	Determining the level of performance that an organization aims to achieve for a particular activity (Bourn 2001).	Wait times and recent work at Health Quality Ontario
Accountability mechanisms	Instruments through which an agent is answerable to another for progress towards meeting defined objectives (Deber 2014).	Contractual arrangements with regional health authorities Cancer Care Ontario
Resource allocation and portfolio management	Processes of (dis)investment of resources and prioritization in pursuit of organizational goals.	Ontario Ministry of Health experience
Financial incentives	Payment incentives intended to promote or discourage certain activities; e.g., Pay for Performance (Oliver 2015).	Activity-based funding (Ontario, Alberta, British Columbia) Quality-based procedures (Ontario)
Non-financial incentives	Non-payment incentives intended to promote or discourage certain activities; e.g., public reporting, professional autonomy (Oliver 2015).	Excellent Care for All Act (Ontario 2010)
Quality improvement	A systematic approach to making changes that lead to better patient outcomes, stronger system performance, and enhanced professional development (Health Quality Ontario n.d.).	Saskatchewan Lean Initiative Wait Times process flow redesign

More generally, the political role of the performance management paradigm in an era of retrenchment, characterized by a political context focussed on budgetary discipline with little financial capacity to make significant new investments, has been questioned. Other criticisms have been typified by skepticism with regard to whether key measures related to public satisfaction will improve, incredulity towards the ability of government to deliver transformative changes, and a lingering hesitancy to "call out" poor performers.

It would be an error, however, to conclude on the basis of the challenges that have been identified that performance management is not an obvious way forward for health system performance improvement in Canada. The challenges, as Eddy (1998) points out, "are a necessary phase in the development of any program to solve a difficult and important social problem." All levels of the health system need performance information to clarify what they are seeking to achieve (aspirations), a method to measure progress against aspirations (management), and to understand whether investments deliver value for money (accountability; Hughes 2013).

From an operational perspective, those who manage and provide health services need detailed performance information to understand which services perform well, and which need to improve. Good performance information is essential for health systems striving to deliver value for money, and improved services, especially in times of scarce resources. In other words, performance measurement is vital for effective performance management and improvement: for creating, maintaining, and demonstrating excellence and for making optimal decisions and use of resources. Measurement is not an end in itself—the purpose, of course, is to improve healthcare quality—but "persistent questions about quality and the tension between quality and cost cannot be resolved without measuring quality" (Eddy 1998). Our collective task with regard to performance measurement and management, as Mannion and Braithwaite (2012) point out, "is to reap the benefits, but beware of the pitfalls."

MAKING PERFORMANCE MANAGEMENT WORK IN CANADA

The nature of healthcare in Canada's federal context means that within the parameters of the Canada Health Act, provincial governments have considerable leeway in shaping their health systems in ways that respond to their population and economic needs. This is one of the system's strengths and a valuable source of innovation. One consequence, however, is that decisions in jurisdictions may not be optimally informed by the experience (both successful and otherwise) of other jurisdictions, and that opportunities for spreading and scaling innovation and best practices are limited, especially in smaller jurisdictions. Although the structure of Canada's health system enables responsiveness to local priorities and contingencies, it does not lend itself easily to the identification and pursuit of shared policy goals and common performance priorities. Despite variations in health system performance, all of Canada's provinces are facing similar challenges when it comes to healthcare and there is much to be gained from a coherent and coordinated approach to health system performance measurement and management. In this context, there are a number of ways forward to be considered to make performance management work in the health sector in Canada.

Create alignment between national and provincial performance measurement frameworks

Driving health system improvement for all Canadians will involve preserving provincial government autonomy and flexibility with regard to delivering health services appropriate to population needs while bringing greater coherence to the relationship between provincial and federal levels. One way to achieve this would be to develop shared strategic goals and objectives through the alignment of federal and provincial frameworks centred on the elaboration of shared health system priorities. Of course, provincial autonomy and flexibility will continue to be a defining hallmark of health services delivery, but the alignment of federal and provincial frameworks would encourage coordination and learning across jurisdictions and lead to a common sense of performance improvement priorities and opportunities for shared progress. The success of the wait-times initiative and recent work by the Council of the Federation and its Innovation Working Group are partial illustrations of the potential for greater alignment.

In addition, addressing the issue of indicator chaos requires processes for establishing priorities and identifying what to measure and report, and to ensure synergy in the institutional landscape that supports performance measurement at the federal and provincial levels. These processes will need to take into consideration the concerns of patients and citizens and input from healthcare providers regarding the importance and usefulness of performance indicators.

Seek a balance between parsimony and actionability of well-designed sets of performance indicators

Different audiences are interested in different aspects of health system performance and require different levels of reporting. A teaching hospital, for example, may require detailed information to pinpoint which surgical programs and care processes require improvements, whereas a provincial policymaker may need to see performance trends at a higher level to understand which parts of the system are working well and not so well. As users and funders of the healthcare system, Canadians also have a vested interest in health system performance and want to know whether they are receiving good care relative to the public expense of providing it. A key challenge, therefore, in advancing the performance measurement agenda is the inherent tension between providing information tailored to the needs of different audiences (the general public, provincial health ministries, regional health authorities and healthcare facilities) while ensuring that reporting is parsimonious and focused on a small number of indicators aligned with the system transformation priorities of jurisdictions.

The vision for the health system reporting initiative currently being implemented by the Canadian Institute for Health Information (http://www. yourhealthsystem.cihi.ca) is to propose a focused set of cascading metrics meaningful to, and useful for, their respective audiences (Figure 1.3). Information is presented at the international, national, provincial/territorial, health region and facility levels, where available. This type of approach would be beneficial also at the provincial level and is already being implemented in Alberta.

Promote cross-provincial learning

In addition to public reporting, CIHI is improving and expanding the functionality of health system reporting tools at the facility level with enhanced benchmarking features and improved analytical capabilities. Ultimately, the goal of this program of work is to be able to provide policymakers and health system managers with an integrated view of health system performance that cuts across sectors of care through an enhanced business intelligence solution called *health system performance insight*. In this system, health system managers and decision support staff can drill down into high level performance indicators reported publicly (such as hospital readmissions rates, mortality from major surgery or wait times for emergency rooms) in a private and secure environment respectful of privacy. This technology enables the use of real time data (the indicators are updated on a monthly basis as data are submitted by hospitals) and the ability to drill down to the patient record level for those who have the authorization to do so, enabling, for example, decision support teams to analyze the data to understand what are the main drivers for the performance results reported publicly (e.g., is a high readmission rate in a given hospital driven by patients admitted on Fridays, or by a specific clinical unit such as an intensive care unit?). In effect, this practice allows reconciling high level performance reporting (a burning platform for change) and analytics to understand underlying drivers of performance patterns. But more fundamentally, it provides the opportunity to compare organizations, health regions, and provinces on a small number of carefully selected performance indicators.

In order to promote cross-provincial learning, it will be important to link rich data platforms with repositories of best practices and innovations linked to key performance indicators, such as those proposed by the Federal Panel on Healthcare Innovation (Health Canada 2015). From this perspective, pan-Canadian organizations such as CIHI, the Canadian Foundation for Healthcare Improvement, the Canadian Patient Safety Institute, and Accreditation Canada among others should be working collaboratively with provincial quality councils, other agencies, and provincial governments to develop an improvement platform that would build on the strengths of these organizations, and would accelerate the spread and scale of performance improvement through the use of performance information and best available evidence about best practices. An alternative proposal, suggested by the Federal Panel on Healthcare Innovation (Health Canada 2015), would be to create an innovation agency for the health-

FIGURE 1.3
Cascading indicators for performance measurement

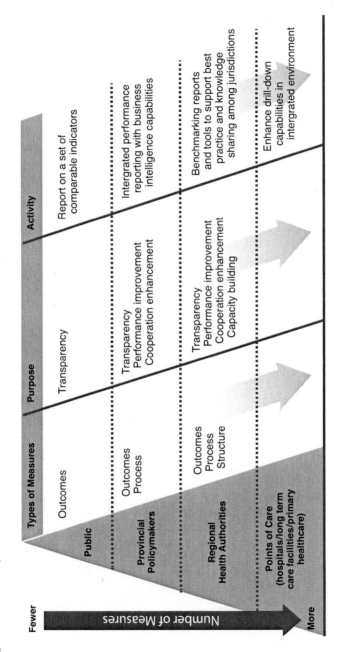

care sector in Canada.

Finally, more research efforts should be made to develop novel methods to identify and study positive outliers, and strengthen established benchmarking networks (such as the Western CEOs Forum) and emerging benchmarking initiatives (such as the Collaborating for Excellence in Health Care Quality).

Fill in performance information gaps

The Canadian Institute for Health Information and Statistics Canada hosted a national consensus conference on indicator development in late 2014, gathering senior representatives from each province and territory in Canada, the federal government, national and international experts, and national organizations. The conference had two objectives. The first was to consider retiring identified CIHI indicators from public reporting that had become less relevant over time, and by doing so, reduce indicator chaos. The second was to identify priorities for future indicator development, focusing on areas of strategic importance for health system performance improvement and on how to fill gaps in performance reporting. Through a modified Delphi process with facilitated working group and plenary discussions, the conference participants identified five theme areas for future development:

- healthcare outcomes;
- value for money;
- care transitions and trajectories, focusing on integration and continuity of care;
- community care and in particular mental healthcare; and
- upstream investments in population health determinants.

Of key importance was the need to fill the gap in indicators that could measure performance in how the health system responds to the needs of multi-morbid patients requiring access to care that is coordinated and integrated across all providers. Conference participants also recognized the need for indicators to reflect the perspectives of patients and caregivers on their needs for, and experiences with, healthcare, as well as their care outcomes.

Investing in better measurement and reporting of outcomes of care and value for money seems, therefore, a priority for the federal and provincial governments, and would offer the opportunity to structure a new Health Accord around sustainable results.

The need for better leadership and governance

Experience demonstrates that, notwithstanding the advantages of the federal model, the sum of the parts does not always amount to more than the whole. Coordination, consistency and standardization do not emerge spontaneously. To move Canada's currently fragmented health system to a performance management model characterized by some degree of harmonization will call for provincial and federal leadership. As noted, there are recent historical precedents for this. There are also opportunities for forms of health system governance more prone to facilitate the development and articulation of performance expectations and priorities and to create clearer, evidence-informed relationships between strategy, targets, and improvement.

There is also a need for forms of governance capable of encouraging a mature conversation with Canadians and professionals about Canada's health sector and what will be required to transform it into a high-performing population health system. This conversation needs to engage multiple players—provider organizations as well as funders, policymakers, and managers. In particular, clinicians can play a key leadership role in driving change at multiple levels of the system and ensuring that performance information produced is meaningful for performance improvement at the clinical level.

A more mature dialogue among policymakers, system managers, clinicians, and patients about performance expectations for example will contribute to the emergence of a health democracy where patients and citizens have a meaningful voice in the governance of the health system. If ways to engage patients and citizens in decision making and system management are not straightforward, experimentations under way such as the appointment of citizens' or patients' representatives on boards of governors of various institutions, and the engagement of patients in the co-design of clinical programs that benefit them, such as Health Links in Ontario, are positive initiatives that should be built upon and evaluated for further spread and scale across the health sector.

CONCLUSION

Performance management is very much focused on quality improvement and health system transformation. But in its insistence on transparency and its focus on results (particularly those valued by patients) it also renders healthcare systems more visible to the scrutiny of the citizens who pay for and use their services. What is more, the need to identify clear goals and objectives that will be used to identify what is to be measured calls for broader engagement of patients and of the general public in discussing performance expectations.

The visibility and accountability ushered in by the performance management model emerging in Canada is an important condition to the emergence of a health democracy that will enable a meaningful dialogue between the ultimate stakeholders of the healthcare system (Canadians and in particular patients) and their elected governors. But how to consolidate the so far timid gains of a fragile, yet emerging, health democracy remains a challenge that confronts us and keeps on calling for greater leadership, governance, and investments in information systems, as well as research that supports the consolidation of health systems capable of adaptation and improvement.

REFERENCES

Agency for Healthcare Research and Quality. 2013. Prioritizing the Public in HHS Public Reporting Measures: Using and Improving Information on Quality, Cost, and Coverage to Support Health Care Improvement. Companion Report to the National Quality Strategy, http://www.ahrq.gov/working-forquality/reports/hhsreporting.htm.

Alberta Health. 2013. Health System Outcomes and Measurement Framework. http://www.health.alberta.ca/documents/PMIS-Outcomes-Measurement-Framework-2014.pdf.

Berwick, D. M., T. W. Nolan, and J. Whittington. 2008. "The Triple Aim: Care, Health, and Cost." *Health Affairs* 27(3): 759–769.

Bevan, G., and C. Hood. 2006. "What's Measured Is What Matters: Targets and Gaming in the English Public Health Care System." *Public Administration*, 84(3): 517–538.

Bourn, J. 2001. "Measuring the Performance of Government Departments." Report to the House of Commons by the Comptroller and Auditor General. The Stationary Office, London, HE, 301, 2000–2001.

Carson, A. S. 2015. "If Canada Had a Healthcare Strategy, What Form Could It Take?" In *Toward a Healthcare Strategy for Canadians,* edited by A. S. Carson, J. , Dixon, and K. R. Nossal. Montreal & Kingston: McGill-Queen's University Press, 255–276.

CIHI. 2014a. *International Comparisons: A Focus on Quality of Care.* Ottawa, ON: CIHI. https://secure.cihi.ca/estore/productFamily.htm?locale=en&pf=PFC2451&lang=en&media=0.

———. 2014b. *HCC Bulletin: Special Issue on Health System Performance.* Ottawa, ON: CIHI, http://www.cihi.ca/CIHI-ext-portal/pdf/internet/BUL_30NOV14_PDF_EN.

CIHI. 2015a. *Report from the Fourth Health Indicators Consensus Conference 2014.* Ottawa, ON: CIHI. Unpublished.

———. 2015b. *Wait Times for Priority Procedures in Canada, 2015.* Ottawa, ON: CIHI, https://secure.cihi.ca/estore/productSeries.htm?pc=PCC395.

Commission on Social Determinants of Health. 2008. *Closing the Gap in a Generation: Health Equity Through Action on the Social Determinants of Health.* Geneva: World Health Organization.

Commonwealth Fund. 2011. *The Commonwealth Fund 2011 International Health Policy Survey of Sicker Adults in Eleven Countries.* http://www.commonwealthfund.org/~/media/files/publications/in-the-literature/2011/nov/ihp-survey/pdf_schoen_2011_survey_article_chartpack.pdf.

Council of Australian Governments. 2011. *National Healthcare Agreement 2011.* Canberra: Council of Australian Governments.

Daniels, A. C. and J. E. Daniels. 2004. *Performance Management: Changing Behaviour that Drives Organizational Effectiveness.* Fourth edition. Atlanta: Performance Management Publications.

Deber, R. 2014. "Thinking About Accountability." *Healthcare Policy* 10(Special Issue):12–24.

Donabedian, A. 1966. "Evaluating the Quality of Medical Care." *Milbank Memorial Fund Quarterly* 44(3, Part 2): 166–206.

———. 1989. "The End Results of Health Care: Ernest Codman's Contribution to Quality Assessment and Beyond." *The Milbank Quarterly* 67(2): 233–255.

Eddy, D. M. 1998. "Performance Measurement: Problems and Solutions." *Health Affairs* 17(4): 7–25.

Exworthy, M. 2011. "The Performance Paradigm in the English NHS: Potential, Pitfalls and Prospects." *Eurohealth* 16(3): 16–19.

Fafard, P. 2013. "Intergovernmental Accountability and Health Care: Reflections on Recent Canadian Experience." In *Overpromising and Underperforming? Understanding and Evaluating New Intergovernmental Accountability Regimes*, edited by P. Graefe, J. M. Simmons, and L. M. White, 31–55. Toronto: University of Toronto Press.

Feng, et al. 2009. "Use of Physical Restraints and Antipsychotic Medications in Nursing Homes: A Cross-National Study. *International Journal of Geriatric Psychiatry*, October; 24(10): 1110–1118. doi:10.1002/gps.2232.

Fierlbeck, K. 2012. "Health Care Governance in Federal Systems: Can Europe's Experimental Governance Models Work in Canada?" Occasional Paper No. 13. Halifax: European Union Centre of Excellence (EUCE), Dalhousie University.

Groot, T. and T. Budding. 2008. "New Public Management's Current Issues and Future Prospects." *Financial Accountability & Management* 24(1): 0267–4424.

Health Care Innovation Working Group. 2012. *From Innovation to Action: The First Report of the Health Care Innovation Working Group*. Ottawa, ON: The Council of the Federation.

Health Canada. 2015. "Unleashing Innovation: Excellent Health Care for Canada." Report of the Advisory Panel on Healthcare Innovation.

Health Quality Ontario. n.d. What is Quality Improvement? http://www.hqontario.ca/quality-improvement.

Hughes, M. 2012. Measure for Measure: Using Performance Information in Tough Times. Manchester, UK: Association for Public Service Excellence. http://www.apse.org.uk/apse/index.cfm/research/current-research-programme/measure-for-measure-using-performance-information-in-tough-times/.

Kaplan, R. S. and D. P. Norton. 1992. "The Balanced Scorecard: Measures that Drive Performance. *Harvard Business Review* 83(7): 71–79.

———. 2001. "Transforming the Balanced Scorecard from Performance Measurement to Strategic Management: Part 1." *Accounting Horizons* 15(1): 87–104.

Klazinga, N. 2011. "Health System Performance Management: Quality for Better or for Worse." *Eurohealth* 16(3): 26–28.

Mannion, R. and J. Braithwaite. 2012. "Unintended Consequences of Performance Measurement in Healthcare: 20 Salutary Lessons from the English National Health Service." *Internal Medicine Journal* 42(5): 569–574.

OECD. 2011. "Mortality Amenable to Health Care in 31 OECD Countries: Estimates and Methodological Issues." OECD Working Paper #55.

————. 2015. "Health at a Glance 2013: OECD Indicators." OECD Publishing http://dx.doi.org/10.1787/health_glance-2013-en.

Oliver, A. 2015. "Incentivising Improvements in Health Care Delivery." *Health Economics, Policy and Law*, 1–17.

Osborne, D. and T. Gaebler. 1992. *Reinventing Government: How the Entrepreneurial Spirit is Transforming the Public Sector*. New York: Addison-Wesley.

Plsek, P. and T. Greenhalgh. 2001. "Complexity Science: The Challenge of Complexity in Health Care. *BMJ* 323: 625–628.

Porter, M. E. 1996. "What is Strategy?" *Harvard Business Review* 74(6): 61–78.

Porter, M. E. and T. H. Lee. 2013. "The Strategy that Will Fix Health Care." *Harvard Business Review*, 91(10): 50–70.

Saskatchewan Health Quality Council. 2011. *Think Big, Start Small, Act Now: Tackling Indicator Chaos; A report on a national summit: Saskatoon, May 30–31*, 2011. http://hqc.sk.ca/Portals/0/documents/tracking-indicator-choas.pdf

Smith, P. C. 2002. "Performance Management in British Health Care: Will It Deliver?" *Health Affairs* 21(3): 103–15.

Smith, P. C., E. Mossialos, and I. Papanicolas. 2008. "Performance Measurement for Health System Improvement: Experiences, Challenges and Prospects." Background document, 2. Copenhagen: World Health Organization.

Smith, P. C., E. Mossialos, I. Papanicolas, and S. Leatherman, eds. 2009. *Performance Measurement for Health System Improvement: Experiences, Challenges and Prospects*. Cambridge: Cambridge University Press.

Totten, A. M., J. Wagner, A. Tiwari., C. O'Haire, J. Griffin, and M. Walker. 2012. "Public Reporting as a Quality Improvement Strategy," In *Closing the Quality Gap: Revisiting the State of the Science*. Evidence Report No. 208. Prepared by the Oregon Evidence-based Practice Center under Contract No. 290-2007-10057-I. AHRQ Publication No. 12-E011-EF. Rockville, MD: Agency for Healthcare Research and Quality. http://www.effectivehealthcare.ahrq.gov/reports/final.cfm.

UK Department of Health. 2014. *The NHS Outcomes Framework 2012/13*. London, UK: National Health Service.

US Congress. 2010. *Patient Affordable Care and Protection Act*, http://www.gpo.gov/fdsys/pkg/BILLS-111hr3590enr/pdf/BILLS-111hr3590enr.pdf.

van den Berg, M., D. S. Kringos, L. K. Marks, and N. Klazinga. 2014. "The Dutch Health Care Performance Report: Seven Years of Health Care Performance Assessment in the Netherlands." *Health Research Policy and Systems* 12(1).

Veillard, J., F. Champagne, N. Klazinga, V. Kazandjian, O. A. Arah, and A. L. Guisset. 2005. "A Performance Assessment Framework for Hospitals: The

WHO Regional Office for Europe PATH Project." *International Journal of Quality in Health Care* 17(6): 487–496.

Veillard, J., T. Huynh, S. Ardal, S. Kadandale, N. Klazinga, and A. D. Brown. 2010. "Making Health System Performance Measurement Useful to Policy-Makers: Aligning Strategies, Measurement and Local Health System Accountability." *Healthcare Policy* 5(3): 49–65.

Veillard, J., A. D. Brown, E. Baris, G. Permanand, N. S. Klazinga. 2011. "Health System Stewardship of National Health Ministries in the WHO European Region: Concepts, Functions and a Framework for Action." *Health Policy* 103: 191–199.

World Health Organization. 2000. *The World Health Report 2000: Improving Health System Performance*. Geneva: WHO, http://www.who.int/whr/2000/en/.

Chapter 2

TARGETING IMPROVEMENTS THROUGH LOCAL HEALTH PERFORMANCE REPORTING: THE AUSTRALIAN EXPERIENCE

ADAM CRESSWELL AND DIANE WATSON

In both Canada and Australia, legislative powers for matters such as taxation and healthcare are assigned to both national and regional levels of government. In the case of Canada, this involves the federal government and the provinces, while in Australia this relates to the federal (also called Commonwealth) government and those of the states and territories. Both nations provide universal health insurance, though the roles and responsibilities of the two main levels of government differ between countries. Despite these differences in governance, both countries face similar challenges addressing the forces that influence general revenue and spending on health. While both nations have experience in performance reporting to improve transparency and accountability, Australia has begun to drive improvements nationally for its population of 24 million through its smart use of health data to compare and report on the performance of its public and private health organizations.

This chapter describes the policy context in which performance reporting became increasingly prevalent in Australia, draws parallels to the evolution of policy in Canada and sheds light on the implementation of recent reforms in Australia that were designed to drive improvements by reporting on the performance of comparable health organizations and local health systems. To this end, it examines the factors that placed health back at the top of the political

Managing a Canadian Healthcare Strategy, edited by A. Scott Carson and Kim Richard Nossal. Montreal and Kingston: McGill-Queen's University Press, Queen's Policy Studies Series. © 2016 The School of Policy Studies, Queen's University at Kingston. All rights reserved.

agenda in Australia in the first decade of the new century. It looks at how a focus on reporting on health organizations came to be part of the response, and the key principles that were devised to guide the implementation of that agenda. We also explore the role of Australia's National Health Performance Authority (established in late 2011) in making the policy objectives a reality.

We devote considerable space to describing the strategies and tactics adopted by the NHPA, as the impacts achieved by the agency in its first three years have been striking. As demand for information about more than 1,000 public and private hospitals and primary healthcare organizations in Australia grew, the Performance Authority focused its 50 staff on creating a narrative about performance and engaging with diverse audiences. It could do so by relying on innovative approaches to using technology and social media to make hundreds and thousands of items of performance information accessible and available in reports, brochures, infographics, and on posters, websites and the development of interactive tools. By the end of the agency's third year of reporting, there had been a cumulative total of more than 3,000 media items published about its 22 reports released to that point. These reports achieved an average audience reach of nearly 4.4 million Australians per report (range: 700,000 to 26.7 million[1]), while the agency's two main websites were by that time attracting about 2 million page views per year. In terms of impact, the agency's third report—which included release of a website interactive with postcode-level information on child immunization rates—resulted in 700 media items within 30 days of its release in early 2013. In turn, it sparked a media campaign in the nation's biggest-selling newspaper that led to new laws both at the national and state levels, and subsequently to the agreement by government health authorities to the introduction of an aspirational target for child immunization rates.

THE STRUCTURAL FOUNDATIONS OF AUSTRALIA'S HEALTH SYSTEM

On 29 November 1973, Bill Hayden, the minister for social security, rose in the federal parliament to introduce the second reading of the Health Insurance Bill that would usher in Australia's first universal health insurance system (Hayden 1973). "The principles of social equity, universal coverage and cost efficiency which form the Government's intention in this legislation are central to our whole philosophy of social progress," he told the House of Representatives. The new system was not a revolution, at least in structural terms. It worked in cooperation with, rather than in opposition to, the management and ownership arrangements that had evolved over many decades, under which public hospitals were owned and run by the state or territory in which they were located. The new system was a hybrid, involving federally funded

---

[1] Audience reach figures are calculated independently based on the audited audience or circulation of the media outlet(s) concerned. In cases of extensive media coverage, this may result in members of the public being counted more than once, as the audiences of large newspapers, radio, and TV stations, etc., often overlap.

public insurance for those not covered by private health insurance or using private hospitals, federal contributions for state-run public hospitals and subsidies for private clinicians. Previously, public hospital patients in most states were usually means tested, but the launch in 1975 of the new system, called Medibank, meant patients in public hospitals would be treated free of charge (unless they had elected to be treated privately). The Bill, passed after a rare joint sitting of the two houses of parliament, also established a system of taxpayer-funded rebates, again available to all without means testing, for subsidized care provided by general practitioners (GPs), who under Australia's arrangements remain private practitioners.

This is the bedrock of Australia's healthcare system to this day, and like any sedimentary rock comprising elements laid down over time, it is veined with structural divisions. In the Australian health system, these divisions are embedded in the country's constitutional arrangements, which go considerably further back in time than 1973; they take the form of different management responsibilities of, and funding commitments from, the two main levels of government.

When the Australian colonies decided to federate in 1901, they sought to ensure that the Commonwealth of Australia would operate under a constitution that strictly defined the powers of the new national government. The matters on which the federal parliament in Canberra is permitted to legislate are listed in Section 51 of the Constitution. Of the 39 "heads of power" enunciated in this list, only one was even remotely connected to health when the Constitution was promulgated: the power to legislate over quarantine (subsection ix). A second power was added following a referendum on social services in 1946, amid an ultimately unsuccessful plan to introduce a United Kingdom–style National Health Service. This gave the federal—or Commonwealth—government power over "the provision of maternity allowances, widows' pensions, child endowment, unemployment, pharmaceutical, sickness and hospital benefits, medical and dental services (but not so as to authorize any form of civil conscription), benefits to students and family allowances" (subsection xxiiiA). This addition provided the legal basis for the creation of Australia's Pharmaceutical Benefits Scheme in 1948, which provides subsidies for pharmaceutical drugs, as well as for the creation of Medibank 25 years later.

In Australia, the states retain "residual powers" for all aspects of healthcare other than those cited in the Constitution, including the running of public hospitals. However, as a result of a long-running shift in revenue-raising activities away from the states, the federal government now raises 80 percent of all tax collected in Australia (ABS, 2013–14), leaving the states with limited resources from which to fund their health system obligations. Under powers granted in Section 96 of the Constitution, the Commonwealth government provides payments to states to help fund their expenditures, including those for hospitals and other health activities through National Health Reform funding. While the states can supplement this funding from other sources, such as the distributions they receive from the Commonwealth-administered Goods and Services Tax (a sales tax introduced in 2000 with proceeds earmarked for use by the states), and from their own revenue sources, such as property taxes, the national government's much greater financial power has given it the means to influence the health policy environment in certain areas, such as public hospitals, that are nominally outside its constitutional preserve.

Although the system Hayden unveiled in 1973 came into existence nearly 30 years after the creation of Britain's National Health Service, and nearly 20 years after Canada's first foray into national standardization of hospital coverage with its Hospital Insurance and Diagnostic Services Act, Australia's universal health insurance arrangements remained a topic of controversy and underwent several further revisions through the 1970s and into early 1980s, as the electoral pendulum successively installed governments of different political stripes (Biggs 2003). Rebranded as Medicare in the mid-1980s, the system by the mid-1990s had won enough popular support that it was no longer under threat of being dismantled. However, from 2000 onwards, increased demand, rising costs, and a number of high-profile controversies involving allegations of poor patient care, put both the hospital and primary care sides of the system under increasing strain, financial stress, and public scrutiny. This led to the health system once again becoming a major focus of the 2007 general election campaign.

Despite the many reforms and changes to Australia's health financing arrangements in the four decades after 1973, only in recent years has a focus been placed on the benefits of performance reporting at the local level. To understand how this has come about, and the parameters within which performance reporting in Australia has been established, a more detailed outline of the events—particularly those that have taken place since 2000—will be required.

HEALTH'S RISE TO THE TOP OF THE AUSTRALIAN POLICY AGENDA

"When it comes to improving Australia's health and hospital system, as Prime Minister if elected, the buck will stop with me," Kevin Rudd, then the leader of the opposition Australian Labor Party (ALP), declared on national TV, shortly before the 2007 general election that would eject the Liberal-National government led by John Howard after 11 years in power. "I'm sick and tired of one level of Government blaming the other" (Brissenden 2007).

While this was plainly part of a political strategy—simply in the sense that it marked a point of difference from the incumbent government's position—Rudd's promise also reflected a widely shared concern over a structural and intrinsic feature of the Australian health system since the early days of Medibank, but one that was becoming increasingly problematic in the first decade of this century. The problem was that the Commonwealth on the one hand, and the states and territories on the other hand, were not (and still are not) equally responsible, either financially or managerially, for all parts of the system. When Medibank was set up, the Commonwealth agreed to pay states and territories 50 percent of the net operating costs of public hospitals on a weighted per capita basis, through formal compacts that by the early 2000s were known as the Australian Health Care Agreements. In return, the states and territories agreed to treat the patients in those hospitals free of charge, without means testing (Australia n.d.). This remained the essential deal after the scheme was rebadged as Medicare in 1984. At the same time, through its responsibility for funding Medicare rebates, the Commonwealth government picked up all the public costs of subsidizing general practitioner (GP) care.

The division of roles and sector responsibilities between the two levels of government remains to this day; in addition, states and territories are also responsible for community health services not covered by Medicare, and for public health. As a Commonwealth Government Green Paper on proposals for updating intergovernmental roles and responsibilities published in 2015 acknowledged, the "division of roles between the Commonwealth and the States and Territories... leads to 'blame shifting,' where each level of government suggests any funding gaps should be met by the other, in an unproductive debate citizens find frustrating" (Australia 2015, 38).

The arrangement results in a number of perverse incentives. If Commonwealth-funded primary health systems are not working well—for example, if patients find GPs too expensive or otherwise difficult to access—the result may be increased demand at state-run emergency departments. On the other hand, all eight states and territories have an incentive to reduce their hospital outpatient and emergency department (ED) costs by encouraging patients to seek treatment from Commonwealth-subsidized GPs and specialists. This also means that for performance reporting, Australia has not one health system, but eight—each of which has evolved its own procedures and practices, including those relating to patient care, coding of that care, and data collection (although it should be noted that considerable effort has been directed towards developing national standards in coding, collection, and reporting since the late 1980s).

This dynamic of finger pointing played out to increased effect from 2000 onwards, as the share of funding provided by the Commonwealth fell well below 50 percent—eventually dipping as low as 37 percent by 2012–13 (Australia n.d., appendix B). At the same time, there was increasing public and professional disquiet from 2000–2007 as perceptions rose that quality, as well as financial sustainability in the Australian hospital system, was under pressure. No fewer than four public inquiries were set up in different Australian states and territories from 2000 to 2005, to investigate persistent concerns about systemic quality issues and adverse events that in one case (that of the Bundaberg Base Hospital in Queensland) had been linked to the deaths of up to 90 patients (Dunbar et al. 2007).

This, then, was the backdrop to Rudd's 2007 promise to stop buck-passing on health. As part of his election campaign pitch, Rudd pledged to invite the states and territories to undertake major reforms of the nation's hospitals; furthermore, he said that if this did not occur, he would seek new powers through a referendum for a Commonwealth takeover of the hospital system. Rudd and the ALP won power in 2007 partly on the basis of this platform, and within three months of taking office, he set up a National Health and Hospitals Reform Commission to develop specific reform proposals. However, events elsewhere were already advancing the agenda outside of this Commonwealth process. These were to become the genesis for Australia's focus on health performance reporting as a mechanism to effect healthcare improvements at the coalface, rather than simply to offer transparency about financial or other inputs and outputs.

In New South Wales, Australia's most populous state, a fresh wave of concern about hospital safety had been triggered in late 2005 after the death of a 16-year-old girl who had been struck on the head by a golf ball, but who had died after receiving doses of opiates later described to a coroner as "excessive" (HETI 2007). The coroner's inquest ran for a year and kept the controversy simmering in the media, which led to an intense focus on, and heightened sensitivity to, other episodes of adverse events in hospitals as they continued to arise. The result was that in early 2008 the NSW Government established its own Special Commission of Inquiry into Acute Care Services in NSW Public Hospitals under the stewardship of a senior lawyer, Peter Garling.

The report of this investigation produced 139 recommendations. Some recommendations were imbued with greater significance than others: Garling himself identified "four pillars of reform" among his proposals, comprising recommendations for four new agencies designed to coordinate the response to the issues the inquiry uncovered. The establishment of one of these agencies in particular, which Garling proposed be called the Bureau of Health Information, he described as being of "the highest priority." "The problem is not collecting information itself but rather gathering it, understanding its meaning and interpreting it for the practitioners down to the ward or clinical unit where the patients are cared for," Garling wrote in his final report in November 2008. "It does not help if data which show a particular clinical procedure is risky are held in a computer at the headquarters of NSW Health in North Sydney until that data is interpreted and explained at the ward or unit level to the very people who carry out the procedure. All of the leading world experts to whom I spoke, told me that understanding, analysing and publishing sensibly [sic] health information will lead to big improvements in healthcare. They are right. Information is the basis for knowing where healthcare in hospitals is at, where it has to go, and when it has arrived" (Garling 2008).

This report was to prove pivotal in the development of health performance reporting in Australia. Health ministers had approved a National Health Performance Framework as early as the 1990s, which involved reporting at the national and state and territory level. As Garling tacitly acknowledged, this sort of reporting did not have the power to provide the kind of feedback that he considered necessary; the scope was too broad and local fluctuations in performance would remain camouflaged in the state and national-level averages.

When Garling's final report was published in November 2008, the tide was now running strongly in favour of using health performance reporting to drive improvement. Eight months later, and just before the NSW Government set up the Bureau of Health Information in 2009 almost exactly according to Garling's vision, the Rudd government's National Health and Hospitals Reform Commission (NHHRC) published its own final blueprint for reform at the national level. This contained its own set of proposals, covering funding and governance, access and equity, rural and remote issues, and a new focus on accountability for performance including a system of national targets covering access and treatment times. Like Garling, this report, too, included a strong emphasis on smart use of health data, with the NHHRC commissioners declaring themselves "keen to promote a culture of continuous improvement through health performance reporting," including systems to "provide comparative clinical performance data back to health services and hospitals, clinical units and clinicians. This is essential to foster continuous quality improvement" (NHHRC 2009). In their discussion of the issues, the NHHRC members went into some detail, saying they "support the use of benchmarking exercises that encourage health services to understand how they are performing relative to their peers," and also specified the need for a "nationally consistent approach to the collection and comparative reporting of indicators which monitor safety and quality of health care delivery," covering national patient experience surveys in addition to clinical quality measures (NHHRC 2009, 133).

Another crucial point for the NHHRC was that health performance reporting should not be kept out of sight as a fusty preserve for data nerds and policy wonks. Instead, it should be liberated by means of "a passionate commitment to measure and improve health and performance outcomes customized for all 'users'—consumers, health professionals, funders and governments." This vision of health reporting as a tool pitched at multiple audiences was to prove influential in the decisions that were to follow.

Since the mid-1980s, the policy contexts of Australia and Canada were converging in relation to the establishment of universal health insurance systems and increased demand for performance information, though the intergovernmental and fiscal drivers of change varied between the two nations. A reasonable conclusion is that in Canada there was a greater focus on ensuring the availability of statistics from its national agencies, and on establishing a separate narrative, by the Health Council of Canada, regarding the performance of provincial health systems (see text box 2.1). The Health Council never reported on—or created a narrative about—health organizations or local health areas. By comparison, Australia increasingly focused on the need for a narrative about performance of all of its health organizations and local health systems.

THE EVOLUTION OF THINKING ON INDICATORS IN AUSTRALIA

As the above chronology of events suggests, the thinking in Australia about what would be the main benefits of health reporting, what measures reporting primarily should focus on, and the audience it should attempt to engage was broadening rapidly from 2008 onwards. Garling's focus was mainly on the clinicians who, in his words, work on the wards and "carry out the procedure" relevant to each measure. For the 10 NHHRC commissioners, reporting just eight months after Garling, health reporting should apply "across all health services—public and private—and across all health settings." Performance reports, the NHHRC held, should be tailored not for one audience but for several, and the Commission's final report quoted approvingly from one submission, from a director of clinical governance at a large metropolitan teaching hospital, that public reporting to consumers "needs a meaningful narrative and should address issues of consumer concern and not just be a by-product of clinical or bureaucratic reporting." This submission argued that "Public reporting should be provided in a way that supports and develops community health literacy ... This can be achieved by making reports accessible and meaningful to consumers, by explaining and contextualising data, using meaningful data, addressing issues of concern to consumers as well as clinicians and engaging clinicians and consumers in the development and production process" (Draper n.d.).

The Commission's enthusiasm for this view had been visible for some time, as the commissioners had been focusing on the criteria that should help identify suitable indicators—and even what the specific indicators might be—from the outset. In April 2008, just two months after the NHHRC was established, the Commission published a discussion paper entitled "Beyond the Blame Game: Accountability and Performance Benchmarks for the next Australian Health Care Agreements" (NHHRC 2008). While reporting against health service performance indicators was already by this time increasingly being undertaken among all levels of government, the focus to this point had been almost exclusively on public hospitals, and the results were very rarely publicly available. The new principles articulated by the NHHRC set out to overturn this conception of what health performance reporting should be about.

The document set out eight guiding criteria for the development and use of performance benchmarks:

- There should be a clear distinction between performance indicators, targets and benchmarks. For example, "performance indicators" would be used to measure an attribute of the health system irrespective of whether a particular level of desirable performance had been identified, whereas some performance indicators would also have "targets" that could be used to attribute good and bad performance and encourage improvements. A "benchmark" would be a subset of targets that would have financial payments attached, or other consequences, according to whether it was hit or missed.
- There should be reciprocal measures to ensure that both tiers of government (Commonwealth, and states/territories) each had accountabilities.
- Indicators should be workable, relevant, applicable to diverse populations, and capable of being understood by those expected to act on the results.
- Regular reporting should occur across all levels of government, across the health system, and at different levels of geography ranging from whole-of-state down to individual hospitals and sub-populations, such as Indigenous Australians.
- Reporting should focus on a small group of meaningful indicators, rather

2.1 Canadians' demand for performance information: 1980 to 2007

The policy context between Australia and Canada was converging in the mid-1980s when the Canada Health Act, enacted in 1984, established the conditions under which provincial and territorial health insurance programs were eligible for federal transfer payments. Branded as Medicare, this system won popular support among Canadians in the late 1980s and early 1990s when public sector health spending was rising 3 percent to 5 percent per annum.

In the early 1990s, Canada underwent major structural changes in health in response to the size of the national debt, substantial government deficits, and unprecedented shrinkage in public sector spending. Between 1990 and 1992, governments slowed growth in health spending to 3 to 4 percent per annum, and between 1993 and 1996 spending was declining 1 percent year on year. By the end of the decade, the economy was booming and governments were reinvesting in healthcare. Between 2001 and 2005, health reviews or commissions were conducted in many provinces to guide reform and reinvestment. Calls for increased transparency and accountability could be heard nationwide, and a number of provinces established small agencies to monitor, report on, and in some instances improve health services. In 1999, the Canadian Institute for Health Information (CIHI) and Statistics Canada launched a collaborative project to report on states and their health regions in relation to health and the health system. These statistics are reported each year in CIHI's flagship product *Health Care in Canada*. CIHI made no explicit attempt to compare and pass judgment on performance across similar hospitals or health regions until its first report on hospital-standardized mortality.

In 2002, a Royal Commission on the Future of Health Care in Canada and the Standing Senate Committee on Social Affairs, Science and Technology each made recommendations to support sweeping changes in the health system. The Commission called for significant increases in funding and the establishment of the Health Council of Canada to establish common indicators and benchmarks and measure the performance of the healthcare system. In 2004, the first ministers signed the 10 Year Plan to Improve Health Care in Canada, and with it agreed to establish the Health Council of Canada to monitor and report on health system performance for the next 10 years. Starting in 2005, the Council's first reports focused on interpreting statistics to create a meaningful narrative about performance and on describing initiatives to drive improvements in order to pass judgment about the speed and direction of health reform as envisioned by first ministers. The Health Council never reported on, or created a narrative about, health organizations or local health areas.

than a longer list, in the Commission's words, to "ensure that the health system does not get 'benchmarked out.'"

- Reporting agencies should, where possible, use linked data and other methods to allow a holistic view of the patient's journey through, and experience of, the health system.
- Performance benchmarks should be selected that have the flexibility to

evolve over time in response to shifting priorities.
- Benchmarks should be set at levels capable of driving real improvement (for example, at the level of the best-performing state).

The NHHRC's document did not merely state these principles; it went further, proposing 56 specific performance benchmarks or tracking indicators that it suggested could be used in the next generation of Commonwealth-state health-care agreements. The list was prescient, with about half of the benchmarks or indicators on the proposed list being either identical or broadly similar to those agreed by all Australian governments four years later. But that is jumping ahead; in 2008 all this was seminal thinking in the context of the Australian health system at the time, and it fed in directly to the focus of the ALP government—begun by Rudd and continued by Julia Gillard after she ousted Rudd in June 2010—on using the billions of dollars of Commonwealth health funding as a lever to drive performance improvements. For the federal government, it was also seen as a means by which Canberra could prise open the lid of state-held hospital system information that had to that point been largely closed to it, and hold states and territories publicly accountable for their performance with Commonwealth funds.

In 2008, the Commonwealth signed a National Healthcare Agreement with the states and territories. This document embedded some of the principles proposed by the NHHRC, notably its stratification of indicators, targets, and benchmarks. However, it evidently took less heed of some of the NHHRC's other points, namely the concern that reporting not be too distracting or burden-some. As a review of the NHA conducted on behalf of governments in 2012 observed, the 2008 agreement contained one overall objective, split into seven long-term objectives, 11 outcomes, 26 progress measures and 15 outputs, all to be tested by means of no fewer than 70 performance indicators. (The review recommended the 70 indicators be more than halved, to just 33.) Out of this National Healthcare Agreement, two other intergovernmental partnership agreements followed. One was a National Partnership Agreement on Improving Public Hospital Services with financial reward funding attached, in the case of indicators such as emergency department access times and elective surgery waiting times (COAG 2011).

Rudd's reformist approach reached its zenith in March 2010, eight months after the delivery of the NHHRC's final report, when the prime minister used an address to the National Press Club in Canberra to announce "the most significant reform of Australia's health and hospital system since the introduction of Medicare almost three decades ago." The plan, or at least the first part of it that Rudd chose to reveal, included the establishment of a National Health and Hospital Network in which the Commonwealth would have the dominant funding role. "For the first time, eight state-run systems will become part of one national network," Rudd told those present. "And there will be one set of tough national standards to drive and deliver better hospital services" (Rudd 2010).

Rudd's original vision was that the Commonwealth would take the majority funding role of state-run public hospitals. However, this later foundered after the states and territories refused to hand back some of the tax revenues that the Commonwealth would require in order to pay for its vision. Still, the Commonwealth retained its focus on ensuring greater transparency on what it was getting for its money. To this point, the Commonwealth's payments to the states towards the running of public hospitals had taken the form of block grants, under which pre-agreed sums were paid regardless of the volume or quality of care delivered. The Commonwealth now sought to modify this approach and encourage greater efficiency and higher performance in two main ways. These were, firstly, the introduction of payments tied to targets related to national standards (e.g., waiting times for surgery and length of time in emergency departments), and secondly, by shifting the method of calculating how much it paid states for public hospital running costs to a system of activity-based funding, based on a national efficient price for each hospital service.

As considerable sums of extra funding were predicated on this new reporting regime, the states and territories were prepared to cooperate. In the 2009–2010 Commonwealth Budget, the Rudd government announced what it described as a record $64 billion boost to health and hospital funding as a result of the newly signed healthcare agreement, a $20 billion or 50 percent increase on the funding allocated under the previous set of agreements signed by the previous federal government (Health 2009).

Building on the recommendations of the NHHRC final report, revisions of the national agreements in 2011 contained the first references to a National Health Performance Authority, which was set up under an Act of Parliament, the National Health Reform Act 2011. The agreements also referred to a Performance and Accountability Framework (PAF), which codified the attempts of all nine governments to agree on a set of indicators that would apply across the health system, covering not just hospitals but also primary and community healthcare. The PAF was finally approved in December 2011 by the Council of Australian Governments (COAG), the peak intergovernmental forum in Australia that includes the prime minister and the premiers and chief ministers of the states and territories. However, the process for agreeing the indicators it contained has been described as challenging. Some of those involved in the process recall that an initial approach from the Commonwealth, state and territory negotiators was not to whittle down the 70 indicators contained in the original National Healthcare Agreement, but to add hundreds of new indicators, despite a tacit acknowledgement from participants that the NHHRC had been right in advocating for restraint and judicious selection of measures.

After much haggling, and driven by an understanding that something had to be done and that an unworkable list was not an option, the list was honed down to a list of 48 indicators, divided into two groups. Crucially, and in contrast to the reporting done to that point, these indicators were to be reported locally for the first time. About one-third (17) were focused on hospitals and the Local Hospital Networks set up by Rudd, while the remaining 31 were focused on Medicare Locals, the new network of 61 organizations also set up under the Rudd reforms to coordinate primary healthcare services (NHPA n.d.). The 48 indicators were allocated into one of three domains: equity, effectiveness, and efficiency. The PAF, which incorporated clauses anticipating future reviews and additions to the list of indicators, also articulated nine selection criteria to guide the inclusion of indicators as follows, many of which bore a strong resemblance to the criteria suggested by the NHHRC (NHPA 2012):

Policy:

1. Relevance and appropriateness for policymakers (the measure covers outcomes and/or an area of health policy focus)
2. Avoidance of perverse incentives
3. Relevance to National Health and Hospitals Network Agreement and National Health Reform Agreement

Scientific soundness:

4. Valid (accurately reflects the event or activity it purports to measure, and changes can be quantified in a scientifically sound manner)
5. Reliable (there are no data gaps, results do not vary because of unrelated factors such as who collected the data, there are no significant data delays and agencies agree the measure can be reliably and accurately measured and reported)
6. Attributable (the measure reflects outcomes that are substantially attributable to the part of the health system being assessed)
7. Comparable (the measure allows for comparisons over time, at the desired level of geographic disaggregation, between target groups, e.g., Indigenous populations, and across public and private sectors)
8. Ability to measure progress over time (indicator is sensitive enough to provide meaningful information about performance between reporting periods)

Efficiency:

9. Administratively simple and cost-effective.

Nearly 40 years after the first moves to introduce Medibank, Australia was starting to catch up with comparable advanced nations that had already been using publicly available local-level performance reporting targeted at clinicians and the public for the previous 10 to 15 years. The nation had a brand new, local-level reporting organization, the National Health Performance Authority, and a new set of indicators. But like all new organizations, its processes were untested and its success unassured. Its founding legislation, the National Health Reform Act 2011, required an independent review of the organization be conducted one year after its establishment. Given the complex intergovernmental responsibilities and funding arrangements in Australia, a number of factors would prove decisive in enabling the new Performance Authority to achieve significant impacts.

IMPLEMENTING THE NEW REPORTING REGIME

Background and Strategy

The National Health Performance Authority began its operations in early 2012. To avoid confusion, the organization is often referred to as the "Performance Authority," while the term "the Authority" tends to be used to refer to the body of seven members, appointed by the federal minister for health. The Authority membership comprises a chairman, deputy chairman and five other members, whose strategic advice and guidance feeds into operational decisions taken by the CEO. The formal appointments of all members are made by the federal minister for health. By convention, the selection of the chairman is approved by the prime minister, while the legislation requires that the appointment of the deputy chairman be approved by the premiers or chief ministers of the states and territories; the appointments of all other members (other than the chairman and deputy chairman) were initially approved by the heads of all governments and subsequently by the Commonwealth minister. Under the terms of its founding legislation, the National Health Reform Act 2011 (Section 72, clauses 1–3: see ComLaw 2011), the Performance Authority's functions are to monitor and prepare reports on local hospital networks, public and private hospitals, primary healthcare organizations, and other bodies or organizations that provide healthcare. Its Strategic Plan 2012–15 explains the mission further, saying it is to "stimulate and inform improvements in the Australian health system, increase transparency and accountability and inform consumers" (NHPA 2015).

The term "primary healthcare organizations" as used in the National Health Reform Act 2011 has always been interpreted as meaning the regionally based bodies funded by the Commonwealth to coordinate GP and allied healthcare services, rather than individual GP practices or individual practitioners. When the Performance Authority was set up, these primary care coordination bodies were known as Medicare Locals, of which there were 61 then being established across the continent. In mid-2015, these were replaced by 31 larger organizations called Primary Health Networks, which then became the prime focus for the Performance Authority's reporting about primary healthcare and the health characteristics of local populations. However, Section 7.1 of the Performance and Accountability Framework limits the Performance Authority's reporting: the "Authority will not report on the performance of individual clinicians." Strong privacy and confidentiality provisions are included in its founding Act.

The Act commits the Performance Authority to publishing reports either in print or online, which it does through its two public reporting websites. MyHospitals (www.myhospitals.gov.au), which carries information for more than 1,000 public and private hospitals across Australia, was set up in 2010 and responsibility for its maintenance was transferred to the Performance Authority in 2012. The website underwent a major upgrade to its navigation and structure in 2014 in order to increase its useability for diverse audiences. The second website, MyHealthyCommunities (www.myhealthycommunities.gov.au), houses the Performance Authority's primary care reporting and was built and launched by the agency in 2013. This website reports against the 61 Medicare Locals (now the 31 Primary Health Networks), and breaks that information down into smaller geographies where possible—either to one of the various "Statistical Areas" used by the Australian Bureau of Statistics (there are 351 Statistical Areas Level 3 covering the whole of Australia, or 106 Statistical Areas Level 4), or right down to the level of 1,500 postcodes for indicators where statistical power is sufficient. The MyHealthyCommunities website now includes more than 140 measures of health and care and the MyHospitals website includes 270 measures. Between them, these two websites are so extensive that a complete update of both would involve the refresh of more than one million items of information.

This wealth of information was achieved despite the fact that a number of the 48 indicators approved by federal, state, and territory governments have not been reported on by the Performance Authority. This is so for a variety of reasons, including the fact that a number of indicators lack a national data collection system to support them. Of the 48 indicators, 26 have been reported; but they have resulted in many more than 26 measures being reported (more than 130 on the MyHealthyCommunities website, and more than 270 on the MyHospitals website) because some indicators are measured in many different ways, such as a single indicator for primary healthcare organizations called "Measures of patient experience." Other indicators proliferate into many measures because the measures are in some cases specific to particular patients or conditions. This is the case for a hospitals indicator called "Relative Stay Index for multi-day stay patients," which is reported on in the context of lengths of stay specific to 16 common procedures and conditions responsible for a large share of bed days, while elective surgery waiting times—again a single indicator—is reported for more than 15 common types of surgery.

In developing its inaugural strategic directions, the Authority members relied on insights about what information would be useful to help local health systems improve performance through consultations with health ministers and key stakeholders. The chief executive established advisory and statutory committees of health policymakers, administrators, clinicians, and consumers to help guide this work.

In its Strategic Plan 2012–15, the Authority committed to pursue five strategic directions:

- Regularly review and assess the Performance and Accountability Framework to ensure that it remains relevant to the needs of the community.
- Build and maintain relationships with stakeholders to support the Authority's role and enhance its impact.
- Design and disseminate comparable information to stimulate and inform efforts to improve the health system, improve transparency and accountability, and inform consumers.
- Regularly monitor and report timely, accurate, and locally relevant information that compares and tracks performance of healthcare organizations and local health systems.

- Develop effective processes and tools to support data availability, collation, analyses, and information management.
- Pursue excellence in the governance, management and operations of the Authority.

Importantly, the Authority also decided against publishing its reports in the form of regular omnibus updates providing information on all 48 indicators, or as many of them that could be reported, at once. It was felt this would not be conducive to the aim of providing information in a way most likely to connect with public and professional audiences, and driving change (and would have risked the outcome warned against by the NHHRC, of audiences feeling "benchmarked out"). Instead, the organization adopted an approach intended to shorten the lag time between the availability of information and action to improve health and care. This involved a different philosophy: to optimize the positive impact of public reporting, the audience and purposes of reporting should be defined prospectively to make good decisions on report content and design. The Authority considered that effective reports and products are designed with those audiences in mind, and that to achieve results, the topics and content must offer information that is useful to target audiences, such as by shedding new light on topics on which there was previously a paucity of information. Part of this calculus was the understanding that reports must also be designed and made available using approaches to communications that align with the audiences' learning styles.

Tactics to Maximize Impact

Within this overarching strategic framework, the CEO and various component units of the Performance Authority used a number of specific approaches to ensure reports had the best prospect of, first, being noticed, and secondly but just as importantly, of connecting with the "right" audiences in order to drive change.

These approaches can be conceptualized in several specific categories:

- Apply vigilance over the wider policy and professional context, and how this might offer opportunities for specific report topics.
- Maximize the accessibility of information (to ensure it is readily understandable by target audiences).
- Maximize the availability of information (using multiple delivery channels to ensure target audiences are aware of it).
- Encourage appropriate stakeholder engagement throughout and after the production of performance information.
- Drive media uptake by leveraging the relevance of local-level results for local communities that would otherwise see little relevance in national or state-level statistics.
- Collaborate with third-party organizations to offer post-release support for the promotion of previously released information.

Many of these approaches were used in each of the Performance Authority's 22 report releases that took place from December 2012 to November 2015; a few were used in a smaller number of releases. To take the first of the above approaches, an example of this occurred just a couple of months after the release of the organization's first report. In the Performance Authority's first year, health ministers placed priority on information about primary healthcare; as a result, the agency released its first Healthy Communities report (its second report overall) in early 2013 (Healthy Communities 2013a). That report examined use of primary healthcare services (such as GP attendances), measures of patient experiences and the self-reported health of populations living in each Medicare Local area, waiting times for GP services and after-hours GP service utilization.

An additional and more telling example of being vigilant to the wider social and policy context came almost immediately after this episode. The immunization rate for children was originally to be included in that first Healthy Communities report, but the Performance Authority's staff noticed that there were low rates in a number of local areas. The differences were larger than had been expected, as previous state- and national-level publications had recorded high and relatively stable rates (exceeding 90 percent) at these much larger levels of geography, and stakeholders believed that rates were high across communities with only a few known exceptions. Accordingly, the immunization information was extracted from the earlier report, and released separately two months later as the Performance Authority's first report comparing immunization rates across local areas. The extra time enabled the Authority to establish an advisory committee with national immunization experts and expand the report and types of information released to support targeted interventions.

This first report on local variation in childhood immunization among one-, two- and five-year-olds found there were nearly 77,000 children nationally who were not fully immunized according to the country's immunization schedule (Healthy Communities 2013b). The report also found that in 32 out of 325 statistical areas across the country, the percentage of children fully immunized was less than 85 percent in at least one of the three age groups—levels clearly low enough to risk the degradation or loss of herd immunity in these low-rate areas, certainly for some of the more contagious pathogens such as measles and pertussis. The report resulted in more than 700 newspaper, radio and television items with a combined estimated audience of 27 million, a campaign by the nation's biggest-selling newspaper to improve rates and rapid changes to public health legislation in New South Wales, Australia's most populous state. Attempts to change legislation in two more states were tabled or mooted, but did not pass at that point. The validity of treating child immunization as a topic in its own right was reconfirmed the following year (2014), when the Performance Authority published its second immunization report. This time the report included new information on the uptake of the human papillomavirus vaccine designed to protect girls against cervical cancer (Healthy Communities 2014a). The report disclosed the number of children in each local community that were not fully immunized, as well as data on the number who have a parent recorded as a conscientious objector. This report prompted a similar pro-vaccination campaign by a second popular newspaper in another state. The result of media engagement processes was a combined estimated audience of 15 million within 30 days of release.

After its second year of reporting, local variation in childhood immunization remained the Performance Authority's most popular topic in terms of continued media attention. The agency's other reports that have most closely followed child immunization in terms of media coverage also show the benefit of reporting on topics likely to strike a chord with the public. Two simultaneously published reports (Healthy Communities 2013c) describing local rates of overweight and obesity and smoking attracted a combined estimated audience of five million within 30 days of release, while the time patients spend in emergency departments was also a popular topic (Healthy Communities 2014b), with a combined estimated audience of five million. Media reports about a report focusing on child and maternal health (Healthy Communities 2014c) had an estimated audience of about four million within 30 days of release.

Maximizing the accessibility of information found expression in a number of different ways. Part of the approach for making information accessible (i.e., comprehensible) has involved teasing out a compelling narrative to help make sense of the findings, rather than leaving them as tables of figures from which audiences are left to draw their own conclusions. To help with this, most report releases focus on a single topic into which a number of performance indicators can be grouped under one unifying theme. An example of this was the above-mentioned report on child and maternal health, which focused on four specific Performance and Accountability Framework indicators (infant and child mortality rate, proportion of babies with low birth rate, prevalence of smoking and the number of women with at least one antenatal visit in the first trimester; Healthy Communities 2014d). This tactic assists in identifying and targeting audiences most likely to benefit from the information, enhances the learning experience and the likelihood it will be memorable, and focuses media engagement.

While some topics are more interesting to public and health audiences than others, the Performance Authority has always taken a second, and parallel, approach to accessibility: that of designing its print and electronic products in a way intended to help target audiences learn relevant information quickly and easily. All statistical agencies use tables and graphs to convey information, but the Performance Authority employs graphic and web designers, as well as cartographers, who are interested in innovation in information graphics and use artistic and visually appealing layouts to attract and retain the attention of health audiences and journalists who are often short of time. Often the focus is on simplifying presentations of information to help them be readily understood by a generic audience; at other times, the focus is on tailoring information to make it accessible for a specific, and sometimes quite narrow, audience.

An example of audience-specific tailoring of information came about a year into the Performance Authority's reporting activities, when it detected a need among community-based health organizations for a summary of information across a number of different measures of performance. By revealing variation in performance, the agency had also learned that each hospital or local area had its own unique health "signature" in relation to its strengths and opportunities. This understanding was used to develop a unique "dartboard" graphic summarizing a wealth of performance and usage data on one chart, which was incorporated into a report that focused on local variation in health outcomes (i.e., amenable mortality and life expectancy; Healthy Communities 2013d). While media engagement focused on the numbers of avoidable deaths, the entire back half of the report also contained a section for professional health audiences comprising one of the new dartboard graphics for each of the 61 Medicare Local primary health organizations. The graphic included comparable performance information on health outcomes, in tandem with comparable performance on measures of prevention, use of health services and experiences with care. These graphics made use of the Performance Authority's peer grouping methodology, under which local areas are allocated to peer groups based on socioeconomic status, rurality and distance to hospitals. Comparing within, rather than across, peer groups allows more informed insights as to where models of care might be operating more successfully, and while this graphic was unlikely to be understood by the public, it allowed health workers in each local area to see at a glance how their area compared to other areas in their own peer group. These graphics were reproduced and distributed to each community organization as posters, and made available on the MyHealthyCommunities website. Many health professionals in local areas had never had this information before, or if they had, had been required to pay significant sums to obtain it from other agencies.

Information has also been tailored for smaller and discrete audiences. In April 2015, the Performance Authority released a Hospital Performance report comparing the costs incurred by more than 80 of Australia's largest and busiest public hospitals to provide equivalent blocks of patient care. The methodological challenges in preparing this report were immense: some 18 months of investigation and prepatory work were required to find acceptable approaches to ensuring that the hospitals from different states and territories could be compared fairly. This involved using two separate but related methodologies, each of which took a slightly different approach: one of these involved calculating the cost at each hospital of completing a "National Weighted Activity Unit," while the other method also focused on activity units but used slightly different arithmetic to reach a "Comparable Cost of Care" for each hospital. One activity unit equates to a notional "average" hospital service (excluding plant, property and equipment costs); the report was the first national comparison of hospital costs that fairly accounted for the fact that some hospitals performed more complicated operations or saw sicker patients.

The report found wide variations in costs: even among major metropolitan hospitals, the costs of providing a single NWAU could vary almost two-fold, from AUD$3,100 (CAD$3,017) to AUD$5,800 (CAD$5,644) in 2011–12. However, due to the necessary reliance on some relatively advanced statistical concepts ("cost per NWAU" being but one), it was recognized early that media outlets would find it difficult to report the findings prominently. This did not prevent the report attracting significant attention in professional circles, and vigorous debate at a number of specialist conferences at which senior Performance Authority staff presented and discussed the findings post-release.

Another example of tailoring information for more specific audiences—as well as an example of the next tactic in the list, that of delivering information through multiple channels—is the provision of interactive tools on the websites. After the agency's second year of reporting, there had been more than 35,000 users of its web-based interactive tool that enables parents and healthcare professionals to look up childhood immunization rates in local communities. Accordingly, the Performance Authority designed a completely new and updated interactive tool featuring enhanced usability and functionality to accompany updated reports on child immunization rates and potentially preventable hospitalizations.

Web-based interactives are an important secondary channel, but they are not the only means of delivering report information besides PDF reports and website data displays. The Performance Authority has gradually built up its activity on social media platforms, primarily Twitter and also LinkedIn, and has seen an increase in follower counts on both platforms in line with this. Twitter, in particular, is a useful platform for supporting report releases through broadcasting supportive contextual information likely to be noticed by journalists and health policy experts. To this end, Performance Authority staff have capitalized on the attention paid to tweets carrying new, original and useful information, by designing customized infographics—each bearing one or two salient statistics from a new report—which are then tweeted starting early in the morning on release day. These are sent out as part of a long list of tweets promoting the report and its contents, many with links to different pages of the websites, which are prepared and cleared two to three days in advance to help drive awareness of the release and engagement with the contents.

These infographics can be recycled, or adapted, for use in other contexts. After a regional branch of Australia's National Heart Foundation expressed interest in using the agency's findings on tobacco smoking rates to support its campaign for a smoke-free policy in a local town, Performance Authority staff liaised closely with the group to design and supply posters illustrating the unusually high smoking rates in the region affected, which were then shipped to the town and used for presentations at the local council and in local newspapers. (This is also an example of the last activity on the list, namely collaborating with third-party organizations where opportunities arise to promote previously released report results.) Similar approaches, involving posters, flyers, and brochures, and even movie reels illustrating the Performance Authority's work and findings, have been used as promotional tools at conference booths.

The Performance Authority has devoted significant resources to the development and refinement of these various graphic presentations (including graphics in PDF reports as well as infographics and on posters) in line with a recognition of the impact these products can have. The designers and cartographers responsible for these graphics consult with report teams and senior staff internally as well as with some external stakeholders about the designs, which, as a result, can progress through five to 20 iterations as refinements are progressively made. Although this process requires some time to complete, staff recognize that the benefits are clear in terms of improved accuracy and more effective promotion of the results.

Again, all this has overlaps with another important part of the Performance Authority's activities related to stakeholder engagement and communications. These activities are apparent in all aspects of the agency's work, but are particularly evident in the final two months of a report's production process. In addition to governance committees that provide advice to Authority members, the chief executive adopted the practice of establishing advisory committees for all reports to provide advice regarding the types of information that target audiences need in order to take action and to ensure appropriate interpretation of data. These technical and topic-specific stakeholders are but one piece of the stakeholder engagement puzzle.

Another important group of stakeholders is the state and territory governments, who are responsible for running the hospital systems in their areas and who supply data custodians with raw data about the measures before that information reaches the Performance Authority in response to a specific data request. A Jurisdictional Advisory Committee, one of the earliest committees set up by the Authority and which is chaired by an Authority member, includes a representative from each state and territory and this body is the main conduit of information from the Performance Authority to state and territory governments about which topics are proposed for future reports, and how those reports are progressing. When data is received for a specific report, and once exhaustive checks are done to ensure comparability and fitness for purpose, the data (in the form of a spreadsheet) is sent back to the relevant jurisdiction for validation. When the report itself is finalized a few weeks later, it is then provided confidentially to state and territory governments, with a specific window (usually five or 10 working days, depending on the novelty and complexity of the report) for providing feedback in time for edits to be made to the report if the Performance Authority's chief executive, a statutory office holder, considers this necessary.

The Authority's communications team co-authors all reports in collaboration with performance measurement staff, and is responsible for procedures and practices in relation to the layout and design of products (including branding), release of reports, and maintenance of the websites. The team includes people who have a background in health journalism, media relations, marketing, and graphic design. Within the week leading up to the release of a report, the communications staff provide a staggered series of briefings to a progressively widening circle of relevant stakeholders. After the jurisdictions, this usually starts with organizations whose performance may be scrutinized in the context of the findings (such as Medicare Locals, and now the Primary Health Networks), and progresses to other interested stakeholders (such as consumer groups, health and medical professional organizations and standards-setting bodies) and ends with health journalists, who are provided the report under embargo 48 hours before public release. It is important for the jurisdictions to have the opportunity to understand the report, liaise with hospitals or other organizations likely to receive media scrutiny, and discuss the detail of the methodology with report teams. General stakeholders also need time to understand the findings and consider if they wish to prepare media statements or materials of their own. Many do, and this tends to increase media coverage of a report when this happens. Interviews with key journalists are arranged one or two days before public release, so they can file a story in advance. These journalists sometimes also use the 48-hour head start created by the embargo period to commission customized interactive graphics from their own website teams. Pre-recordings with radio occur the day before public release, so that radio can run the story at the same time as the first reports begin to appear in the morning papers and other news outlets.

On the day of release, the Authority closely monitors all media to ensure accuracy of information, particularly statistics. Media outlets have usually been responsive on the rare occasion they have been notified of a major error. This risk management strategy is employed to minimize the risk of inaccurate portrayal of information on health and care in local communities. Because stakeholder engagement is so extensive and resource intensive to support awareness of and knowledge about the findings, reports are only released every four to eight weeks.

Finally, the Authority's Communications staff have promoted the Authority's brand and awareness of its information by attending select professional seminars and conferences and by pitching tailored editorial commentaries and interview opportunities to selected media outlets in three distinct ways.

The first involved placing an "op-ed" commentary in the national daily newspaper *The Australian* the day before the publication of the Authority's very first report. This timing was designed to heighten awareness of and raise anticipation for the first report, and to disseminate understanding of the Authority's role and purpose without diverting attention from the report's contents. This approach appeared to pay off, as the report was covered in a front page lead story in the same newspaper when it was released the next day.

The second approach involved communications staff working with the CEO to support specific report releases through targeted newspaper commentaries focusing on specific report topics. One, which concerned a report about regional variation in rates of stories about infant and young child mortality and some measures of maternal health, was published in the *Sydney Morning Herald* on the report's release day, and illustrated how one specific lower- to middle-income regional area had bucked the normal trend by achieving lower infant and young child mortality rates than many other higher-income city areas.

Meanwhile, the third approach has involved communications staff pitching newspaper commentaries outside report release cycles in response to opportunities created by other running issues. An example was a focus on "big data" by the *Australian Financial Review*, which ran an op-ed by the CEO explaining how big data techniques had already been, and could continue to be, used to unlock health performance improvements.

Of course, there have been plenty of other lessons aside from those learned in the course of implementing and refining particular tactics such as these. Without local information on performance, health professionals often use state-level statistics and make decisions about improvement priorities based on them. Importantly and unexpectedly, the agency's reports enabled health professionals, often for the first time, to know more about what they did not need to work on, or what they did not need to improve. For example, the Performance Authority's report on rates of overweight and obesity, and a separate report on smoking rates in local areas, highlighted communities where interventions might not be considered a high priority (because rates were low). Another report on infant and child mortality highlighted a low-income regional area where existing interventions were resulting in exemplary outcomes (as revealed by the report which showed the area having the best performance in its peer group, better than in some high-income metropolitan areas) that had not been previously known to health professionals in that area. Other health professionals, for example, learned that their local area had overweight and obesity rates twice the state-level statistic that had hitherto been the best source of local information. Finally, new information about health and care in local communities can, if communicated and promoted effectively, command large audiences. The number of users of the Performance Authority's first interactive tool on immunization rates, for example, was equal to more than half the number of GPs in the nation and likely includes public health nurses, parents and daycare workers.

On occasion, events have unfolded in unexpected ways, requiring the Performance Authority to change its approach. In 2013 work commenced on statistical work intended to result in a Hospital Performance report on rates of hospital mortality, for which there are three separate indicators in the Performance and Accountability Framework. As experience in countries other than Australia, such as the UK, has shown, such work is highly sensitive as well as highly complex, and had to be undertaken with a high degree of rigour. Extensive consultations were held over a period of many months involving statistical as well as clinical experts from Australia and elsewhere. Many consultations and teleconferences to discuss the progress of investigations were convened, some of them involving experts in different continents.

Although progress necessarily had to be deliberative, much was achieved: the Performance Authority partnered with Flinders University in South Australia to develop a new method of calculating hospital standardized mortality ratios, called the Australian Composite Model. This represented a major advance on the previous methodology that Flinders staff had previously developed in conjunction with another Australian government agency, the Australian Institute of Health and Welfare, and which had been incorporated by the Australian Commission for Safety and Quality in Health Care into a measure called the core hospital-based outcome indicator (CHBOI). The CHBOI resulted in one hospital-level mortality result, with limited opportunities for disaggregation to allow better understanding of which areas of a hospital's operations might be performing well or less well. The Australian Composite Model addressed this, by adopting the innovations from worldwide experts and institutions, including the Dr Foster Unit at Imperial College, London, and producing a method that can calculate hospital standardized mortality ratios (HSMRs) and risk of mortality for each of the 70 diagnostic conditions that make up 80 percent of the most frequent causes of death in Australian public and private hospitals.

However, the mortality work also encountered methodological challenges that proved harder to solve. In particular, differences in coding practices between states (and sometimes even between hospitals within states) have required more time to work through. These include differences in coding for admissions: in some Australian hospitals, patients who attend emergency departments (including those who die) are recorded as admitted patients, while in other hospitals such patients are recorded in a different dataset for emergency department patients only. Different practices in this area can distort results between hospitals and make fair comparison problematic. Other differences relate to palliative care; the Performance Authority found extensive variation between states and territories, and sometimes between the hospitals in the same jurisdictions, in the way that palliative care is coded and also in interpretation of the national coding standards. As palliative care patients have a greater likelihood of death as an outcome of an episode of care when compared to other types of patients, decisions on whether to include or exclude palliative patients therefore have a material impact on hospital mortality measures. Meanwhile, Performance Authority staff also encountered widespread variation across states and territories in the models of care around inter-hospital transfer of patients, in particular for conditions such as acute myocardial infarction, hip fracture surgery, and stroke, factors that again can alter the mortality ratios in ways that may distort fair comparisons. Taken together, these issues meant the agency's CEO took the view that it was not possible to proceed to publication without further work to ensure more reliable comparability.

The emphasis on reliability and on sound methodology was, and remains, paramount across the agency's reporting activities. The creation and release of valid and reliable information at small areas of geography is reliant on well-developed information systems and the use of technological innovation. The degree to which health audiences, particularly professional audiences, take heed of report findings depends on their faith in the results and confidence in the robustness of the calculations. Accordingly, in all report releases the Authority makes available technical supplements to disclose its measurement and peer group methodologies, describe its data suppression protocol for each report and cite information on which it relies.

Confidence in the accuracy and utility of report findings is essential in order for the publications to command the attention of key audiences, particularly the health managers, planners and clinicians whose everyday decisions have the potential, as Garling recognized, to bring improvements in healthcare services. In line with this reasoning, the Performance Authority in the third quarter of 2015 commenced a public consultation exercise to review the indicator set included in the Performance and Accountability Framework. This is also in accordance with the original scope of the Framework, which stipulated a number of outputs for which indicators were "to be developed": these included (for hospitals) access for special needs patients, appropriateness of care, capability and sustainability, and (for primary healthcare organizations) access for special needs patients, capability and sustainability, and continuity of care. The two-month consultation period involved an invitation to any organizations, groups or individuals to contribute their suggestions for proposed changes that could include amending existing indicators, adding new indicators or deleting existing indicators from the initial set, with any changes requiring agreement from all ministers for health (sitting as the COAG Health Council). At the time of writing, the Performance Authority was due to collate the feedback received as part of the consultation and use this to inform its own recommendations to ministers to be submitted in the first half of 2016.

As the material above illustrates, the impacts and successes of the Performance Authority from 2012 to 2015 have been considerable. However, all this is not to say the path towards an effective implementation of local-level health performance reporting in Australia has proved straightforward. In 2013, the general election resulted in a change of government in Canberra. The new Liberal-National Coalition-led administration in mid-2015 announced it would wind up the Performance Authority effective from 30 June 2016, and transfer its performance reporting functions to two existing government organizations: the Australian Institute of Health and Welfare and the Australian Commission for Safety and Quality in Health Care. This move was consistent with the new government's Smaller Government reform agenda (Finance 2015), but the commitment to preserve the Performance Authority's reporting functions confirmed that the benefits of performance reporting by this point had been recognized on both sides of the political divide. This apparent bipartisan support to local level reporting is important, and it will be interesting to note if the other element of the success enjoyed so far—establishing a narrative—is sustained.

EPILOGUE: LESSONS FOR CANADA

Australia and Canada have much to learn from each other, given similarities in their health governance structures and universal health insurance schemes. Over the past 30 to 40 years, shifts in the health economies and policy context in both countries have increased demand for performance information. While both countries have a long history of publishing health statistics, a reasonable conclusion is that Canada over time had more focus on ensuring the availability of statistics from its national agencies. Between 2004 and 2014, the Health

Council of Canada was established to engage Canadians and health professionals in a narrative about the performance of provincial health systems and the speed and direction of health reform as envisioned by first ministers. The Health Council never reported on, or created a narrative about, health organizations or local health areas.

By comparison, Australian policymakers increasingly focused on the need for a narrative, supplied through the interpretation and presentation of statistics, about the relative performance of more than 1,000 public and private hospitals and primary healthcare organizations and of local health systems. The intention was that the smart use of data would make information meaningful so consumers, patients and health professionals might better understand their health system and identify, through the illumination of variation between similar hospitals and local areas, where action should be taken. Commissioner Peter Garling had argued in his 2008 inquiry report that this approach would instill confidence among the public that information was being used to instil improvements in health and care.

What lessons might there be for Canada? First, the establishment of a small agency dedicated to monitoring and reporting on health organizations in Australia was a product of intergovernmental health policy and aligned with advice to emerge from more than one commission of inquiry (one state, one national). The degree to which board and chief executive need to be statutory office holders to ensure editorial independence is unknown, though it was used in Australia. Next, an organization dedicated to creating a narrative about performance needs a different mix of staff than one dedicated to health statistics, particularly in relation to the number or portion of staff dedicated to communications. Furthermore, a small agency established to create a narrative about performance of thousands of health organizations was only able to achieve this by capitalizing on the opportunities, only available recently, to introduce more automation processes in relation to data collection, calculations, verification and visualization. Finally, the size and growth in the use of information published by the Performance Authority suggests that health information audiences may value a narrative about performance as much as, or more than, availability of health statistics. Indeed, such a narrative may have the power to increase the size of these audiences and the number of people ready to take action to improve health and care.

REFERENCES

ABS (Australian Bureau of Statistics). 2013–14. Taxation Revenue, Australia, 2013–14. http://www.abs.gov.au/ausstats/abs@.nsf/Latestproducts/5506.0Main%20Features72013-14?opendocument&tabname=Summary&prodno=5506.0&issue=2013-14&num=&view

Australia. n.d. [2015]. *Reform of the Federation White Paper, Issues Paper 3: Evolution of Government Involvement in Health Care.* https://federation.dpmc.gov.au/evolution-government-involvement-health-care.

Australia. 2015. *Reform of the Federation: Discussion Paper.* https://federation.dpmc.gov.au/sites/default/files/publications/reform_of_the_federation_discussion_paper.pdf

Biggs, Amanda. 2003. "Medicare—Background Brief." Parliamentary Library. http://www.aph.gov.au/About_Parliament/Parliamentary_Departments/Parliamentary_Library/Publications_Archive/archive/medicare.

Brissenden, Michael. 2007. "Rudd announces hospital takeover plan." *The 7.30 Report,* 23 August. http://www.abc.net.au/7.30/content/2007/s2013516.htm.

COAG (Council of Australian Governments). 2011. *National Health Reform Agreement,* July. http://www.federalfinancialrelations.gov.au/content/npa/health_reform/national-workforce-reform/national_partnership.pdf.

ComLaw (Australian Legislation). 2011. *National Health Reform Act 2011.* https://www.comlaw.gov.au/Details/C2014C00363/Download.

Draper, Mary. n.d. Submission to NHHRC. http://www.health.gov.au/internet/nhhrc/publishing.nsf/Content/265/$FILE/Submission%20265%20-%20Mary%20Draper%20Submission.pdf.

Dunbar, James A., Prasuna Reddy, Bill Beresford, Wayne P. Ramsay and Reginald S.A. Lord. 2007. *Medical Journal of Australia* 186(2). https://www.mja.com.au/journal/2007/186/2/wake-hospital-inquiries-impact-staff-and-safety.

Finance (Australian Department of). 2015. "Efficiency through Contestability Programme." http://www.finance.gov.au/resource-management/governance/contestability/.

Garling, Peter. 2008. *Final Report of the Special Commission of Inquiry, Acute Care Services in NSW Public Hospitals,* 27 November. http://www.dpc.nsw.gov.au/__data/assets/pdf_file/0003/34194/Overview_-_Special_Commission_Of_Inquiry_Into_Acute_Care_Services_In_New_South_Wales_Public_Hospitals.pdf.

Hayden, Bill. 1973. House of Representatives, *Commonwealth Parliamentary Debates.* http://parlinfo.aph.gov.au/parlInfo/genpdf/hansard80/hansardr80/1973-11-29/0143/hansard_frag.pdf;fileType=application%2F.pdf.

Health (Australian Department of). 2009. *A New Partnership—A New Era in Health and Hospital Reform,* http://www.federalfinancialrelations.gov.au/content/npa/health_reform/national-workforce-reform/national_partnership.pdf.

Healthy Communities. 2013a. http://www.myhealthycommunities.gov.au/our-reports/australians-experiences-with-primary-health-care/march-2013.

_____. 2013b. http://www.myhealthycommunities.gov.au/our-reports/immunisation-rates-for-children/april-2013.

_____. 2013c. http://www.myhealthycommunities.gov.au/our-reports/overweight-and-obesity-rates/october-2013 and http://www.myhealthycommunities.gov.au/our-reports/tobacco-smoking-rates/october-2013.

_____. 2013d. http://www.myhealthycommunities.gov.au/our-reports/avoidable-deaths-and-life-expectancies/december-2013.

_____. 2014a. http://www.myhealthycommunities.gov.au/our-reports/immunisation-rates-for-children/march-2014.

————. 2014b. http://www.myhospitals.gov.au/our-reports/time-in-emer-gency-departments/may-2014/report.

————. 2014c. http://www.myhealthycommunities.gov.au/our-reports/child-and-maternal-health/july-2014.

————. 2014d. http://www.myhealthycommunities.gov.au/our-reports/child-and-maternal-health/july-2014.

HETI (Health Education and Training Institute, New South Wales). 2007. *Inquest into the Death of Vanessa Anderson.* http://www.heti.nsw.gov.au/Global/District-HETI/Westmead_coroners_court_inquest_Vanessa_Anderson.pdf.

NHHRC (National Health and Hospitals Reform Commission). 2008. *Beyond the Blame Game: Accountability and Performance Benchmarks for the Next Australian Health Care Agreements,* April. http://www.health.gov.au/internet/nhhrc/publishing.nsf/Content/504AD1E61C23F15ECA2574430000E2B4/$File/BeyondTheBlameGame.pdf.

NHHRC. 2009. *A Healthier Future for All Australians: Final Report June 2009.* http://www.health.gov.au/internet/nhhrc/publishing.nsf/content/1AFDEAF1FB76A1D8CA257600000B5BE2/$File/Final_Report_of_the%20nhhrc_June_2009.pdf.

NHPA (National Health Performance Authority). n.d. http://www.nhpa.gov.au/internet/nhpa/publishing.nsf/Content/1CF48F88798490D8CA257B1A0013576F/$File/121105-PAF-for-web.pdf.

NHPA. 2012. *Performance Indicators.* http://www.nhpa.gov.au/internet/nhpa/publishing.nsf/Content/PAF~PAF-Section-6

NHPA. 2015. *Strategic Plan: 2012–15.* http://www.nhpa.gov.au/internet/nhpa/publishing.nsf/Content/Strategic-Plan.

Rudd, Kevin. 2010. "Better Health, Better Hospitals." 3 March. http://www.federalfinancialrelations.gov.au/content/npa/health_reform/national-work-force-reform/national_partnership.pdf.

Chapter 3

INTERNATIONAL EXPERIENCE WITH HEALTH SYSTEM PERFORMANCE ASSESSMENT

PETER C. SMITH

Health system performance assessment (HSPA) is becoming a central instrument in the governance of modern health systems. The idea of a "health system" was first given concerted attention in the *World Health Report 2000* (World Health Organization 2000), and further developed in the WHO report *Everybody's Business: Strengthening Health Systems to Improve Health Outcomes* (WHO 2007). It defined the health system as "all the activities whose primary purpose is to promote, restore or maintain health." The WHO defines HSPA as "a country-specific process of monitoring, evaluating, communicating and reviewing the achievement of high-level health system goals based on health system strategies" (WHO 2012a). The prime objectives of HSPA are

- to set out the goals and priorities for a health system;
- to act as a focus for policy making and coordinating actions within the health system;
- to measure progress towards achievement of goals;
- to act as a basis for comparison with other health systems; and
- to promote transparency and accountability to citizens and other legitimate stakeholders for the way that money has been spent.

HSPA was given a further stimulus in the WHO European Region by the sign-

Managing a Canadian Healthcare Strategy, edited by A. Scott Carson and Kim Richard Nossal. Montreal and Kingston: McGill-Queen's University Press, Queen's Policy Studies Series. © 2016 The School of Policy Studies, Queen's University at Kingston. All rights reserved.

ing of the Tallinn Charter on Health Systems for Health and Wealth in 2008. The 53 ministers of health from the European region made a commitment "to promote transparency and be accountable for health systems performance to achieve measurable results." HSPA is seen as an important mechanism for fulfilling that commitment. As envisaged by the WHO, it is primarily a country-specific process for which there is no single accepted template, although there are many generally accepted principles of best practice in developing a specific HSPA (World Health Organization 2012a). Some of these include:

- HSPA should focus on the health system as a whole, including health promotion and public health as well as health services;
- health systems goals should be expressed in terms of outcomes such as improved health and reduced exposure to financial risk, rather than inputs such as workforce size or numbers of treatments;
- wherever feasible, progress should be quantified using reliable metrics and associated analytic techniques;
- HSPA should be a regular process, embedded in all aspects of health policy making; and
- the exact form of HSPA should be a matter of choice for individual systems, although its effectiveness is likely to be maximized by the adoption of metrics and methods that enjoy widespread international use.

Despite differences in how objectives are expressed and measured, there is almost universal agreement that any HSPA should reflect health system goals related to the following:

- the improvement in health that can be attributed to the health system as a whole;
- the health system's responsiveness to citizens' preferences;
- the financial protection offered by the health system; and
- the productivity, or value-for-money, of the health system.

Furthermore, many formulations of HSPA make reference to the issue of fairness, or equity, in how attainment of its goals is distributed across different population groups.

There is less consensus on how to incorporate health system functions into HSPA. These might include service delivery; workforce; information resources; medical products, vaccines and technologies; financing; and stewardship. Such functions are the fundamental building blocks of any health system, and how they are deployed can have a major influence on health system outcomes. However, they are often difficult to compare across different types of health system, and a focus on functions can sometimes inhibit progress towards new ways of promoting the ultimate goals of the health system, such as a shift away from treatment towards prevention of disease. It is for this reason that HSPA should focus primarily on outcomes. Assessment of functions may be an important diagnostic tool for understanding reasons for progress (or lack of progress) towards health system goals, but should not be the prime focus of HSPA.

Text box 3.1 summarizes the key features of HSPA, as envisaged by the WHO (WHO 2009).

3.1: Key features of HSPA

Health system performance assessment is regular, systematic and transparent. Reporting mechanisms are defined beforehand and cover the whole assessment. It is not bound in time by a reform agenda or national health plan endpoint, although it might be revised at regular intervals better to reflect emerging priorities and to revise targets with the aim of achieving them.

HSPA is comprehensive and balanced in scope, covers the whole health system, and is not limited to specific programs, objectives or levels of care. The performance of the system as a whole is more than the sum of the performance of each of its constituents.

HSPA is analytical and uses complementary sources of information to assess performance. Performance indicators are supported in their interpretation by policy analysis, complementary information (qualitative assessments), and reference points: trends over time, local, regional, or international comparisons or comparisons to standards, targets, or benchmarks.

In meeting these criteria, health system performance assessment needs to be transparent and promote the accountability of the health system steward.

Source: WHO (2009, 141).

PROGRESS WITH HSPA

Since the *World Health Report 2000* there have been several international efforts to promote the principles of HSPA, primarily in the form of internationally comparable report cards. Most notably, in its most recent *Health at a Glance* report, the OECD has published a series of dashboards that seek to compare 34 OECD countries in five dimensions of health system performance: health status of the population, underlying health risk factors, access to care, quality of care, and healthcare resources. These dashboards draw heavily on the long-standing OECD health database and its more recent series of healthcare quality indicators (OECD 2015). In a similar vein, the Commonwealth Fund has published a comparison of 11 countries that participate in its international survey of patients (Davis et al. 2014), and the Health Consumer Powerhouse publishes a regular scorecard of European health systems (Björnberg 2014).

There have been an increasing number of efforts to implement HSPA in individual countries. In the United States, the Commonwealth Fund has developed a report card for comparison of states (Radley et al. 2012). Nordic states are seeking to develop common approaches to HSPA. England has developed a series of national performance reporting frameworks. The Netherlands was an early adopter of the principle of HSPA. The World Health Organization (WHO 2012b) summarizes experiences in seven contrasting countries of their Europe region.

It is important to distinguish between the objectives of HSPA and those of the many other approaches to performance measurement that exist in the health system. The focus of HSPA is on accountability to populations, identifying priorities, developing strategy, and tracking progress. It is not intended to offer operational guidance on individual providers or treatments, but is rather a high-level instrument of health system governance. Implementations of HSPA can nevertheless have a variety of strategic objectives. The World Health Organization (WHO 2012b) identifies the following for the seven countries it surveys.

- *Armenia*: enhance stewardship; accountability; transparency; identify policy priorities.
- *Belgium*: transparency and accountability; comparisons with other countries; performance monitoring over time.
- *England*: performance management of public sector organizations.
- *Estonia*: enhance accountability and stewardship; provide a monitoring scheme for the National Health Plan.
- *Kyrgyzstan*: monitor progress and impact of health sector programs; accountability to donors; identify potential policy problem areas.
- *Portugal*: accountability; inform policy.
- *Turkey*: provide a monitoring and evaluation scheme for the Health Transformation Program; transparency and accountability; support the development of evidence-based policy making; guide governmental policy development; identify policy priority areas.

It is noteworthy that while these WHO case studies place quite different emphases on the various possible objectives of HSPA set out above, promoting accountability and transparency is a common theme.

RESOURCES FOR HSPA

A cornerstone of HSPA is the comparison of different health systems, either through the use of quantitative indicators or using more qualitative descriptions. HSPA can be used for international comparisons, comparisons of regions, or for comparing a single system's trends over time, or even subsystems within that single system. If undertaken persuasively, such comparisons can be a powerful instrument for securing media interest, engaging policymakers, and encouraging reform. However, such comparison can be contentious and analytically complex for a number of reasons. These include: non-comparability of concepts (e.g., different definitions of disability), different data collection mechanisms, and the need to adjust for different contextual factors (e.g., the age distribution of the populations).

A variety of information system resources have been developed to facilitate comparison and support HSPA. The longest established dataset for high income countries is the OECD Health Data, which includes data series from 1961 covering health outcomes, health service resources, utilization, and workforce (OECD 2013a). More recently, the OECD has established a Health Care Quality Indicator (HCQI) project that is identifying and collecting a series of comparable indicators of the quality of specific aspects of health services (OECD 2014a). The OECD has also been instrumental in developing the System of Health Accounts (SHA), the standard framework for producing consistent and internationally comparable financial data on health systems. Various perspectives on the OECD data sources are presented in the OECD *Health at a Glance* publications, which include a publication dedicated to the situation in OECD and EU States (OECD 2014b; OECD 2015).

The European Commission has created the European Core Health Indicators (ECHI) initiative, which assembles 88 indicators relevant to HSPA, for over 50 of which data are readily available and reasonably comparable. The indicators are grouped into five broad areas: demographic and socio-economic factors, health status, determinants of health, health services, and health promotion. The ECHI indicators can be analyzed using the web-based HEIDI tool (European Commission 2014). This prepares graphs, maps, or bar charts, showing trends in indicators, or allowing comparison between chosen countries or groups of countries.

Other data repositories include the World Bank's World Development Indicators, the World Health Organization's Global Health Observatory, and Institute of Health Metrics and Evaluation's Global Health Data Exchange. However, the coverage, completeness and reliability of these series varies greatly. The European Commission has also funded several projects under its FP7 program that identify and analyze health data from the perspective of cross-country comparisons. These include EuroREACH, EuroHOPE and ECHO. EuroREACH developed a "Health Data Navigator" that helps potential users to secure access to, and analyze, comparable data sources across Europe (Hofmarcher and Smith 2013).

Within Europe, the prime source for informed and comparable descriptions of health systems is the European Observatory on Health Systems and Policies, a partnership between the European Commission, the World Bank, the WHO, and certain member states (European Observatory on Health Systems and Policies 2014). Its Health Systems in Transition (HiT) series offers comprehensive descriptions of health systems (including some outside Europe) according to a standardized template. The series includes reports on Canada and the USA. The Observatory also publishes books on important policy issues, including a volume on the principles and practice of performance measurement in health (Smith et al. 2010) and a volume specifically examining the issues associated with health system performance comparison (Papanicolas and Smith 2013).

In 2011 the Council of the European Union set up "a reflection process ... to identify effective ways of investing in health, so as to pursue modern, responsive, and sustainable health systems." A survey of the use of HSPA by member states found that amongst 17 respondents, fully 13 (Austria, Belgium, Croatia,

Denmark, England, Finland, Greece, Lithuania, Portugal, Slovakia, Slovenia, Spain, and Sweden) reported having some sort of HSPA in place at a national or regional level. The European Commission now places a high priority on further development of HSPA, and has developed a template for health system performance assessment (Social Protection Committee Indicators Sub-group 2013). The intention is to develop a "first-step screening device to detect possible challenges in [countries'] health systems, with a specific focus on issues related to access, quality and equity." The Commission's health directorate SANTE has established an expert group to act as a forum for sharing experiences and ideas.

SOME EXAMPLES OF HSPA

This section briefly summarizes four contrasting HSPA endeavours from Belgium, Estonia, Netherlands, and the United States. The intention is to draw out the differences and commonalities between the initiatives. Each description highlights the objectives of the HSPA, the analytic framework adopted, and the mode of presentation.

Belgium

The Belgian HSPA report was released in 2012, building on publication of an earlier report in 2010 entitled "A first step towards performance assessment." The 2012 report was commissioned from an external team of independent experts (Vrijens et al. 2012). The stated strategic objectives of the Belgian HSPA process were

- to inform the health authorities of the performance of the health system and to be a support for policy planning;
- to provide a transparent and accountable view of the Belgian health system performance, in accordance with the commitment made in the Tallinn Charter; and
- in the longer term, to monitor the health system performance over time.

The specific operational objectives of the 2012 report were

- to review the core set of 55 indicators of the previous report, with a special focus on the 11 indicators for which there were no data in 2010;
- to enrich the core set with indicators from the domains of health promotion, general medicine, mental health, long-term care, end-of-life care; and to add indicators on patient-centeredness and continuity of care (two sub-dimensions of quality); and, finally, to propose indicators on equity in the health system;
- to measure the selected indicators, when possible, or to identify gaps in the availability of data; and
- to interpret the results in order to provide a global evaluation of the performance of the Belgian health system by means of several criteria, including international benchmarking when appropriate.

The report presented a "conceptual framework" that formed a basis for the HSPA, as shown in Figure 3.1. This embraced five dimensions of performance: quality, accessibility, efficiency, sustainability, and equity. A total of 74 indicators were then chosen to assess levels of performance at the national level. Considerable attention was paid to accessible presentation of the results, and Belgian results were assessed in relation to the other EU-15 countries. Many of the indicators were disaggregated according to factors such as gender, region, and socio-economic status. Where they existed, data gaps and weaknesses were acknowledged. The presentation of data concluded with an overall assessment of the strengths and weaknesses of the Belgian health system based on the reported indicators.

The final section of the report reflected on the contribution of the report itself. It suggested that the major contributions since 2010 were improved data availability, a more extensive set of indicators offering a more comprehensive view of the system, simplification of the structure of the indicators to facilitate easier understanding, more systematic analysis of the data, better use of existing information, and improved communication of results. The acknowledged weaknesses relate principally to continued data shortcomings, including data coverage, timeliness and reliability.

Netherlands

The Netherlands HSPA is reported every four years by RIVM, the Dutch National Institute for Public Health and the Environment (van den Berg, Kringos, Marks, and Klazinga 2014), with the most recent report in 2014 (van den Berg, de Boer, Gijsen, et al. 2014). The Dutch Health Care Performance Report (DHCPR) is presented to parliament as a means of holding the health ministry to account for its stewardship of the health system, and therefore plays a role similar to national audit reports in many other countries and parts of the public sector. The stated objective is "to make a contribution to the strategic decision-making of the Ministry of Health in the area of health care." The 2014 report comprised 140 indicators organized according to the three strategic objectives for which the ministry bears statutory responsibility: quality, accessibility, and affordability. The indicators were organized according to a conceptual framework developed for the OECD (Arah et al. 2006) and illustrated in Figure 3.2.

The 2014 report contained an extensive discussion on the findings, with an assessment of the performance of the Dutch system relative to previous levels of attainment, international comparators, quality standards, and legal entitlements. It found generally good and improving standards of care quality, though with some concern about care for the elderly. There were generally good levels of access to needed care, although the report notes concerns about increasing financial barriers. "Affordability" addresses the financial sustainability and efficiency of the system. The report was cautiously optimistic that recently introduced policies may have served to temper expenditure rises, and stimulated improved efficiency. A separate chapter focused on equity, mainly in the form of variations in access to care for different social groups; some evidence of

FIGURE 3.1
Conceptual Framework for Belgian HSPA Report

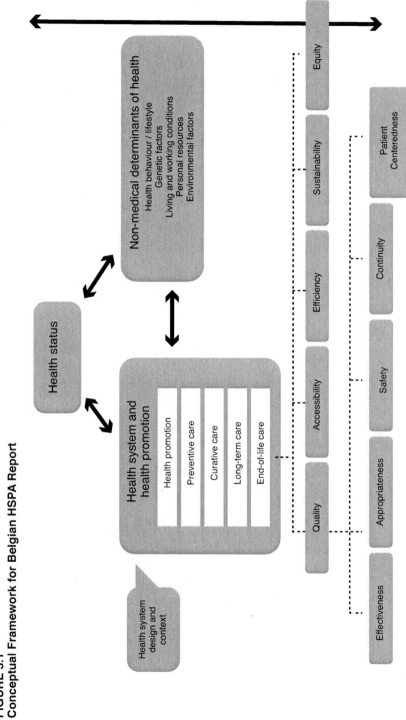

FIGURE 3.2
Conceptual Framework for Netherlands Health Care Performance Report

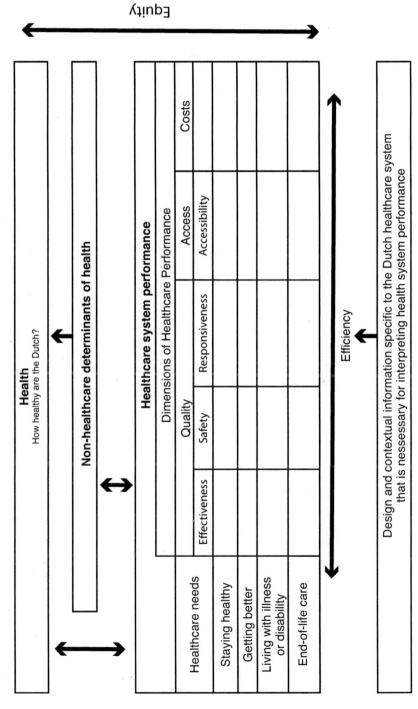

inequity, especially relating to those with lower levels of education, was found.

The 2014 report ended with an assessment of data gaps and limitations and priorities for development. Particular data weaknesses were highlighted, for example, in the areas of disease prevention, linking patient data across all modes of care, and disparities in access to services, especially for vulnerable groups. In the curative sector, there was an absence of measures of the outcomes of treatment (as opposed to the processes of care). The discussion noted the importance of comparison and discussed three main methods: comparison across countries, comparison across time, and comparison with a policy standard. The OECD quality indicators played an especially important role in international comparisons. Table 3.1 replicates an assessment of the basis for comparison in the previous reports, underlining the heavy reliance on time trends. The Dutch report for 2010 asserted that the "most important reference point" of the performance reports was "its usefulness for strategic policymaking" (Netherlands 2010, 239). To improve this, the 2010 report declared a need for "strengthening the analytical, diagnostic and future-oriented function of the DHCPR, strengthening discussions on the findings of the DHCPR within and outside the Health Ministry, [and] if need be, interim (annual) updates of a series of key indicators" (Netherlands 2010, 240).

TABLE 3.1
Percentage of indicators that allow comparison between countries, over time and with policy standards, in successive editions of the Dutch Health Care Performance Report

Comparison	Percentages of indicators that allow comparison in four editions of the DHCPR			
	DHCPR 2006	DHCPR 2008	DHCPR 2010	DHCPR 2014
International	20	26	24	24
Time trend	50	61	71	73
Policy standard	<5	21	18	17

Sweden

Sweden has a decentralized health system in which the responsibility for health services is devolved to 21 democratically elected county councils. An annual comparison of the performance of the counties is prepared jointly by the Swedish National Board of Health and Welfare and the Swedish Association of Local Authorities and Regions (2013). The report compares the performance of counties using 169 different indicators, including a considerable volume of hospital-specific data. The report takes advantage of the especially rich health information infrastructure available in Sweden, much of it derived from the national quality registers for specific diseases. Many of the data are routinely available in the public domain, but are collected together under the umbrella of the annual report. The stated objectives are

- to make the publicly financed healthcare system more transparent;
- to advance the cause of healthcare management and control; and
- to promote quality and availability [of] data about healthcare performance and outcomes.

There is no conceptual framework for the organization of the indicators, and the contents appear to reflect readily available indicators rather than any special new data collection efforts. The first 39 indicators are general measures of system performance, such as mortality, avoidable hospital use, prescribing, patient experience, and costs. The remainder of the report presents indicators for specific disease areas such as cancer, diabetes, and mental health. They include indicators of process (such as proportion treated according to guidelines), outcomes (including patient-reported outcomes), patient experience (including waiting), and costs.

The 2012 report showed that virtually all of the indicators of survival and mortality were improving. The results for some indicators were broken down by the educational level of patients, and demonstrated that those with the least education generally have lower survival rates, higher mortality rates and a greater incidence of avoidable hospitalization. Growing disparities between women and men were also apparent. The results on "confidence and patient experience," based on a National Patient Survey, were particularly extensive—and unusual in HSPA. The results in this domain suggested relatively little variation between counties, although the report indicated that there was some general room for improvement in certain dimensions, especially relating to the patient receiving adequate information about their condition and adequate involvement in treatment decisions. Although it contained a wealth of information, the report did not draw any overall conclusions about the state of Swedish healthcare.

United States

The Commonwealth Fund, a private New York foundation that aims to promote high performing healthcare systems, with a particular focus on vulnerable and minority populations, has for some time been producing scorecards of various aspects of health systems in the United States. The last national scorecard was produced in 2011; the latest edition of a series of scorecards for the 50 states was published in 2014 (Commonwealth Fund Commission on a High Performance Health System 2011). The state scorecard compares jurisdictions on 42 performance indicators of healthcare access, quality, costs, and outcomes over the 2007–2012 period (Radley et al. 2014). The purpose is to track and compare healthcare experiences and recent trends in key areas of performance to help policymakers and health system leaders identify opportunities for improvement. The intention is that, by comparing the level of performance in each state to that in the top-performing states, the scorecard should offer attainable benchmarks.

The 42 key indicators are grouped into four dimensions:

- Access and affordability (consisting of six indicators, including rates of insurance coverage, out-of-pocket expenses for medical care and cost-related barriers to receiving care)

- Prevention and treatment (16 indicators, including measures of the quality of care in ambulatory, hospital, long-term and postacute settings)
- Potentially avoidable hospital use and cost (nine indicators, including indicators of per-capita spending and insurance costs)
- Healthy lives (11 indicators, including indicators of premature death and health risk behaviours)

There are also equity indicators of variations in performance according to patients' income level (nine indicators), or race or ethnicity (10 indicators) that span the four other dimensions of performance. The indicators drew on publicly available data sources, including government-sponsored surveys, registries, publicly reported quality indicators, vital statistics, mortality data, and administrative databases.

The report highlighted large variations among the states on many indicators, reflecting the great diversity of health systems within the United States. A particular feature of the scorecards is the effort to measure change over time. The Fund was able to construct a time series for 34 of 42 indicators. There was generally five years between a historical and current year data observation, although the starting and ending points varied between indicators. The general findings were disappointing, in the sense that little progress was detected on many indicators. However, there was some evidence that targeted national policies did have a beneficial impact in some domains.

COMPARISON OF APPROACHES

Table 3.2 summarizes some of the approaches taken in the HSPA reports of the four countries under discussion. There is some variation in objectives. Notably, the focus of the Netherlands is on helping the health ministry (and possibly enabling it to be held to account) whilst the other reports have a broader objective of promoting transparency and accountability to citizens. They are each part of an ongoing process of HSPA. The reports are organized in a variety of ways. Most notably, the Netherlands, Swedish, and US reports focused strongly (but not exclusively) on health services, while the Belgian report focused slightly more on broader population health, with a particularly strong emphasis on equity. The US report is hampered by the data limitations created by its uniquely heterogeneous set of health system institutions.

There are very strong commonalities among all reports, most notably in the treatment of health services. Moreover, they all employ similar conceptual frameworks, either explicitly or implicitly. However, there are important differences. These, in part, reflect differences in the target audiences. For example, the Netherlands report is clearly aimed at those with responsibility for stewardship of the health services. The variations also reflect differences in priorities. Perhaps the weakest general areas of all reports are the limited availability of data relating to the two areas of equity and efficiency.

The basis of comparison varies markedly among the reports. Key decisions to be made include

- whether to focus on trends over time or on cross-sectional international comparison;
- whether to maintain a consistent basis for comparison across all indicators (as in the use of EU-15 in Belgium), or to vary comparators depending on the availability and usefulness of data;
- whether to focus on individual countries or some average level of attainment as a basis for comparison; and
- whether to use regional variations as a basis for identifying best local practice within a country.

Whatever the basis for comparison, it is important that the comparator health systems are considered to be genuinely comparable, with no major differences in factors beyond the control of the health system (such as diet or income levels) that are likely to influence performance. This is an area on which little research has been done, and further thinking may be fruitful. Likewise, the indicators used for international comparison have, in general, been chosen opportunistically rather than systematically. Wherever feasible they should be prepared on a consistent basis, relatively free from influences external to the health system, and available across a reasonable number of health systems, over a number of years. These are very demanding requirements, and further work might offer more systematic guidance on choice of indicators, and how best to make decisions when data are of limited quality. Increased systemization of such considerations is important not only because it improves the technical reliability of the HSPA, but also because it increases confidence that reporting is not influenced by arbitrary or biased choices regarding the basis for comparison.

HSPA IN CANADA

The chapter by Veillard and his colleagues describes the progess that has been made in performance measurement in Canada at the federal and provincial level. The discussion highlights the additional complexities that arise in seeking to implement HSPA in a federal country compared with its unitary counterparts. However, there is a sense in which the demands of decentralization, intrinsic in federal systems, places even more reliance on comparisons among systems. One of the strengths of a federal system should be that it facilitates experimentation in how services are organized, delivered, and governed. However, such experimentation can only yield its full benefits if there is adequate comparative evidence with which to assess the impact of different models. Standardization of performance metrics is always likely to be a fundamental part of such comparison.

Paradoxically, therefore, increased decentralization leads to a heightened need for standardized information resources—for comparison purposes. Such standardization can be achieved only at a national level, either through fed-

TABLE 3.2
Comparison of HSPA reports

	Belgium	Netherlands	Sweden	United States
Objectives	To help with policy planning and to promote transparency and accountability.	To inform the strategic decision-making of the Ministry of Health.	To improve transparency; to help management and control; to improve quality and availability of data.	To help policymakers and health system leaders identify opportunities for improvement.
Part of continuing process of HSPA?	Yes (since 2010)	Yes (since 2006)	Yes (since 2006)	Yes (since 2006)
Number of indicators	74	140	169	42
Basis of comparison	EU-15 average Trends over time	Trends over time Selected OECD countries EU-15 average	Trends over time County Councils Hospitals	Trends over time US States
Organization of HSPA report	Health status Accessibility Quality of care Efficiency of the health-care system Health promotion Equity and equality	Quality of care Access to care Affordability	Mortality and avoidable hospitalization Drug therapy Confidence and patient experience Availability Costs Specific diseases	Access and affordability Prevention and treatment Avoidable hospital use and cost Healthy lives Equity

eral actions, or through collaboration between provinces. Because of the large grant-in-aid transferred to provinces from the national government, federal authorities have a legitimate interest in requiring consistent performance reports from provinces. Such reports are an essential accountability requirement to reassure Canadian citizens that their federal taxes are being used well by all provinces in receipt of federal funding. Yet hitherto it seems that Canadian national governments (in common with many other federal countries) have been reluctant to require such reporting.

Moreover, a far more satisfactory approach toward standardization in principle is to secure a national consensus on data specification and performance metrics, agreed to by all relevant decentralized entities, which can serve as the basis for regular, consistent performance reporting. It is likely that the participatory nature of such action will make it more enduring, encourage adherence, and increase the reliability of information provided. The OECD health quality indicators initiative is an example of how voluntary collaboration can yield major gains in information scope and quality. Whilst Veillard and colleagues note some hopeful signs of progress towards consensus in the Canadian context, to an outside commentator, progress appears to be somewhat slow and limited, and it may be the case that some federal intervention is needed to secure resolution.

The Canadian wait-time initiative shows that collaboration between provinces can lead to meaningful standardization, consistent reporting, heightened government and managerial attention, and consequent benefits for patients and taxpayers. The challenge is to convert that energy and determination to the broader scope of the entire health system. It is not feasible to develop concrete metrics of the effectiveness of an HSPA initiative. However, in undertaking that task, a peer review of the Belgian HSPA initiative (Smith 2014) identified the following questions that need to be addressed:

- Does the HSPA have clear objectives that guide those charged with undertaking the analysis and organizing dissemination?
- Is there a clear process for commissioning the HSPA, with guidance on who is accountable for each stage of preparation?
- Is there a clear conceptual framework for the HSPA?
- Does the HSPA focus on the health system as a whole, including health promotion and public health as well as health services?
- Are systems goals appropriate? Are they expressed in terms of outcomes such as improved health and reduced exposure to financial risk, rather than processes such as workforce size or numbers of treatments?
- Is progress quantified using reliable metrics and associated analytic techniques? Are the chosen international benchmarks appropriate?
- Does the HSPA use metrics and methods that enjoy widespread international acceptance?
- Is the HSPA adequately disseminated and promoted?
- Is the HSPA a regular, sustainable process, with suitable arrangements for reviewing and updating?

- Is HSPA fully embedded in health policy making?

Explicit consideration of such criteria is likely to be essential for any Canadian HSPA initiative. It is clear that the work of CIHI and others described by Veillard et al. has secured a great deal of progress in addressing many of the analytic questions asked. Furthermore, it has facilitated some progress in addressing the specifically Canadian phenomenon of "indicator chaos." What remains is for the federal and provincial governments and other relevant authorities to determine the governance arrangements for HSPA; for example, who should prepare the reports, how will they disseminate the reports, and to whom will they be accountable?

DISCUSSION

It is important to underline that HSPA is not merely a technical accounting process. By helping to assess the governance of systems, and the effectiveness of system reforms, HSPA seeks to improve the health of citizens by exposing wasteful, poor quality, or unnecessary practices. At its best, it should focus the attention of governments, oppositions, managers, and clinicians on the fundamental objectives of the health system. HSPA is therefore an important undertaking that should provide a framework for assessing how a health system is performing, improving transparency, providing accountability for the money spent, and identifying priorities for action. It is difficult to see how publicly funded health systems can justify their expenditure to finance ministries, parliaments and the general public without seeking to demonstrate that the money for which they are responsible is well spent. This principle has become even more important in light of the financial challenges currently facing many countries. In decentralized or federal countries, it applies both at the national level and at the local level. Local administrations in decentralized countries are almost always in receipt of some element of federal or central government funding, and so should provide accountability both to their own population, and also to those of other states, provinces, or local jurisdictions.

While there are compelling arguments in favour of HSPA, it is without question a complex undertaking. Modern health systems represent one of the most complicated sectors of the economy, seeking to address a huge diversity of health needs using many types of interventions. Furthermore, although improved health and reduced inequalities are a prime objective of all health systems, there is a continuing debate about the extent to which health outcomes can be attributed to health system actions. This uncertainty has led to some debate about the correct definition of the health system, and the extent to which it should embrace broad social determinants of health such as diet and other health-related behaviour.

Notwithstanding the challenges, HSPA can help to frame our thinking about health systems, and what they are seeking to achieve. In making HSPA operational, it is crucial that there should be consistent data sources both within and between countries, since comparisons are fundamental to all HSPA exercises.

These may look at international or regional differences. Such comparisons can help identify problems and inefficiencies within national or local healthcare provision. Comparison of trends over time can also help to identify the impact of reforms. The efforts of OECD, the European Union, the World Health Organization, the Commonwealth Fund, and others are rapidly increasing the coverage, quality, and longevity of relevant data sources.

Data weaknesses nevertheless remain a common constraint, with information on certain areas of activity either absent, weak, unreliable, or out-of-date. Certain thematic areas such as mental illness present special difficulties. However, HSPA is in itself a means of improving the quality and scope of data. In a number of countries, HSPA has stimulated new data collection efforts. In particular, use of international datasets may draw attention to gaps in national data. Particular concerns noted in previous HSPA initiatives have included the absence of useful indicators of system efficiency, and the technical difficulty of developing appropriate indicators of inequalities among social groups. A further constraint in some countries has been the real or perceived threats to privacy posed by use of some health data sources.

A number of technical challenges remain. The concept of equity in health provision is difficult to capture in metrics. Access to care is an important concern, notably the coverage of health insurance systems and whether or not co-payments are required from patients. The measurement of efficiency also raises questions. Should inefficiencies be treated simply as money badly spent, or should an effort be made to measure low-value outputs? Nor is it always easy to determine whether health outcomes, such as life expectancy, are attributable to the health system or to other causes. Some progress is being made on this latter issue, through the development of concepts such as "avoidable mortality" and "avoidable hospital admissions." In addition, patient-reported outcome measures (PROMs) can assist the reporting of outcomes other than mortality. For example, instruments such as the generic EQ-5D outcome measure could be used to determine whether people with chronic long-term conditions, such as diabetes, enjoy a different quality of life in different systems.

Accountability is key to the success of HSPA. But who is to be accountable, and to whom? And how? Is it the accountability of governments to parliaments? Or of governments to citizens? Or of healthcare providers to patients? Such questions need careful consideration, as the answers will determine the nature and content of HSPA. The precise format for HSPA is generally considered to be a matter for individual countries, as there are variations in institutional arrangements, and therefore legitimate variations in the perspective to be adopted and the goals of the HSPA.

Finally, it should be noted that—by its nature—HSPA passes judgment on governments and other accountable entities, and may result in uncomfortable and controversial findings. Therefore, to the extent that it is possible, the financing and processes of HSPA should be independent of direct stakeholders. In many systems, parliaments may be the most appropriate guardians of the HSPA process, but federal and devolved systems are likely to present differing models. Whatever form it takes, however, the transparency inherent in HSPA is an intrinsic part of good governance and the accountability demanded by citizens. Rigorous, ongoing HSPA is becoming standard international practice.

Ultimately, the failure of health systems to be properly accountable for the use of their resources may lead to a reluctance on the part of governments and citizens to continue to support publicly funded health services. The breakdown of solidarity in the health domain could lead to many adverse consequences: reduced health, increased exposure to financial risk, and diminished equity. Undertaken effectively, HSPA has the potential to contribute significantly to that need for accountability, and there is a compelling argument to promote the principles of HSPA and support best practice.

ACKNOWLEDGEMENTS

This chapter has benefited greatly from the comments of participants at the Queen's Conference, and in particular from the advice of Scott Carson and Jeffrey Dixon at Queen's University. Some of the material formed the basis of a European Union peer review of the Belgian Health System Performance Assessment initiative in May 2014.

REFERENCES

Arah, O., G. Westert, J. Hurst, and N. Klazinga. 2006. "A Conceptual Framework for the OECD Health Care Quality Indicators Project." *International Journal for Quality in Health Care* 17(1): 5–13.

Björnberg, A. 2014. *Euro Health Consumer Index 2014*. Stockholm, Health Consumer Powerhouse.

Commonwealth Fund Commission on a High Performance Health System. 2011. *Why Not the Best? Results from the National Scorecard on U.S. Health System Performance, 2011*. Washington, DC: The Commonwealth Fund.

Davis, K., K. Stremikis, C. Schoen, and D. Squires. 2014. *Mirror, Mirror on the Wall, 2014 Update: How the U.S. Health Care System Compares Internationally*. New York: The Commonwealth Fund.

European Commission. 2014. "European Core Health Indicators (ECHI)." http://ec.europa.eu/health/indicators/echi/index_en.htm.

European Observatory on Health Systems and Policies. 2014. "European Observatory on Health Systems and Policies." Retrieved 4 March 2014, from http://www.euro.who.int/en/about-us/partners/observatory.

Hofmarcher, M. M. and P. Smith, Eds. 2013. *The Health Data Navigator. A Toolkit for Comparative Performance Analysis. A EuroREACH Product*. Vienna: European Centre for Social Welfare Policy and Research.

Netherlands. 2010. *Dutch Health Care Performance Report 2010*. Bilthoven: National Institute for Public Health and the Environment. http://www.doctorsandmanagers.net/adjuntos/262.1-10298_dhCPR2010.pdf

OECD (Organisation for Economic Co-operation and Development). 2013a. *OECD Health Data 2013*. Paris: OECD.

————. 2013b. *Health at a Glance 2013: OECD indicators*. Paris: OECD.

————. 2014a. "OECD Health Care Quality Indicators." http://www.oecd.org/health/health-systems/healthcarequalityindicators.htm.

————. 2014b. *Health at a Glance: Europe 2014*. Paris: OECD.

————. 2015. *Health at a Glance 2015: OECD indicators*. Paris: OECD.

Papanicolas, I. and P. Smith, Eds. 2013. *Health System Performance Comparison: An Agenda for Policy, Information and Research*. Maidenhead: Open University Press.

Radley, D., S. How, A. Fryer, D. McCarthy, and C. Schoen. 2012. *Rising to the Challenge: Results from a Scorecard on Local Health Performance, 2012*. New York: The Commonwealth Fund.

Radley, D., D. McCarthy, J. Lippa, S. Hayes, and C. Schoen. 2014. *Aiming Higher: Results from a Scorecard on State Health System Performance, 2014*. Washington, DC: The Commonwealth Fund.

Smith, P. (2014). *Peer Review in Social Protection and Social Inclusion: Health System Performance Assessment*. Brussels: European Commission.

Smith, P., M. Mossialos, I. Papanicolas, and S. Leatherman, Eds. 2010. *Performance Measurement for Health System Improvement: Experiences, Challenges and Prospects*. Cambridge: Cambridge University Press.

Social Protection Committee Indicators Sub-group. 2013. *Developing an Assessment Framework in the Area of Health Based on the Joint Assessment Framework Methodology: Final Report to the SPC on the First Stage of Implementation*. Brussels: European Commission Social Protection Committee.

Swedish National Board of Health and Welfare, and the Swedish Association of Local Authorities and Regions. 2013. *Quality and Efficiency in Swedish Health Care—Regional Comparisons 2012*. Stockholm.

van den Berg, M., D. de Boer, R. Gijsen, R. Heijink, L. Limburg, and S. Zwakhals, Eds. 2014. *Dutch Health Care Performance Report 2014*. Bilthoven: National Institute for Public Health and the Environment.

van den Berg, M., D. Kringos, L. Marks, and N. Klazinga. 2014. "The Dutch Health Care Performance Report: Seven Years of Health Care Performance Assessment in the Netherlands." *Health Research Policy and Systems* 12(1): 1.

Vrijens, F., F. Renard, P. Jonckheer, K. Van den Heede, A. Desomer, C. Van de Voorde, D. Walckiers, C. Dubois, C. Camberlin, J. Vlayen, H. Van Oyen, C. Léonard, and P. Meeus. 2012. *Performance of the Belgian Health System. Report 2012*. Brussels: Belgian Health Care Knowledge Centre (KCE).

WHO (World Health Organization). 2000. *The World Health Report 2000. Health Systems: Improving Performance*. Geneva: World Health Organization.

————. 2007. *Everybody's Business: Strengthening Health Systems to Improve Health Outcomes*. Geneva: World Health Organization.

————. 2009. *The European Health Report 2009. Health and Health Systems*. Copenhagen: World Health Organization Regional Office for Europe.

————. 2012a. *Pathways to Health System Performance Assessment: A Manual to Conducting Health System Performance Assessment at National or Sub-National Level.* Copenhagen: World Health Organization Regional Office for Europe.

————. 2012b. *Case Studies on Health System Performance Assessment. A Long-Standing Development in Europe.* Copenhagen: World Health Organization Regional Office for Europe.

Part 2

STAKEHOLDERS AS AGENTS OF CHANGE

Chapter 4

HARNESSING PATIENTS' VOICES FOR IMPROVING THE HEALTHCARE SYSTEM

SABRINA T. WONG AND JULIA M. LANGTON

Patients define the care that meets their needs. What they report from their experiences tells the system something important about the quality of healthcare delivery. In considering the transformative roles of evaluation and research, also referred to as performance measurement and reporting, this chapter explores the incorporation of patients' voices in contributing to health reforms, specifically in the area of primary healthcare.

Strong community-based primary healthcare (PHC) leads to a more equitable system of care with better population health outcomes at reduced cost (WHO 1978; WHO 2008a; WHO 2008b; Martin-Misener et al. 2012; Starfield 1998). We use the term PHC to represent the various community-based first-contact healthcare models that deliver general medical services, as well as those incorporating health promotion and community development to address the social determinants of health. Over the last decade, in response to various commissions (Clair 2000; Fyke 2001; Mazankowski 2001), and reports of poor PHC performance (Blendon et al. 2001; Schoen et al. 2005; The Commonwealth Fund 2011), Canada has seen extensive reforms and investments in PHC totalling over $1 billion (Aggarwal and Hutchison 2012). This has unleashed a myriad of innovations, only some of which have been evaluated.

In 2000, Canada's first ministers produced the Action Plan for Health System

Managing a Canadian Healthcare Strategy, edited by A. Scott Carson and Kim Richard Nossal. Montreal and Kingston: McGill-Queen's University Press, Queen's Policy Studies Series. © 2016 The School of Policy Studies, Queen's University at Kingston. All rights reserved.

Renewal, which identified the need to monitor the impact and effectiveness of PHC investments. They promised regular, comprehensive, public reporting to Canadians using agreed upon indicators of health status, outcomes, and service quality. Yet the Canadian Institute for Health Information's (CIHI) review of 10 years of healthcare system performance reporting describes PHC as a black box (CIHI 2009b). The Conference Board of Canada (2008) has found little credible PHC performance data. A report by Don Drummond (2012) found that Ontario health professionals face unclear objectives and weak accountability. There are ongoing calls for better transparency and reporting on these renewal initiatives (Drummond 2012; Cohen, McGregor, Ivanova, and Kinkaid 2012). After extensive consultation with many stakeholders, the Canadian Working Group for Primary Healthcare Improvement published a PHC Strategy for Canada (Aggarwal and Hutchison 2012), which, citing research linking performance measurement to high-performing systems, recommended such practices as a strategic priority.

PERFORMANCE MEASUREMENT AND PRIMARY HEALTHCARE

Performance measurement provides information on the quality of care to relevant stakeholders, such as clinicians, policymakers, and patients, for accountability and quality improvement in healthcare (Adair et al. 2006a; Adair et al. 2006b; Smith, Mossialos, Papanicolas, and Leatherman 2009). It is one mechanism to evaluate the extent to which health systems meet their objectives (Institute of Medicine 2006). Information about performance can be used in many ways, including public reporting, pay for performance programs, accreditation/ benchmarking, or for internal use within healthcare organizations (quality improvement; Panzer et al. 2013, Stange et al. 2014). Importantly, the provision of timely, high quality, relevant performance information is central to a continuously learning health system (Etheredge 2014). Over the last 20 years, there has been growing experience with, and recognition of, the benefits of healthcare performance measurement and reporting (Chassin, Loeb, Schmaltz, and Wacther 2010; Larsson et al. 2012; McGlynn 2003; Okun et al. 2013; Powell et al. 2014; Sinha et al. 2013; Stelfox and Straus 2013), including consumer/patient awareness and improved quality of care (Boivin et al. 2014; Powell et al. 2014).

Performance in PHC refers to the extent to which this sector meets its objectives. Though patients, clinicians, and decision makers have multiple (at times competing) objectives for PHC, most agree that we need responsive first-contact care for emerging problems, capacity to resolve common health problems, ongoing care for most chronic conditions, routine delivery of preventive and health promotion services, timely coordination with other actors concerning specific diseases, and action on social determinants of health (Haggerty and Martin 2005; Kringos et al. 2010). Moreover, Canadians expect an ongoing relationship with a trusted clinician or team, respectful treatment, and empowerment to achieve their health goals (Wensing et al. 2011; Wong, Peterson, and Black 2011).

In addition to improving the health of populations, an important goal of PHC is achieving healthcare equity: care that is delivered in response to a health need, without systematic variations related to the social, economic, demographic, or geographic characteristics of groups (Browne et al. 2012). Targeting the delivery of PHC to groups who are made vulnerable due to multiple intersecting determinants of health, can reduce health inequities. Thus, PHC performance for complex vulnerable patients is itself a test of health system performance. Our experience suggests that, far from being a small minority, up to one quarter of patients in the waiting room of a PHC clinician (e.g., family physician, nurse practitioner) could be considered complex vulnerable.

Given the breadth of the goals of PHC, it is not suprising that despite some efforts (see next section), no single data source can capture or represent its performance in Canada. There is a need to develop capacity in data collection to enhance the capabilities of performance measurement and reporting in this area of healthcare.

What is Already Known

Reporting is the immediate goal of performance measurement. In a democracy, transparency and public accountability are goals that have inherent worth, and there are growing demands for performance reporting in PHC from many stakeholders, including patients (Berta, Barnsley, Brown, and Murray 2008; Shortell and Casalino 2008). However, PHC performance reporting is challenging because of the dearth of concise and synthesized information, and because many clinicians prefer to be accountable only for their individual role and do not view themselves as elements within a larger system (Veillard et al. 2010). Despite uncertainty about how best to report PHC performance results (Gardner, Sibthrope, and Longstaff 2008; Health Council of Canada 2012; Marshall, Shekelle, Letterman, and Brook 2000; Powell, Davies, and Thomson 2003), regional case studies of performance reporting (Smith, Wright, Queram, and Lamb 2012; Young 2012), and evidence from the hospital sector (Tu et al. 2009) indicate these results can influence quality improvement agendas and improve performance. Past work shows that public performance reporting may improve performance (Faber et al. 2009; Hibbard et al. 2012; Smith, Wright, Queram, and Lamb 2012; The Commonwealth Fund 2011; Watson 2009), as it has the potential to improve the quality of care, increase accountability, facilitate public participation in healthcare (Ellins and McIver 2009; Powell, Davies, and Thomson 2003), impact societal and professional values, and direct attention to issues not currently on the policy agenda (Oxman, Lavis, Lewin, and Fretheim 2009; Oxman, Lewin, Lavis, and Fretheim 2009). It may also facilitate collaboration among stakeholders as they set a common agenda (van Walraven et al. 2010). While performance reporting in the hospital sector grows, performance reporting in PHC lags behind.

There are examples of national public reporting of PHC performance in other countries such as the National Health Performance Authority in Australia (NHPA 2014; NHPA 2015), National Ambulatory Medical Care Survey in the United States (CDC 2015), the Quality and Outcomes Framework in the United Kingdom (HSCIC 2014; Roland 2004) and the Healthcare Effectiveness and Data Information Set (HEDIS) in the United States. In Canada, by contrast, public reporting is limited. There has been some provincial PHC reporting by provincial health quality councils (e.g., Health Quality Ontario 2015; BC Patient Safety and Quality Council), mainly in Ontario, Quebec and British Columbia. The only significant national effort to date in Canada was the joint CIHI/Health Council of Canada report of a 2008 population survey (CIHI 2009a). The most commonly referenced performance information about PHC in Canada is from The Commonwealth Fund's patient and clinician surveys in industrialized nations (The Commonwealth Fund 2011). The surveys are based on samples of one thousand patients or clinicians per country in independent surveys, and show that PHC performance in Canada is poor compared to other countries. These disappointing results have helped put PHC on Canada's policy radar. Yet, the Commonwealth Fund surveys have limitations. Notably, the small sample size does not permit meaningful analysis at the regional level, where policy decisions are often made. Currently, data that would enable a better understanding of which regional features of PHC in Canada can be improved upon are nascent, with most data sets lacking the view of patients or those with limited access to PHC.

Beyond surveys, most analyses that help us understand PHC performance depend on using provincial administrative data. For example, a report on the various models of primary care in Ontario used some data from electronic records held at community health centres as well as administrative data from Ontario's Ministry of Health and Long Term Care held at the Institute for Clinical Evaluative Sciences (Glazier, Zagoriski, and Rayner 2012). Another example comes from the Manitoba Centre for Health Policy where Katz and colleagues (2014) used administrative data collected by Manitoba Health to examine 23 indicators of primary care that could have been attributed to the introduction of a physician integrated network. Yet, performance measures based only on administrative data cannot address core PHC dimensions such as health promotion, interaction with social sectors, or interpersonal processes of care. Not only is the PHC portrait of performance incomplete, there is no national level information since each system is provincially based and produces different data. For instance, administrative data usually includes only activity for physicians and omits contributions of other PHC team members. As increasing numbers of physicians are paid by salary or capitation, the quality of the administrative billing data are reduced and these data become less representative of service delivery and use.

PHC is very complex, managing as many as 450 conditions, including chronic conditions and complex care needs. Therefore, examining PHC performance requires an information system linking contextual, organizational, clinician, and patient level data to administrative and clinical data. Beyond assessing the variation within and across jurisdictions in PHC performance, a measurement system has the additional dividend of making it possible to identify innovations and combinations of innovations that are associated with better PHC performance and healthcare equity. We must assess and report on these variations so decision makers can respond to regional performance gaps and select which investments to maintain, expand, or discard.

THE ROLE OF PATIENTS' VOICES

Increasingly, patients' voices—an overarching term that includes individuals with personal experience of a health issue and informal caregivers, including family and friends (see Abelson 2015)—are recognized as a necessary part of monitoring PHC performance. Patients can offer valuable contributions toward the improvement of their own care as well as that of their loved ones. More than 20 years ago, Donabedian (1992) and others pointed out that patients could be definers of good quality, evaluators of healthcare delivery, and reporters of their experiences (Hadorn 1991; Wensing et al. 1998). As participants in healthcare delivery, they can also influence the quality of care in more direct ways, such as through involvement in treatment decisions. Using patients' perspectives for assessing the quality of care focuses on aspects of service delivery that are important for consumers (Hadorn 1991; Wensing et al. 1998). Ongoing, routine feedback to PHC providers using patient self-report surveys can lead to practice improvements and internal quality control (Cleary and Edgman-Levitan 1997).

Active engagement of patients in their own care increases their adherence to a recommended treatment and better understanding of their condition. Thus, it is more likely that they can achieve a better quality of life and satisfaction with PHC (Davis, Schoenbaum, and Audet 2005). Outcomes of patient engagement include adherence to medical advice (Golin, DiMatteo, and Gelberg 1996), fewer complaints (Taylor, Wolfe, and Cameron 2002), fewer grievances (Halperin, 2000), reductions in the level and seriousness of malpractice claims (Hickson et al. 2002), and improved functional health outcomes (Houdsen, Wong, and Dawes 2013; Maly, Bourque, and Engelhardt 1999).

Significance of Patients' Voices

Capturing patients' experiences faciliates the development of clear definitions of the desired goals of PHC and the ability to measure and monitor goal achievement, both of which are important elements of accountability (Denis 2014). Moreover, a democratic accountability goal is based on the principle that users of the healthcare system have a right to contribute to determining what publicly funded PHC services are delivered and how they are delivered (Abelson 2015). In meeting patients' healthcare needs, funders of PHC services (federal and provincial) should be able to provide rationale to patients for a specified decision or set of actions such as which services or procedures are covered by a provincial or regional health authority. That is, democratic accountability is met through answerability (Abelson & Gauvin 2004). Relationships, defined as trust, responsiveness, and agreed-upon expectations between patients and the funder of healthcare services, are another dimension of social accountability (Abelson & Gauvin 2004). Capturing patients' voices and incorporating their reports regularly into performance measurement and monitoring is a way to meet both answerability and relationship accountability dimensions. It also begins to make visible to PHC clinicians, most of whom are contracted by the government, whether patients' healthcare needs and jurisdictional service delivery needs are being met.

Abelson's (2015) work also points out that engaging patients in PHC performance measurement and reporting naturally leads to a second goal which is developmental: patients are able to learn about the goals of PHC and what to expect from PHC. In other words, this dialogue strengthens patients' ability to make decisions for themselves and their families. Moreover, when patients engage in dialogue with other PHC stakeholders (e.g., policymakers, service delivery organizations, their regular place of care), public understanding of the PHC system increases.

Taking patients' experiences in PHC seriously for the purposes of performance measurement and reporting enables a diversity of perspectives to inform the delivery and organization of health services. Their lived experience of accessing and using (or not using) PHC, as well as living with an ill-health episode, or one or more chronic conditions, positions patients well to contribute to making the PHC and other parts of the system more effective and efficient. Patient reports can capture valuable information beyond the scope of other data collections. For example, patients are considered the best source of information for judging management continuity and person-oriented dimensions such as interpersonal communication, respectfulness, and whole-person care (Haggerty et al. 2007).

Patients' Views of The Desired Goals of PHC

A valid system of quality assessment is essential for effective functioning of the PHC sector. As noted previously, no one data source (e.g., administrative, surveys from patients, providers, organizations, electronic medical record) can be used for assessing the performance of PHC on its own. Instead, creating a comprehensive performance measurement system in PHC requires combining data sources so they include patients, provider, and health system payer views. Currently, the majority of indicators used in PHC are about the technical quality of care, and the measurement of many indicators relies on proxy measures rather than outcome measures. (Langton et al. n.d.).

Most evidence- and consensus-based quality indicators (Barnsley et al. 2005; Healthcare Commission 2006; Kerr, Asch, Hamilton, and McGlynn 2000; Performance Measurement Coordinating Council 1999) that are relevant to PHC include only some of the dimensions of PHC most important to patients. An emerging body of research attempts to learn more directly from patients using PHC to find out what healthcare quality means to them (Coulter 2005; Gerteis, Edgman-Levitan, Daley, and Delbanco 1993; Ngo-Metzer et al. 2003). These studies report patient-defined goals in terms of the quality of PHC in six dimensions.

- Patient-centred/Whole Person Care: Patients would like to have their physical and emotional needs met. They would like to receive individualized care; have providers who have personalized knowledge of the whole person and who respect and know about their health beliefs, including alternative health practice beliefs; and be able to involve family and friends, if requested.

- Access: Patients are concerned about accessibility of services. They would like to have convenient places and times for visits; spend enough time with the provider; and receive assistance in navigating the health system.
- Interpersonal Processes: Patients are interested in quality of communication, shared decision making, and interpersonal style of staff and providers. This includes open communication and information flow; prompt communication of test results; involvement in decision making, if appropriate; elicitation of concerns; interpersonal style of the staff and providers, such as listening, explaining medical information in lay terms, and showing respect.
- Continuity: Patients define three types of continuity: relational—the ongoing therapeutic relationship between a consumer and provider; informational—the use of information on past events and personal circumstances to make care appropriate; and management—a consistent and coherent approach to the management of a health condition.
- Technical Effectiveness: Patients, for the most part, assume their provider is technically competent. They expect PHC to provide effective treatments, accurate diagnoses, and diligent and efficient services.
- Efficiency of Care: Patients expect efficient care with the appropriate type of provider, depending on the health issue, and coordination between the individuals and organizations involved in their care. They also expect accurate billing, efficient referral and prescription refill processes, short wait times for appointments, co-location of ancillary services, such as lab and pharmacy services, and increased personal ability to manage their own illness episodes.

Capturing Patients' Experiences

There are multiple ways to capture patients' experiences with their care. Determining the method to capture their experiences depends on the goal at hand. Within performance measurement, qualitative data (e.g., patients' stories of their experiences, deliberative consultations) can be used to identify areas that matter to patients such as past work by Wong and colleagues (2008). In the example below, one can determine that measuring transitions in care and coordination between healthcare providers is important. Qualitatively capturing whether care coordination is being achieved can tell us whether the current approach is working and provide information to guide development of performance indicators.

Take for example a family member's account of a recent healthcare experience:

Mr. P, a 75-year-old male with a diagnosis of dementia, was seen in the emergency room because he had fallen. He was admitted and medicated because he started having seizures. While in hospital A, he was catheterized because there was some discussion amongst the providers about his prostate and whether he would be a candidate for surgery. Because of his dementia, he kept pulling the catheter out, trying to get up to go to the bathroom. A referral was made for Mr. P to see the urologist. During his hospitalization, the urologist did not see him. Mr. P remained catheterized and was subsequently discharged to a "short term" stay program at hospital B.

After two weeks in his placement at hospital B, his wife was called to let her know that Mr. P would need to be discharged and go home the following week. Mrs. P stated that her husband could not come home because she was unable to care for him alone, given his dementia, with his added inability to walk and catheter still in situ. Mrs. P asked for hospital B to arrange home support as she had no idea how to assist him with walking or do catheter care. The hospital called a few days later and declared they were discharging Mr. P but did not have home supports in place. Mrs. P called her daughter as she realized she is unable to advocate for herself or her husband. The daughter called hospital B and strongly stated that Mr. P could not be discharged home. After several phone calls between the daughter and the hospital, Mr. P was discharged to a residential care home. After one day of being in the residential care home, Mr. P's catheter bag was filled with blood; the staff at the care home were having difficulty with the catheter.

Mr. P was transported back to hospital A. A referral to the urologist was made again, and his daughter witnessed this referral being made. The urologist stated he had received the referral but would follow up with Mr. P via outpatient (and not in the emergency room). Mr. P was discharged from the ER with his catheter still in situ to the residential care facility. He spent a total of two and a half months shuttling between hospitals A and B. He was still waiting to be seen by the urologist. Mrs. P is now living alone and the daughter has taken time off work to sort through her father's healthcare needs and work with her mother.

Prior to entering the ER, Mr. P was an avid walker and biker. Afterwards, he remained in a residential care home, unable to walk without help, and with a urinary catheter. His daughter had to take time off work and his wife's functional and mental health declined because of the interrelated string of events. There was no single provider or place that was most responsible or accountable for Mr. P's care. Mr. P's decline in health meant he could not advocate for himself, and his family was unable to navigate the healthcare system successfully. Mr. P, his wife, and daughter have spent countless hours in the hospital, trying to navigate the healthcare system, and have not received the support they need from the PHC clinician or other community-based PHC services.

Mr P's case vividly demonstrates that care remains fragmented. Primary healthcare clinicians may not know their patients are hospitalized, and when patients are discharged from the hospital they (or their families) are left to navigate the system themselves as healthcare sectors have little or no incentive, motivation, or capacity to coordinate with each other. This is especially problematic for those who are unable to advocate for themselves, and who may or may not have family in close proximity to assist.

Another way to capture patient experiences is by using deliberation methods. The PHC system benefits from patients being involved in deliberating on and prioritizing healthcare decisions affecting the population. In some recent work, Boivin and colleagues (2014) conducted the first randomized controlled trial assessing the impact of patient involvement on establishing PHC improvement priorities at the community level. They compared the agreement between patients and professionals on healthcare improvement priorities when professionals were consulted alone with consultation involving both patients and professionals. When patients were involved in priority settings, PHC priorities for quality indicators were more aligned with the core components of the Medical Home and Chronic Care Model. This includes access to PHC, self-care support, patient participation in clinical decisions, and partnership with community organizations. In contrast, priorities established by professionals alone placed a greater emphasis on the technical quality of single disease management indicators. Involving patients improved the agreement between professionals and patients on priorities for PHC indicators.

The most common way to capture patients' experiences is through the use of self-report surveys. While patient surveys have been part of measuring and monitoring the quality of the acute care healthcare system for many decades, incorporation of self-report surveys in PHC is more recent (Totten et al. 2012). Indeed there is international interest in the use of patient-reported outcome measures (PROMs) to monitor the effectiveness of healthcare services and interventions. Regulatory agencies, including the U.S. Food and Drug Administration and the United Kingdom's National Health Service, now require the use of PROMs (Devlin and Appleby 2010) and patient-reported experience measures (PREMs). This interest in incorporating PROMS or patients' experiences is driven by the fact that, in most situations, individuals, or those who can advocate for individuals, are the best judges of their own health and well-being (Bryan et al. 2014). Moreover, incorporating patient-reported data fills a gap where more common data such as mortality and hospitalization fail to capture many important aspects of their lives (Bryan et al. 2014; Bryan, McGrail, and Davis 2012; McGrail, Bryan, and Davis 2012).

MOVING PERFORMANCE MEASUREMENT FORWARD IN PRIMARY CARE

Patients can be agents of change in the area of performance measurement and reporting by sharing their experiences through qualitative (e.g., stories, deliberative methods) and quantitative (e.g., surveys) methods that are used to collect information in a rigorous and systematic way. Patients can also allow and advocate for linked clinical and administrative data generated about them to be used in rigorous research that will inform health services delivery.

An example of clinical data that could be linked to administrative data in primary care comes from the Canadian Primary Care Sentinel Surveillance Network (CPCSSN). The CPCSSN is a pan-Canadian network of networks where clinical data are extracted from about 10 different electronic medical record systems. These anonymous clinical and utilization data are from a national sample of patients who have a family physician. Currently, CPCSSN provides standard feedback reports every three months to its over 800 sentinels, representing over one million patients across Canada. The CPCSSN aims to generate and use knowledge to improve the quality of care for Canadians suffering from chronic conditions such as hypertension, osteoarthritis, diabetes, depression, and Parkinson's disease. The CPCSSN has completed pan-Canadian data validation as well as several manuscripts that outline the extent to which these chronic conditions are seen in primary care (Godwin et al. 2015; Williamson et al. 2014; Wong et al. 2014). Linking clinical data from CPCSSN and administrative data has recently taken place in Ontario, Manitoba, and Newfoundland. Studies using these linked data have the potential to inform health service delivery across primary and tertiary care.

Role of Stakeholders

The role of PHC stakeholders is to ensure information that is best reported by patients is incorporated into decision-making processes. Information from patients is likely to be best incorporated at the interface between patients and their regular primary care clinicians. A major challenge is that different stakeholders require different information; for example, aggregated information from patients may be challenging to incorporate at a practice level but may be useful for higher level decisions such as resource allocation, (e.g., division of family practice in British Columbia, health authority).

Developing and maintaining a pan-Canadian PHC information system that includes patients' reports of their experiences and outcomes, and their clinical and administrative, as well as other relevant data (such as provider and organizational information), would provide a valuable asset for Canadians. This system could be used to inform the work of individual providers with a practice panel, whereby patients are assigned to a physician/nurse practitioner within a practice, but may be treated at any given time by any number of clinicians. A robust information system could produce information to be used for targeting health promotion, communicable disease prevention, chronic disease management, and even end-of-life care.

Worldwide, there is an interest in improving the science of comparative health system reporting (Smith, Mossialos, Papanicolas, and Leatherman 2009; Smith and Papanicolas 2012). One of the 12 Community Based Primary Health Care innovation teams funded by the Canadian Institute for Health Research provides an example of researchers, decision makers, clinicians, and patients working together to create a comprehensive performance portrait. They are using data from the most appropriate sources (e.g., administrative, provider, organizational, and patient surveys) to measure and report on dimensions of primary healthcare, and these dimensions are driven by what is most important to stakeholders, instead of simply relying on easily available data or expert opinion (Wong et al. 2013). This kind of work could help to make Canada a leader in evaluating the effectiveness of PHC innovations. The goal of this program of research is to demonstrate the feasibility and usefulness of comparative and comprehensive PHC performance measurement and reporting in regions, as a foundation to inform innovation in the delivery and organization of the Canadian PHC system. As health service researchers, clinicians, and stewards (e.g., health authorities, decision makers) of the healthcare system, our role is to ensure we have information on patient experiences and, importantly, outcomes, and that we investigate what systems or structures produce performance.

Acknowledgement and Reconciliation between Paradigms

It has been argued that there is a need to reconcile competing paradigms of patient-centred PHC and new public management (NPM; Lavoie, Boulton, and Dwyer 2010; Tenbensel, Dwyer, and Lavoie 2014). Within the PHC paradigm, the international community has highlighted key characteristics that must be met in order for PHC to be effective, especially when serving vulnerable populations:

- Services must focus on, and be responsive to, existing and emerging health needs
- Providers must establish trust-based and enduring personal relationships
- Services must be comprehensive, continuous, and provide person-centred care
- PHC services must be responsible for the health of all in the community
- PHC services must take responsibility for tackling determinants of ill-health, and be prepared to act as advocates
- PHC providers must consider that the community and individuals seeking care are partners in managing their own health and that of their community (World Health Organization 2008a).

Indeed, the "patient-centred" approach, which emerged in the late 1960s, is a foundational piece in today's movement of the medical or primary care home. Mead and Bower's (2000; 2002) reviews of the literature identified the following key criteria for a patient-centred clinical encounter: (1) exploring both the disease and the illness experience (biopsychosocial perspective); (2) understanding the whole person (patient-as-person); (3) finding common ground regarding management (sharing power and responsibility); (4) incorporating prevention and health promotion (the therapeutic alliance); and (5) enhancing the doctor-patient relationship (the doctor-as-person; 2000, 1087–88). Within this framework, clinicians are called upon to understand the social and family context, culture, and history of their patients. Clinicians and patients are expected to interact in ways that are non-biased, demonstrating understanding and acceptance of the other's potentially diverse background (Barlow and Reading 2008).

On the other hand, the new public management paradigm, which emerged in the 1970s, focuses attention on competition among clinicians. PHC is reduced to a collection of programs and services that can be tendered separately to different clinicians (Lavoie, Boulton, and Dwyer 2010). Within NPM, there is a conceptualization of health services users as "consumers" who navigate between interchangeable health providers. In some situations, this is contrary to PHC objectives, which emphasize the importance of long-term trust-based relationships between services users and clinicians, and determinants of health.

Internationally, contractual relationships have been influenced by the NPM paradigm, and its language of "empowering consumers," which translated into the contracting out of public services. The NPM has unintended effects such as the promotion of competition between clinicians with the stated intent to increase consumer choices, and an increased emphasis on private (often for-profit) investments in capital and financial incentives (Diefenbach 2009; Dunleavy, Margretts, Bastow, and Tinkler 2005). In Canada, NPM did not result in a wholesale contracting out of health services as seen in New Zealand or the UK (Petsoulas et al. 2011); however, it was nevertheless discussed extensively within the federal public service, by the auditor general of Canada, the Office of the Comptroller General, the Treasury Board Secretariat, and all offices with a regulatory mandate over public administration (Aucoin 1995; Savoie 1994).

An awareness of the PHC and NPM paradigms by stakeholders is needed. Careful attention to the purpose for which we use data collected on patients' experiences and other performance measures is necessary. Measures in isolation of context, which are used to evaluate performance for accountability purposes, promotes isolation rather than helpful conversation (Jordan et al. 2009). Organizations that use metrics to foster reflection, experimentation, and assessment help providers to advance knowledge, rather than simply delivering knowledge that was advanced elsewhere (Saba et al. 2012). As Stange and colleagues (2014) point out, organizations that focus on effectiveness, not just efficiencies, emphasize long-term goals over short-term productivity. These kinds of organizations attempt to navigate between the two paradigms, trying to find a balance between achieving the goals of PHC and the realities of contractual relationships.

CONCLUSION

In summary, patients' voices are important in examining where we can improve PHC in order to better meet patients' needs. Their voices can be harnessed using a variety of different approaches, ranging from having patients tell their healthcare experience stories, to having them fill out surveys and provide self-reporting information, to getting their consent to link their clinical and other data that is already being collected. The role of all PHC stakeholders is to incorporate patients' experience data into an information system that can provide the data for a performance measurement and reporting environment that is meant to stimulate and evaluate innovations in care delivery. Incorporating patients' reports of their experiences also serves to meet important dimensions of democratic accountability that include relationships and answerability. Stakeholders need to be aware of two overarching paradigms, PHC and new public management, in determining the purpose for which performance measures are used. Balancing the use of measures to improve quality and effectiveness of care with efficiency will enable organizations to meet long-term goals.

REFERENCES

Abelson, J. 2015. "Patient Engagement and Canada's SPOR Initiative: A Resource Guide for Research Teams and Networks." For the Ontario SPOR SUPPORT Unit, March (version 1.0).

Abelson, J. and F. Gauvin. 2004. "Engaging Citizens: One Route to Health Care Accountability." Ottawa, ON: Canadian Policy Research Networks.

Adair, C. E., E. Simpson, A. L. Casebeer, J. M. Birdsell, K. A. Hayden, and S. Lewis. 2006a. "Performance Measurement in Healthcare: Part I—Concepts and Trends from a State of the Science Review." *Health Policy* 1(4): 85–104. Accessed 29 September 2014. http://www.pubmedcentral.nih.gov/articlerender.fcgi?artid=2585357&tool=pmcentrez&rendertype=abstract.

―――. 2006b. "Performance Measurement in Healthcare: Part II—State of the Science Findings by Stage of the Performance Measurement Process." *Health Policy* 2(1): 56–78. Accessed 29 September 2014. http://www.pubmedcentral.nih.gov/articlerender.fcgi?artid=2585424&tool=pmcentrez&rendertype=abstract.

Aggarwal, M., and B. Hutchison. 2012. *Toward a Primary Care Strategy for Canada*. Ottawa, ON: Canadian Working Group for Primary Healthcare Improvement.

Aucoin, P. 1995. *The New Public Management: Canada in Comparative Perspective*. Ottawa: Institute for Research on Public Policy.

Barlow, J. K., and C. Reading. 2008."Relational Care." In *A Guide to Health Care and Support for Aboriginal People Living with HIV/AIDS. Final report*. Canadian Aboriginal AIDS Network (CAAN).

Barnsley, J., W. Berta, R. Cockerill, J. MacPhail, and E. Vayda. 2005. "Identifying Performance Indicators for Family Practice." *Canadian Family Physician* 51: 700–701.

Berta, W., J. Barnsley, A. Brown, and M. Murray. 2008. "In the Eyes of the Beholder: Population Perspectives on Performance Priorities for Primary Care in Canada." *Healthcare Policy* 4(2): 86–100.

Blendon, R. J., C. Schoen, K. Donelan, R. Osborn, C. M. DesRoches, K. Scoles, K. Davis, K. Binns, and K. Zapert. 2001. "Physicians' Views on Quality of Care: A Five-Country Comparison." *Health Affairs* 20(3): 233–43.

Boivin, A., P. Lehoux, R. Lacombe, J. Burgers, and R. Grol. 2014. "Involving Patients in Setting Priorities for Healthcare Improvement: A Cluster Randomized Trial." *Implementation Science* 9: 24. http://www.implementationscience.com/content/9/1/24.

Browne, A. J., C. Varcoe, S. T. Wong, V. Smye, J. Lavoie, D. Littlejohn, D. Tu, O. Godwin, and M. Krause. 2012. "Closing the Health Equity Gap: Strategies for Primary Healthcare Organizations." *International Journal of Health Equity* 11:59. doi:10.1186/1475-9276-11-59

Bryan, S., J. Davis, J. Broesch, M. M. Doyle-Waters, S. Lewis, K. McGrail, M. J. McGregor, J. M. Murphy, R. Sawatzky, K. Dalzell, M. Dawes, and M. Smith. 2014. "Choosing Your Partner for the PROM: A Review of Evidence on Patient-Reported Outcome Measures for Use in Primary and Community Care. *Healthcare Policy* (Nov) 10(2): 38–51.

Bryan, S., K. M. McGrail, and J. Davis. 2012. "In God We Trust; All Others Must Bring Data." *Healthcare Papers* 11(4): 55–8.

Canadian Institute for Health Information (CIHI). 2009a. *Experiences with Primary Health Care in Canada*. Ottawa, ON: Canadian Institute for Health Information, 1–23.

———. 2009b. *Health Care in Canada 2009: A Decade in Review*. Ottawa, ON.

CDC (Centers for Disease Control and Prevention). 2015. "Ambulatory Health Care Data. Survey Instruments: NAMCS Survey Instruments." Last modified 6 April 2015. http://www.cdc.gov/nchs/ahcd/ahcd_survey_instruments.htm.

Chassin, M. R., J. M. Loeb, S. P. Schmaltz, and R. M. Wachter. 2010. "Accountability Measures—Using Measurement to Promote Quality Improvement." *New England Journal of Medicine* 363: 683–88. doi:10.1056/NEJMsb1002320

Clair, M. 2000. *Commission d'étude sur les services de santé et les services sociaux: Les Solutions émergentes, Rapport et recommandations*. Gouvernement du Québec.

Cleary, P., and S. Edgman-Levitan. 1997. "Health Care Quality: Incorporating Consumer Perspectives." *Journal of the American Medical Association* 278(19): 1608–11.

Cohen, M., M. McGregor, I. Ivanova, and C. Kinkaid. 2012. *Beyond the Hospital Walls: Activity Based Funding Versus Integrated Health Care Reform*. Vancouver, BC: Canadian Centre for Policy Alternatives.

Commonwealth Fund, The. 2011. *Commonwealth Fund International Health Policy Survey*. New York, NY: The Commonwealth Fund.

Conference Board of Canada. 2008. *Healthy People, Healthy Performance, Healthy Profits: The Case for Business Action on the Socio-Economic Determinants of Health*. Ottawa, ON.

Coulter, A. 2005. "What Do Patients and the Public Want from Primary Care." *British Medical Journal* 331: 1199–1201.

Davis, K., S. Schoenbaum, and A-M. Audet. 2005. "A 2020 Vision of Patient-Centered Primary Care." *Journal of General Internal Medicine* 20: 953–57.

Denis, J. L. 2014. "Accountability in Healthcare Organizations and Systems." *Healthcare Policy* (Sept. 10, Special issue): 8–11.

Devlin, N., and J. Appleby. 2010. *Getting the Most Out of PROMs: Putting Health Outcomes at the Heart of NHS Decision-Making*. March. London: The King's Fund. https://www.kingsfund.org.uk/sites/files/kf/Getting-the-most-outof-PROMs-Nancy-Devlin-John-Appleby-Kings-Fund-March-2010.pdf.

Diefenbach, T. 2009. "New Public Management in Public Sector Organizations: The Dark Sides of Managerialistic 'Enlightenment.'" *Public Administration* 87(4): 892–909.

Donabedian, A. 1992. "Quality Assurance in Health Care: Consumers' Role." *Quality in Health Care* 1: 247–51.

Drummond, D. 2012. *Commission on the Reform of Ontario's Public Services*. Ottawa, ON: Government of Ontario.

Dunleavy, P., H. Margretts, S. Bastow, and J. Tinkler. 2005. "New Public Management is Dead—Long Live Digital-Era Governance." *Journal of Public Administration Research and Theory* 16: 467–94.

Ellins, J. L., and S. A. McIver. 2009. *Supporting Patients to Make Informed Choices in Primary Care: What Works?* Birmingham: University of Birmingham Health Services Management Centre.

Etheredge, L. M. 2014. "Rapid Learning: A Breakthrough Agenda." *Health Affairs* (Millwood) 33(7): 1155–62. doi:10.1377/hlthaff.2014.0043

Faber, M., M. Bosch, H. Wollersheim, S. Leatherman, and R. Grol. 2009. "Public Reporting in Health Care: How Do Consumers Use Quality-of-Care Information? A Systematic Review." *Medical Care* 47(1): 1–8.

Fyke, K. J. 2001. *Caring for Medicare: Sustaining a Quality System*. Regina, Saskatchewan: Government of Saskatchewan.

Gardner, K. L., B. Sibthorpe, and D. Longstaff. 2008. "National Quality and Performance System for Divisions of General Practice: Early Reflections on a System Under Development." *Australia and New Zealand Health Policy* 5(1): 8.

Gerteis, M., S. Edgman-Levitan, J. Daley, and T. Delbanco. 1993. *Through the Patient's Eyes: Understanding and Promoting Patient-Centered Care*. San Francisco, CA: Jossey-Bass.

Glazier, R. H., B. M. Zagorski, and J. Rayner. 2012. *Comparison of Primary Care Models in Ontario by Demographics, Case Mix and Emergency Department Use, 2008/09 to 2009/10: ICES Investigative Report*. Toronto, ON: Institute for Clinical Evaluative Sciences.

Godwin, M., T. Williamson, S. Khan, J. Kaczorowski, S. Asghari, R. Morkem,

M. Dawes, and R. Birtwhistle. 2015. "Prevalence and Management of Hypertension in Primary Care Practices with Electronic Medical Records: A Report from the Canadian Primary Care Sentinel Surveillance Network." *Canadian Medical Association Journal* Open 3(1): E76–E82. doi:10.9778/cmajo.20140038

Golin, C., M. DiMatteo, and L. Gelberg. 1996. "The Role of Patient Participation in the Doctor Visit: Implications for Adherence to Diabetes Care." *Diabetes Care* 19: 1153–64.

Hadorn, D. 1991. "The Role of Public Values in Setting Health Care Priorities." *Social Science and Medicine* 32(7): 773–81.

Haggerty, J., and C. M. Martin. 2005. *Evaluating Primary Health Care in Canada: The Right Questions to Ask!* Ottawa: Health Canada, Primary and Continuing Healthcare Division.

Haggerty, J., F. Burge, J. F. Levesque, D. Gass, R. Pineault, M. D. Beaulieu, and D. Santor. 2007. "Operational Definitions of Attributes of Primary Health Care: Consensus Among Canadian Experts." *Annals of Family Medicine*. 5(4):336–44.

Halperin, E. 2000. "Grievances Against Physicians: 11 Years' Experience of a Medical Society Grievance Committee." *Western Journal of Medicine* 173: 235–38.

Healthcare Commission. 2006. "The 'Better Metrics' Project." Version 7. Better Metrics Project Team. London: Healthcare Commission. Accessed 7 September 2006. http://www.healthcarecommission.org.uk/_db/_documents/Healthcare_Commission_7th_version_better_metrics_28July06.pdf.

Health Council of Canada. 2012. *Progress Report 2012: Health Care Renewal in Canada*. Toronto, ON: Health Council of Canada.

Health Quality Ontario. 2015. Website. Last modified 2015. http://www.ohqc.ca/en/index.html.

Hibbard, J. H., J. Greene, S. Sofaer, K. Firminger, and J. Hirsh. 2012. "An Experiment Shows That a Well-Designed Report on Costs and Quality Can Help Consumers Choose High-Value Health Care." *Health Affairs* (Project Hope) 31(3): 560–68.

Hickson, G. B., C. Federspiel, J. Pichert, C. Miller, J. Gauld-Jaeger, and P. Bost. 2002. "Patient Complaints and Malpractice Risk." *Journal of the American Medical Association* 287: 2951–57.

Housden, L., S. T. Wong, and M. Dawes. 2013. "Are Group Medical Visits for Diabetes Effective? A Systematic and Meta-Analytic Review of the Literature." *Canadian Medical Association Journal* (August) (e-pub). doi:10.1503/cmaj.130053

HSCIC (Health and Social Care Information Centre). 2014. "QOF 2013/14 Results." The Quality and Outcomes Framework. http://www.qof.hscic.gov.uk.

Institute of Medicine (IOM). 2006. *Performance Measurement: Accelerating Improvement. Pathways to Quality Health Series*. Committee on Redesigning Health Insurance Performance Measures, Payment, and Performance Improvement Programs. http://www.nap.edu/catalog/11517.html.

Jordan, M. E., H. J. Lanham, B. F. Crabtree, P. A. Nutting, W. L. Miller, K. C. Stange, and R. R. McDaniel, Jr. 2009. "The role of Conversation in Health Care Interventions: Enabling Sensemaking and Learning. *Implementation Science* (March) 4: 15.

Katz A., D. Chateau, B. Bogdanovic, C. Taylor, K-L. McGowan, L. Rajotte, J. Dziadek. 2014. *Physician Integrated Network: A Second Look*. Winnipeg, MB: Manitoba Centre for Health Policy.

Kerr, E., S. Asch, E. Hamilton, and E. McGlynn. 2000. *Quality of Care for General Medical Conditions: A Review of the Literature and Quality Indicators*. Santa Monica, CA: RAND.

Kringos, D. S., W. G. W. Boerma, A. Hutchinson, J. van der Zee, and P. P. Groenewegen. 2010. "The Breadth of Primary Care: A Systematic Literature Review of its Core Dimensions." *BMC Health Services Research* 10: 65. http://www.biomedcentral.com/1472-6963/10/65.

Langton, J., S. T. Wong, K. McGrail, W. Hogg, J. L. Haggerty, J. Campbell et al. n.d. (under review). "Primary Care Performance Measurement and Reporting at a Regional Level: Could a Matrix Approach Provide Actionable Information for Policymakers and Clinicians?"

Larsson S., P. Lawyer, G. Garellick, B. Lindahl, and M. Lundström. 2012. "Use of 13 Disease Registries in 5 Countries Demonstrates the Potential to Use Outcome Data to Improve Health Care's Value." *Health Affairs* (Millwood) 31 (1): 220–27. doi:10.1377/hlthaff.2011.0762.e

Lavoie, J. G., A. F. Boulton, and J. Dwyer. 2010. "Analysing Contractual Environments: Lessons from Indigenous Health in Canada, Australia and New Zealand." *Public Administration* 88(3): 665–79.

Maly, R. C., L. B. Bourque, and R. F. Engelhardt. 1999. "A Randomized Controlled Trial of Facilitating Information Giving to Patients with Chronic Medical Conditions: Effects on Outcomes of Care." *Journal of Family Practice* 48: 356–63.

Marshall, M. N., P. G. Shekelle, S. Leatherman, and R. H. Brook. 2000. "Public Disclosure of Performance Data: Learning from the US Experience. Quality in Health Care." QHC 9 (1): 53–7.

Martin-Misener, R., R. Valaitis, S. Wong, M. MacDonald, D. Meagher-Stewart, J. Kaczorowski, L. O-Mara, R. Savage, and P. Austin. 2012. "A Scoping Literature of Collaboration Between Primary Care and Public Health." *Primary Health Care Research & Development*, 1–20.

Mazankowski, D. 2001. *A Framework for Reform: Report of the Premier's Advisory Council on Health*, , 1–75. Edmonton, AB: Government of Alberta.

McGlynn, E. A. 2003. "Introduction and Overview of the Conceptual Framework for a National Quality Measurement and Reporting System." *Medical Care* 41: I1–17.

McGrail, K. M., S. Bryan, and J. Davis. 2012. "Let's All Go to the PROM: The Case for Routine Patient-Reported Outcome Measurement in Canadian Healthcare." *Healthcare Papers* 11(4): 8–18.

Mead, N., and P. Bower. 2000. "Patient-Centredness: A Conceptual Framework and Review of the Empirical Literature." *Social Science & Medicine* 51: 1087–1110.

———. 2002. "Patient-Centred Consultations and Outcomes in Primary Care: A Review of the Literature." *Patient Education Counseling* 48: 51–61.

National Health Performance Authority (NHPA). 2014. *Healthy Communities: GP Care for Patients with Chronic Conditions in 2009–2013*. Canberra: Government of Australia.

National Health Performance Authority (NHPA). 2015. *Healthy Communities: Frequent GP Attenders and Their Use of Health Services in 2012–13*. Canberra: Government of Australia.

Ngo-Metzger, Q., M. P. Massagli, B. R. Clarridge, M. Manocchia, R. B. Davis, L. I. Iessoni, and R. S. Phillips. 2003. "Linguistic and Cultural Barriers to Care: Perspectives of Chinese and Vietnamese Immigrants." *Journal of General Internal Medicine* 18: 44–52.

Okun, S., D. McGraw, P. Stang, E. Larson, D. Goldmann, J. Kupersmith, R. Filart, R. M. Robertson, C. Grossmann, and M. Murray. 2013. *Making the Case for Continuous Learning from Routinely Collected Data*. Discussion paper. Washington, DC: Institute of Medicine.

Oxman, A. D., J. N. Lavis, S. Lewin, and A. Fretheim. 2009. "SUPPORT Tools for Evidence-Informed Health Policymaking (STP) 1: What is Evidence-Informed Policymaking?" *Health Research Policy and Systems* 7 Suppl. 1: S1.

Oxman, A. D., S. Lewin, J. N. Lavis, and A. Fretheim. 2009. "SUPPORT Tools for Evidence-Informed Health Policymaking (STP) 15: Engaging the Public in Evidence-Informed Policymaking." *Health Research Policy and Systems* 7 Suppl. 1: S15.

Panzer, R. J., R. S. Gitomer, W. H. Greene, P. R. Webster, K. R. Landry, and C. A. Riccobono. 2013. "Increasing Demands for Quality Measurement." *Journal of the American Medical Association* 310(18): 1971–80. doi:10.1001/jama.2013.282047

Performance Measurement Coordinating Council. 1999. "Desirable Attributes of Performance Measures." A Consensus Document from the AMA, JCAHO, and NCQA. *American Medical Association*. Accessed 8 September 2006. www.amaassn.org/ama/pub/category/2946.html

Petsoulas, C., P. Allen, D. Hughes, P. Vincent-Jones, and J. Roberts. 2011. "The Use of Standard Contracts in the English National Health Service: A Case Study Analysis." *Social Science & Medicine* 73(2): 185–92.

Powell, A. A., K. M. White, M. R. Partin, K. Halek, S. H. Hysong, E. Zarling, S. R. Kirsh, and H. E. Bloomfield. 2014. "More than a Score: A Qualitative Study of Ancillary Benefits of Performance Measurement." *BMJ Quality & Safety* 23 (8): 651–58. doi:10.1136/bmjqs-2013-002149

Powell, A. E., H. T. Davies, and R. G. Thomson. 2003. "Using Routine Comparative Data to Assess the Quality of Health Care: Understanding and Avoiding Common Pitfalls." *Quality & Safety in Health Care* 12(2): 122–28.

Roland, M. 2004. "Linking Physicians' Pay to the Quality of Care—A Major Experiment in the United Kingdom." *New England Journal of Medicine*

351(14): 1448–54.

Saba, G. W., T. J. Villela, E. Chen, H. Hammer, and T. Bodenheimer. 2012. "The Myth of the Lone Physician: Toward a Collaborative Alternative." *Annals of Family Medicine* 10: 169–73.

Savoie, D. J. 1994. *Thatcher, Reagan, Mulroney: In Search of a New Bureaucracy.* Pittsburgh: University of Pittsburgh.

Schoen, C., R. Osborn, P. T. Huynh, M. Doty, K. Zapert, J. Peugh, and K. Davis. 2005. "Taking the Pulse of Health Care Systems: Experiences of Patients with Health Problems in Six Countries." *Health Affairs*: 509–25.

Shortell, S. M., and L. P. Casalino. 2008. "Health Care Reform Requires Accountable Care Systems." *Journal of the American Medical Association* 300(1): 95–7.

Sinha, S., G. Peach, J. D. Poloniecki, M. M. Thompson, and P. J. Holt. 2013. "Studies Using English Administrative Data (Hospital Episode Statistics) to Assess Health-Care Outcomes—Systematic Review and Recommendations for Reporting." *European Journal of Public Health* 23(1): 86–92. doi:10.1093/eurpub/cks046

Smith, M. A., A. Wright, C. Queram, and G. C. Lamb. 2012. "Public Reporting Helped Drive Quality Improvement in Outpatient Diabetes Care among Wisconsin Physician Groups." *Health Affairs* (Project Hope) 31(3): 570–77.

Smith, P. C., and I. Papanicolas. 2012. *Health System Performance Comparison: An Agenda for Policy, Information and Research. Policy Summary 4.* Copenhagen, Denmark: WHO Regional Office for Europe: iv–41.

Smith, P. C., E. Mossialos, I. Papanicolas, and S. Leatherman. 2009. *Performance Measurement for Health System Improvement: Experiences, Challenges and Prospects,* 707. Edited by E. Mossialos. Cambridge: Cambridge University Press.

Stange, K. S., R.S. Etz, K. Gullett, S. A. Sweeney, W. L. Miller, C.R. Ja´en, B. F. Crabtree, P. A. Nutting, and R. E. Glasgow. 2014. "Metrics for Assessing Improvements in Primary Health Care." *Annual Review of Public Health* 35: 423–42.

Starfield, B. 1998. *Primary Care: Balancing Health Needs, Services, and Technology.* New York: Oxford University Press.

Stelfox, H. T., and S. E. Straus. 2013. "Measuring Quality of Care: Considering Measurement Frameworks and Needs Assessment to Guide Quality Indicator Development." *Journal of Clinical Epidemiology* 66(12): 1320–27. doi:10.1016/j.jclinepi.2013.05.018

Taylor, D., R. Wolfe, and P. Cameron. 2002. "Complaints from Emergency Department Patients Largely Result from Treatment and Communication Problems." *Emergency Medicine* 14: 43–9.

Tenbensel, T., J. Dwyer, and J. G. Lavoie. 2014. "How Not to Kill the Golden Goose?: Reconceptualising Accountability Relationships in Community-Based Third Sector Organizations." *Public Management Review* 16(7): 925–44. doi:10.1080/14719037.2013.77005

Totten, A., J. Wagner, A. Tiwari, C, O'Haire, J. Griffin, and M. Walker. 2012.

Closing the Quality Gap: Revisiting the State of the Science. Vol. 5: Public Reporting as a Quality Improvement Strategy. Evidence Reports/Technology Assessments, No. 208.5. Portland: Oregon Evidence-based Practice Center. Rockville, MD: Agency for Healthcare Research and Quality.

Tu, J. V., L. R. Donovan, D. S. Lee, J. T. Wang, P. C. Austin, D. A. Alter, and D. T. Ko. 2009. "Effectiveness of Public Report Cards for Improving the Quality of Cardiac Care. The EFFECT Study: A Randomized Trial." *Journal of the American Medical Association* 302(21): 2330–37.

van Walraven, C., I. A. Dhalla, C. Bell, E. Etchells, I. G. Stiell, K. Zarnke, P. C. Austin, and A. J. Forster. 2010. "Derivation and Validation of an Index to Predict Early Death or Unplanned Readmission After Discharge from Hospital to the Community." *Canadian Medical Association Journal* 182(6): 551–7.

Veillard, J., T. Huynh, S. Ardal, S. Kadandale, N. S. Klazinga, and A. D. Brown. 2010. "Making Health System Performance Measurement Useful to Policy Makers: Aligning Strategies, Measurement and Local Health System Accountability in Ontario." *Healthcare Policy* 5(3): 49–65.

Watson, D. E. 2009. "For Discussion: A Roadmap for Population-Based Information Systems to Enhance Primary Healthcare in Canada." *Healthcare Policy/Politiques de Santé* 5 (Spec. No): 105–20.

Wensing, M., H. P. Jung, J. Mainz, F. Olesen, and R. Grol. 1998. "A Systematic Review of the Literature on Patient Priorities for General Practice Care. Part 1: Description of the Research Domain." *Social Science and Medicine* 47(10): 1573–88.

Wensing, M., M. van der Eijk, J. Koetsenruijter, B. R. Bloem, M. Munneke, and M. Faber. 2011. "Connectedness of Healthcare Professionals Involved in the Treatment of Patients with Parkinson's Disease: A Social Networks Study." *Implementation Science* 6(1): 67.

Williamson, T., M. E. Green, R. V. Birtwhistle, S. Khan, S. Garies, S. T. Wong, N. Natarajan, D. Manca, and N. Drummond. 2014. "Expanding Opportunities for Using Electronic Medical Record Data: Validation of Eight Case Definitions for Chronic Disease Surveillance in the Canadian Primary Care Sentinel Surveillance Network Database." *Annals of Family Medicine.*

Wong, S. T., W. Hogg, F. Burge, K. McGrail, S. Johnston, R. Martin-Misener, C. Scott, J. L. Haggerty et al. 2013. "Transforming CBPHC Delivery through Comprehensive Performance Measurement and Reporting." Team Grant: Community-Based Primary Healthcare. Canadian Institutes for Health Research. http://www.transformationphc.ca/

Wong, S. T., D. Manca, D. Barber, R. Morkem, S. Khan, J. Kotecha, T. Williamson, R. Birtwhistle, and S. Patten. 2014. "The Diagnosis of Depression and Its Treatment in Canadian Primary Care Practices: An Epidemiological Study. *Canadian Medical Association Journal* Open 2(4): E337–42. doi:10.9778/cmajo.20140052

Wong, S. T., S. Peterson, and C. Black. 2011. "Patient Activation in Primary Healthcare: A Comparison Between Healthier Individuals and Those with a

Chronic Illness." *Medical Care* 49(5): 469–79.

Wong, S. T., D. Watson, S. Regan, and E. Young. 2008. "Public Perspectives of Primary Health Care." *Healthcare Policy* 3(3): 89–104.

World Health Organization (WHO). 1978. *Declaration of Alma Ata.* Geneva: WHO.

———. 2008a. *The World Health Report 2008. Primary Health Care: Now More Than Ever.* Geneva, Switzerland: World Health Organization.

———. 2008b. *Closing the Gap in a Generation: Health Equity through Action on the Social Determinants of Health. Commission on Social Determinants of Health.* Geneva, Switzerland: World Health Organization.

Young, G. J. 2012. "Multistakeholder Regional Collaboratives Have Been Key Drivers of Public Reporting, But Now Face Challenges." *Health Affairs* (Project Hope) 31(3): 578–84.

Chapter 5

PATIENT ENGAGEMENT FOR HEALTHCARE SYSTEM CHANGE

MONICA C. LABARGE, JAY M. HANDELMAN, AND ALEX MITCHELL

In this chapter, we address the ways that patients attempt to influence health-care system change through individual and collective advocacy, and consider how healthcare organizations can harness that patient involvement to create systems and structures that genuinely place the patient at the centre of care. We examine individual level advocacy by first exploring some of the existing tensions between the current physician-centred care system and the newer approach of patient-centred care. We then draw on perspectives of individual complaining behaviour and (dis)satisfaction from the marketing literature to understand how, within a patient-centred healthcare context, health organizations can benefit by effectively tending to this dynamic.

Having established these individual level dynamics, we then investigate the broader socio-political collective dynamics that facilitate this patient-centred trend. Last, we present a case study of a mid-sized healthcare organization that has effectively tended to both individual and collective level issues in order to arrive at lessons learned. The chapter demonstrates that patient-centred care leads to a number of benefits for patients and for healthcare providers. For patients, patient-centred care leads to greater levels of satisfaction which is associated with improved medical outcomes as satisfied patients are more likely to comply with treatment advice as well as be more actively engaged in their

Managing a Canadian Healthcare Strategy, edited by A. Scott Carson and Kim Richard Nossal. Montreal and Kingston: McGill-Queen's University Press, Queen's Policy Studies Series. © 2016 The School of Policy Studies, Queen's University at Kingston. All rights reserved.

own care. For the healthcare organizations, practicing patient-centred care attunes these organizations to important societal trends that have come to legitimize the patient's experience. By skillfully engaging in the societal dialogue about healthcare, rather than ignoring this dialogue, refuting it, or trying to "correct" it, healthcare providers win greater trust and legitimacy from societal stakeholders.

UNDERSTANDING PATIENT-DRIVEN ADVOCACY

Patient-centred care has rapidly become the new paradigm within healthcare organizations. The concept pervades practical discussions about quality and efficiency of care and the organizational structure necessary to enact such a patient focus, as well as more philosophical deliberations about the roles of, and relationships between, patients and doctors. The definition of patient-centred care seems simple enough: It is care that is centred around the patient, a model in which healthcare providers partner with patients and families to identify and satisfy the full range of patients' needs and preferences (Frampton et al. 2008). A broader perspective argues that the originators of the concept were driven primarily by moral arguments based on a deep respect for patients as "unique living beings, and the obligation to care for them on their own terms; thus patients are known as persons in context of their own social worlds, listened to, informed, respected, and involved in their care—and their wishes are honored … during their health care journey" (Epstein and Street 2011).

Accompanying the rise of patient-centred medicine, with its goals of improved quality, safety, and efficiency—together with an expanded role for the patient in the equation of healthcare delivery—has been a concurrent transformation of the individual, who was previously simply a member of society, into a "consumer"—of commercial products, of public goods and services, and also of healthcare. As identified by Bardes in an editorial in the *New England Journal of Medicine* (2012, 782–83), "if the patient is reconceived as a consumer, new priorities take center stage: customer satisfaction, comparison shopping, broad ranges of alternatives, choice, and unimpeded access to goods and services." While perhaps overly simplistic in his description of the priorities of a patient in a healthcare "service" encounter, Bardes is nonetheless correct when he identifies that this shift towards "patient as consumer" sets up a conflict between "a Ptolemaic universe revolving around the physician [against] a Copernican galaxy revolving around the patient" (2012, 782–83), and that the favouring of one party over another fails to recognize the need for an ongoing, functional, and trust-based relationship between the two in order to achieve both patient goals as well as broader societal health goals.

And yet, this conflict between the desire of physicians to dispense treatment in the way that they feel is superior versus the happiness (or lack thereof) of the patient with that treatment is not new. What is new is the increasing visibility of patients who feel the need to express displeasure at (real or perceived) substandard care, at the same time as there has been an explosion in the media that shares that sentiment, ranging from within small social groups to a broader, sometimes global, scale. In order for organizations to cope with and manage this feedback, it is important to understand what we have learned from years of studying both consumers and organizations about how and why individuals behave the way they do when they are unhappy with the provision of a service, and the implications of those behaviours for the service-providing organization. To arrive at this understanding, we will first examine the individual level dynamics that surround patient-centred care.

INDIVIDUAL LEVEL PATIENT-DRIVEN ADVOCACY

Patient Complaining

In marketing, we have always known that consumers complain when they are unhappy and, in fact, that complaining is an important part of social life. Accordingly, marketing research can help to explain in healthcare the role of complaining in individual patient-driven advocacy. Complaining can be broadly defined as "a behavioral expression of dissatisfaction" (McGraw, Warren, and Khan 2015), and in the context of marketing has typically either been expressed as direct communication of that dissatisfaction to the service provider via in-person complaints, calls, or letters, or word-of-mouth conversations with friends and family. Over the years, however, the reach of negative experiences and dissatisfaction has expanded, through both traditional media interested in airing (and sometimes obtaining redress for) major service failures, and digital forms like social media and websites where consumers (including patients) can expound at length about their dissatisfying encounter with a service provider. Depending on the forum, these complaints can be directed at a small number of people an individual knows personally, or at a wider range of individuals they may want to "warn" about their interactions with a service provider, through to a disclosure of appalling treatment that receives national or international attention and widespread media coverage.

A variety of reasons or purposes for such complaining behaviours emerged in a recent review of consumer complaining behaviour (McGraw, Warren, and Khan 2015). People may complain to simply make small talk or to vent frustrations, which can help reduce the detrimental emotional effects of coping with negative thoughts and feelings as a result of a product failure or negative service encounter. People also complain in order to influence the perception and behaviour of others, either for their own or others' benefit. Complainers may want to warn people about a negative experience so that they may avoid a similar fate, they may want to obtain redress, which could range from a simple apology to something more material such as a refund, or they may simply want to receive sympathy and/or moral support.

However, complaining is not always beneficial for the complainer. Moreover, it can have unintended consequences. People who complain frequently or about what others perceive as "trivial" matters are frequently viewed negatively—as grumpy, argumentative, or boring. At other times, people believe that complaining will not have the effect that they are hoping for, or they do not have time to seek redress. Due to these costs of complaining, people sometimes do not complain even when they are greatly dissatisfied (McGraw, Warren, and Khan 2015).

Patient Complaining in a Healthcare Environment

It is important to recognize, however, that much of our understanding about consumer complaining, as described above, comes out of a context that is not at all similar to that experienced by patients in a healthcare environment. First, a commercial context is frequently characterized by competition: If consumers are unhappy, they will first complain, and if that complaint is not addressed then they will take their business elsewhere. As a result, organizations are primarily motivated by self-interest, as they must make consumers happy or risk financial loss. In healthcare, however, and particularly in Canada, it is rare for patients to have the flexibility of being able to choose healthcare providers. In many cases, patients are aware that they are lucky to have a primary healthcare provider who will see them on a somewhat timely basis and provide regular care; switching to another provider is often difficult, if not nearly impossible, and this has been made more so with governmental systems (e.g., in Ontario) that require patients to un-enroll from one provider before being able to switch to another. For patients who have ongoing health issues that may need regular or emergency care, the risk of having a period of time without a regular provider is often too great to bear, and thus patients are essentially forced to stay with a provider regardless of their level of satisfaction.

Secondly, while occasionally expensive and certainly frustrating, the vast majority of marketplace transactions that stimulate complaining behaviour are not critical to consumers' immediate or long-term emotional and physical well-being. The same cannot be said for a healthcare environment, in which many patients only engage in interactions with their healthcare provider when they are unwell. That provider is, at least in some sense, what stands between a patient continuing to feel unwell or being provided with some immediate relief (or hope for some future relief as a result of further testing and consultation with a specialist) from the discomfort they are experiencing. As a result, it is reasonable to assert that a patient may feel that they have to maintain a positive relationship with that provider at all costs, regardless of their desire to complain about their treatment. In this way, the costs of complaining about some aspect of treatment may be very salient to the patient, and extreme dissatisfaction may need to occur before the patient is willing to risk a deterioration in the physician-patient relationship by expressing dissatisfaction with some aspect of care. They may fear being labelled a "difficult patient," and having their future healthcare concerns affected as a result. Since the physician acts as a gatekeeper to specialists and advanced forms of testing that the patient would not otherwise be able to access, these are not unreasonable concerns. The author of an essay on the impact of doctor disillusionment with our current medical system recounts hearing countless stories of patients in pain who worry that asking for more pain medication "will be construed as entitled meddling" (O'Rourke 2014).

It is therefore not altogether surprising that if patients are dissatisfied with some element of their care and feel that they are unable to secure redress from the provider, they will want to vent that frustration to other people, either face-to-face or via social or traditional media, as a way of coping with the negative thoughts and feelings that McGraw, Warren, and Khan (2015) have identified as one of the causes of complaining behaviour. Depending on the severity of the perception of mistreatment, such negative feelings may range from simple frustration and disappointment to anger, humiliation, worthlessness, and even abandonment, and have deep and lasting psychological effects (Boodman 2015).

But this increased likelihood that an unhappy patient will engage in indirect, rather than direct, complaining is ultimately bad for the provider, because it fails to allow providers to address problems as they occur and instead forces them to be reactive when those problems get a broader airing. At that point, an organization is more likely to be engaging in crisis management, rather than working to address the original issue, and very often the focus on the patient is lost in favour of managing impressions among a larger community of stakeholders. It is due in no small part to the hope of becoming proactive rather than reactive to patient complaints that more and more healthcare organizations are attempting to measure patient satisfaction, through tools such as the Patient Experience Survey being developed by Health Quality Ontario to assist primary care providers in assessing potential problems within their practices. In the United States, Medicare has taken the lead in requiring hospitals to collect information about patient satisfaction, with the federal government and some private insurers considering these survey results when setting reimbursement levels for hospitals (Boodman 2015). It is to the topic of patient satisfaction and how it relates to patient experience that we next turn.

Patient Satisfaction and Patient Experience

In marketing, customer satisfaction (and lack thereof) has been examined since the late 1970s. It is now well recognized that satisfaction has both cognitive and affective components, each of which contribute to a consumer's global judgment of (dis)satisfaction. The cognitive component is most often described in terms of expectation disconfirmation theory, which explains how individuals compare expectations against perceived performance to both directly and indirectly (through disconfirmation of beliefs) affect judgments of satisfaction. The emotional component of dissatisfaction arises as a result of an assessment of what that shortfall between expectations and reality means for the consumer's values, goals, and beliefs, and possibly also from attributions made as to why that shortfall occurred (Giese and Cote 2000). The more central those values, goals, and beliefs are to the individual, and the more impact the shortfall has on their well-being, the stronger the emotional response generated in response to that dissatisfaction is likely to be. In the context of healthcare, given the centrality of physical well-being to overall well-being, the experience of dissatisfaction as a result of a healthcare encounter is likely to be emotionally acute.

Using the principles of expectation disconfirmation theory, we can approach management of patient satisfaction from two possible routes: attempting to increase patient perceptions of performance, and/or managing patient expectations. If we assume that improved performance (which in the healthcare context can reasonably be interpreted as "curing" a patient, or at least improving their well-being as much as possible) is the goal regardless of concerns about patient satisfaction, then we can put that aside and focus on managing patient expectations. It is in the latter area that the greatest change has occurred in recent years. In particular, there has been a marked increase in patients who want to feel empowered in their healthcare choices and involved in decisions about their care, rather than simply receiving wisdom dispensed to them from doctors, often with little explanation. A common expectation of this new breed of empowered patients is that they are partners in their healthcare, and when that expectation is not met or they are made to feel that that expectation is unreasonable, it is not surprising that they are disappointed and ultimately dissatisfied with their care—and they are more likely to complain as a result.

The measurement of patient satisfaction has taken several routes. Some organizations focus on what can be termed "process" or "operational" concerns, such as in-clinic wait times, the friendliness of reception and nursing staff, the comfort of reception area, the cleanliness of exam room, and so on. Still others concern themselves with broader "relational" questions that are more in line with measuring patient expectations of a positive healthcare experience, such as the physician listening to a patient's concerns and treating them with respect, spending enough time with them, and encouraging them to ask questions. A recent study indicates that patients' care experiences will shape their perceptions of the relationship with their provider, independent of simple satisfaction measures, and that the stronger the relationship with the provider, the better the interpersonal continuity of care (repeated visits to the same provider), which is often considered a major goal of primary care (Beeson 2006; Tabler et al. 2014). Anecdotal data also suggest that satisfied patients are more likely to comply with treatment plans suggested by their doctor, to assume an active role in their care (i.e., be more empowered), and to continue medical care with their current physician. This echoes the results of the study described previously with respect to the relationship between satisfaction and continuity of care (Beeson 2006). While discussion of how to best assess, measure, and deliver a superior patient experience is still in its infancy, it is clear that there are likely to be both organizational and medical benefits to determining how to best engage a patient in care in ways that more closely address their varied medical, social, and personal needs.

Patient-centred care reduces patient complaining behaviour, which would typically occur behind the backs of healthcare providers as patients voice their displeasure to a broader audience. With patient-centred care, better channels of communication are forged between the patient and healthcare provider. Further, patient-centred care leads to higher levels of patient satisfaction that will lead to better interpersonal continuity of care, greater patient compliance with treatment plans, and improved patient engagement in their own care. In addition to these important benefits, embracing patient-centred care also benefits healthcare organizations in the more macro-political environment. We will now examine the collective level issues that arise, contrasting it with the foregoing discussion of how patients as individuals approach healthcare advocacy.

COLLECTIVE LEVEL PATIENT-DRIVEN ADVOCACY

It is important to note that the dynamic surrounding patient complaining behaviour and dissatisfaction does not only concern the patient-healthcare provider relationship. Healthcare organizations have come to be immersed in a social and political environment that comprises a growing number of diverse social actors with an array of interests. The Internet and social media have given rise to a form of communication that empowers individual patients to connect to a network of social actors made up of individuals, small groups, and formal organizations, all of which present various narratives surrounding the nature of healthcare provision. Empowered by digital communication, this wide spectrum of social actors poses new challenges to healthcare providers. As one illustration, healthcare providers not only must track and report on formal government mandated measures of patient satisfaction, but must also consider patient satisfaction measures and reports from a growing and diverse list of "informal" but influential websites that might seemingly be unrelated to healthcare. Increasingly, patients turn to Facebook pages, hospital reputation websites, and even "Trip Advisor," all of which provide patient-driven commentary on experiences with various healthcare providers.

More traditional perspectives of activism regard organizations as typically confronted by politicized and organized social activists who see themselves as "outsiders" in relation to the target system. These organized activists protest what they consider to be problems within the dominant economic, political, and ideological systems with which they see traditional organizations, such as healthcare providers, as being complicit (Glickman 2009). Traditional tools of activism involve lobbying governments, boycotting, and engaging in formal protests as activists seek to trigger change to the dominant system. This traditional perspective regards change to dominant institutions, such as healthcare, as being triggered by activists who have a particular passion for, and concern about, a given social and political arrangement. These activists are seen to mobilize people into a collective effort to change the current social order so as to bring about a more desirable state of the world (den Hond and de Bakker 2007; Fligstein and McAdam 2012).

However, digital technology has enabled a democratization of communication, challenging some of the basic assumptions underlying the traditional view of activism and change in the healthcare system. The "average" patient is now able to access information from any part of the globe with an ease never before possible. Likewise, the online environment provides this patient with the ability to find an audience for their views in a forum previously only accessible to an elite few. For instance, an individual patient's blog espousing some concern about the healthcare system can attract an audience of a size and form never possible before the digital age. These democratized forms of communication challenge the more centralized and unified structure of past activist movements.

What emerges is considered a "field" of social actors who take each other into account in their attempts to achieve both instrumental ends (such as specific changes to certain healthcare practices) as well as existential ends (such as individual meaning making and identity building). All of these ends are achieved through a confluence of actions between social actors within the field. However, rather than a "consensual frame that holds for all actors [there are] different interpretive frames reflecting the relative positions of actors within the strategic action field" (Fligstein and McAdam 2012, 89). The field comes to comprise a diverse range of social actors and roles, bringing a range of interests, perspectives, experiences, and expertise. In this field, the line between the "experts" and the "average person" tends to become blurred, since all social actors share the same tools of communication. What differentiates the voice of one social actor from another is not necessarily expertise, but rather the skill to navigate this social media space. The social actor with the best blog or Facebook page and the ability to distribute and share commentary using the Internet and social media may arise as an influential player in the field. Furthermore, these social actors may not necessarily be driven by well-defined instrumental objectives, but rather by self-identity building projects, such as the pursuit of recognition for one's own points of view, and the corresponding social status that recognition affords within a given field.

Therefore, the healthcare organization is not being confronted by a unified and elite class of activists demanding some common end. Instead, organizations find themselves as but one social actor having to navigate a complex field of a whole range of social actors, presenting healthcare providers with a complex and even confusing social terrain. While the diffused and seemingly confusing nature of this terrain may tempt healthcare providers to ignore this space, there are reasons that emerge as to why this may be a perilous choice when one considers the underlying social change that inadvertently arises from this social dynamic. We next consider this dynamic in more detail.

As noted previously, patients turn to social media to present their complaints about their healthcare experience to a broader audience. In order not to come across simply as a "complainer," these patients will instead work to construct themselves as worthy of having a voice to be heard. Therefore, patients will want to legitimate their voice over that of healthcare "experts." As such, patients will work to present themselves as insightfully aware of the intricacies of some aspects of the healthcare system. These knowledge claims may be based on their own direct experiences with healthcare providers, on their own "research" as they search for information online from other contexts, or on their examination of the experiences of others combined with their own research.

Either way, the field comes to be characterized by patients who are working to construct themselves as "in-the-know," and insightfully aware of the arrangements underlying the healthcare system. In this identity pursuit of the "in-the-know" citizen worthy of their voice being heard, these "patient activists" will inevitably and inadvertently not only confront healthcare organizations, but also end up informing and confronting each other with their diverse range of views and opinions. Healthcare organizations that follow these field-level narratives may experience great frustration as they hear vast amounts of "misinformation" being espoused. It would be understandable for these organizations to be tempted to jump into the field in an effort to "set the record straight" and "educate" patients as to the "facts." To do so, however, is to miss an unexpected and seemingly stealth form of social change that is occurring.

As patients present and debate their positions based on their own "research" and experiences, a social trend towards the legitimacy of "local knowledge" and a simultaneous refutation of "expert knowledge" is emerging. Local knowledge refers to the knowledge claims that arise from an individual's own experiences, perspectives, and insights into a given situation, which is contrasted against the "expert knowledge" that is handed down from authoritative sources. In this context, there are two problems with this expert knowledge. First, the acceptance of this hierarchical knowledge would be completely counter to the social actor's intention to portray themselves as a knowledgeable individual whose own claims are worthy of legitimacy. To accept expert knowledge claims would present the social actor as a cultural dupe, hoodwinked by the "system," and thus violate the identity of an in-the-know individual whose own knowledge is worthy of attention. Second, these hierarchical, expert knowledge claims are often met with suspicion and presumed to be tainted with agendas and interests of control. Therefore, the fundamental nature of the social change that emerges from this field dynamic is the increasing legitimacy of "local knowledge" claims and the simultaneous de-legitimation of "expert knowledge."

Healthcare providers must re-examine their roles within the fields to which they unwittingly belong. To ignore the field is perilous, since patient activists construct narratives and views which can leave healthcare providers completely out of touch and uninformed. To attempt to dominate the field by seeking to "educate" or "correct" what providers view as misinformation will simply violate the core nature of the social movement in such attempts to supersede local knowledge with expert knowledge. Such domineering actions will also subvert the legitimacy of an individual's complaints and therefore further contribute to the healthcare provider-patient problems raised above. This can only be met with more resistance by the patient. However, to understand and work within this field dynamic can present a tremendous opportunity for healthcare providers. Patient-centred care can not only involve lowering complaint behaviour while increasing rates of satisfaction, it can also involve engagement with, rather than refutation of, the "local knowledge" of patient activists.

With this discussion of the individual and the collective approaches to advocating for a patient-centred healthcare system as backdrop, the following case study presents one healthcare organization that has enacted system-wide reforms to create a patient-centred environment, not only at the level of the individual patient, but also in the broader field.

CASE: TRANSFORMING PATIENT EXPERIENCES THROUGH PATIENT-CENTRIC CARE

Putting patients at the core of the service delivery model overturns conventional healthcare approaches in which the patient is often considered as separate from the healthcare delivery team. In the same way that commercial organizations seek to understand and satisfy customers' wants and needs, considering patients as customers pushes healthcare organizations to develop a deeper understanding of patient needs in order to provide experiences that are valuable from the patient's perspective.

Over the last few years, a large regional healthcare institution in Eastern Ontario embarked on a program to develop a patient- and family-centric healthcare service delivery approach in line with a customer-oriented philosophy. Conceptually, the patient- and family-centred initiative establishes patients and families as co-creators of healthcare outcomes by including them as partners in the decision-making process. In addition to reinterpreting the role of patients and families in individual healthcare delivery, the organization also created a new voluntary position: the patient experience adviser. A unique and multi-faceted position, the advisers are recruited from individuals in the local community who have direct knowledge of the patient experience at the healthcare institution, either as patients themselves, or as family, friends, or acquaintances of patients. These advisers volunteer to serve in a decision-making capacity within the institution, to provide a patient perspective on organizational issues that have material impact on the experience of patients, including the hiring of new staff. The creation of these new positions legitimizes the value of the "local" knowledge of patients and their advocates, as well as acknowledges the role of the patient as a partner in their own healthcare. Through the patient advisers, the organization is able to integrate informal feedback within its institutional structure so as to proactively address patient needs as well as legitimize patients as important stakeholders within the organization.

The changing stakeholder relationships amongst healthcare staff and patients in response to the patient-centric model of care reveal the challenges associated with organizations that are implementing customer-centric transformational practices. We outline some of these challenges below.

Challenging Existing Power Structures

The move to patient-centric care, as well as the creation of the patient adviser role, was a direct challenge to existing power hierarchies within the organization. Many of these hierarchies were legacies of the healthcare sector as a whole, while others were particular to the individual departmental arrangements. In these hierarchies, physicians occupy a privileged position relative to nurses, who in turn often saw themselves as having greater authority than social workers, respiratory therapists, and other members of the organization. The movement towards a patient-centric model shifted these power dynamics because the emphasis was not placed on status claims linked to healthcare roles, but rather on the degree to which those roles provided value as determined by the patient. No particular provider role was privileged relative to others, and non-provider roles such as religious figures or family members may have held greater influence.

As a result of these changes, key members of the healthcare decision-making team, patients, their families, and patient advisers now all have a voice in the ways in which the organization delivers healthcare services. This presents challenges to traditional, often paternalistic, modes of healthcare delivery and organizational decision making, in which patients and families are assumed to be passive and deferential to the authority of physicians, nurses, and other healthcare staff. Patient advisers sit on internal committees that deal with all aspects of the organization's operations. This involves more than just transparency; by bringing voice to their experiences at the decision-making table, patient advisers attune the organization to patients' values and concerns in ways that focus-groups, feedback-forums, and surveys simply cannot achieve. The trade-off is that entwining patients and families in such an intimate way with organizational decision making means the organization must be willing to work effectively with those individuals to achieve common goals, and to determine how to reconcile and manage patient goals that may not align with organizational priorities. Healthcare staff in this organization report that they increasingly view their conversations with patients, families, and patient advisers as negotiations in which all sides present their case, and outcomes are driven through mutual understanding and compromise. While in some cases this is not different from traditional dialogue between healthcare providers and patients, increasingly the pathway to agreement is a fluid approach in which evidence-based medicine and processes act as only one pathway to achieving goals. This approach is atypical, given the evidence that many patients futilely seek to be more engaged in decisions related to their care, but are often rebuffed by their medical care providers (O'Rourke 2014).

Patient-Focused Outcomes

Healthcare has been focused on reducing risk and preserving life, but patients are voicing their preference, in some cases, to pursue riskier courses of treatment in the hopes of achieving outcomes that they deem preferable. In one case, a young mother diagnosed with early-stage cancer opted to pursue alternatives to Westernized medical approaches, only to return later with an advanced form of the disease that was no longer treatable. By including patients and families in the decision-making process, the healthcare provider has to adjust their interpretations of, and expectations for, success. The healthcare staff had been trained to follow courses of treatment that would minimize risk to patients, particularly of death, and so often limited the options presented to reflect this training bias.[1] In contrast, a patient-centred approach would require including the patient in the decision-making process, and accepting that patients, as in this case, will sometimes prefer riskier courses of action. Some healthcare providers will react by distancing themselves from the decision-making process by making treatment choices entirely the patient's responsibility. However, if providers choose to dissociate themselves from patient choices rather than opting to delve into the deeper meanings patients associate with courses of treatment, then patient experiences have not been improved, and patient empowerment (which implies truly informed consent) has not been achieved. True patient-centric approaches involve all staff associated with healthcare delivery actively listening to understand a patient's desired outcomes as representative of a patient's value system, and resisting the temptation to layer on value systems based on professional education or training.

Communication Flows and Transcending Boundaries

Management and operations practices have infiltrated healthcare institutions as these organizations seek to become more efficient and effective, as well as accountable to their key stakeholder groups. One consequence of this operational focus is the silo structure that many healthcare organizations employ. In this model, departments are structured as distinct from one another, and separated within the physical space the organization occupies. This structuring extends to the various boundaries, both physical and virtual, that exist between healthcare organizations such as hospitals and primary care providers, such as family physicians. As patients traverse the boundaries within and between healthcare organizations, the patient-centric focus requires that the organization with which the patient interacts be constantly providing feedback to all other members of the service delivery chain. Within the organization studied, healthcare staff found that there were significant communication breakdowns at the points where patients transcended these boundaries. These breakdowns are now identified as missing or incomplete records of care or treatment. A patient-centric model focused on patient experiences and outcomes will attune the healthcare organization to ensure these trans-boundary barriers are removed.

One role within the organization that appears to be underutilized in assisting with boundary issues is the social worker. Individuals in this role are frequently engaged with patients at multiple points during the service delivery process, and have a holistic perspective on patient values and concerns, including those that transcend purely health-related issues. For example, one social worker discussed how a severely ill patient was more concerned with the administration of their disability insurance payments than with following their treatment conditions. This concern was due to the financial situation of the patient's depen-

---

[1] This tendency to privilege medical preferences over other patient concerns and the attendant negative effects it can have on quality-of-life (especially in the case of terminal diseases) is discussed eloquently and extensively in physician Atul Gawande's best-selling book *Being Mortal*.

dent family members. Once the administration of payments was coordinated by the social worker, the patient was able to focus on the treatment plan and the patient's health subsequently began to improve. Despite this patient-centric focus, the degree to which other healthcare staff within the service delivery chain engage with information provided by the social workers is variable, and there are disproportionately few social workers working within the organization relative to other healthcare positions.

BROADER IMPLICATIONS FOR HEALTHCARE ORGANIZATIONS

Day and Moorman (2010) urge organizations, public and private, not-for-profit and for-profit, to engage in what they call an "outside-in" strategy. This involves the organization's leadership coming to understand the value sought by their key stakeholders and then structuring the organization to ensure the ability to deliver this value to those stakeholders. The fundamental argument is that an organization that is unable to deliver value to its key stakeholders will be constantly sidetracked by issues that deflect attention away from the organization's core purpose. Therefore, an outside-in–driven healthcare organization would be a patient-centred organization. However, it is important to recognize that a patient-centred care system does not necessarily mean a patient-"driven" system; as one writer comments, "the patient, unlike the customer, can't always be right, though few of us want to hear that" (O'Rourke 2014). It is important to recognize and legitimize the "local" knowledge of patients, while balancing it with the "expert" knowledge that the patient is unlikely to have.

To become outside-in–driven, the organization must tend to three imperatives: its structure, culture, and metrics. We will examine each one of these imperatives in the healthcare sector context, drawing on the above case study to illustrate.

Organizational Structure

An "outside-in" organization first looks to its key stakeholders to understand the needs that they have and the problems they are looking to solve. To achieve this understanding, the organizational structure must be focused on, and attuned to, understanding stakeholders' needs rather than focused on internal organizational arrangements. The key structural imperative to achieving this is for the organization to break down its internal silos and allow for cross-functional team coordination. As demonstrated in the case study above, the needs of patients do not necessarily fit into predefined organizational silos. A patient's medical needs, social needs, spiritual needs, life goals, financial concerns, family dynamics, and so on, all interact. Many healthcare organizations, however, are structured around internally driven arrangements that most likely mirror professional hierarchies. Consciously breaking down these internally driven structural constraints in order to design healthcare systems that reflect the inter-related dynamics of each patient would be a major step towards delivering patient-centred care.

A second important structural consideration is establishing those organizational roles that help to facilitate an integrated approach to patient care. In the case study above, the role of the social worker was emphasized as a key player in helping the healthcare organization transcend professional boundaries in order to ensure the patient receives value in all aspects of their healthcare concerns. Beyond social workers, the organizational structure must formally include those whose role is specifically designed to transcend these internally driven professional boundaries.

A third structural consideration is having formal organizational mechanisms that integrate the patient's voice into all aspects of organizational decision making and operations. The organization outlined in the above case study used patient advisers. There are, of course, many other roles and mechanisms that can be used to ensure the integration of the patient's voice throughout the organization. Some for-profit organizations are increasingly turning to "Chief Cultural Officers" (McCracken 2011), people trained and tasked with the job of scanning and engaging the social media environment to understand the kinds of social changes (such as the trend from expert knowledge to local knowledge) that may provide opportunities for the way in which the healthcare organization delivers value to patients.

Organizational Culture

Organizational culture refers to the beliefs and norms that guide day-to-day activity within the organization. A patient-driven organization would have a culture in which organizational members firmly believe in and embrace the core principle that decisions about organizational practices must be made from the patient's perspective, and that everyone in the organization, regardless of their position and rank, has a role in delivering this value. But it is not only changes in patient empowerment and the increased impact of patient satisfaction measures on financial performance that are driving this cultural shift. Physicians are also experiencing a crisis that spans their profession: According to a 2012 survey, nearly eight out of 10 American physicians rated themselves as somewhat, or very pessimistic, about the future of the medical profession, and only 6 percent of doctors surveyed in 2008 rated their morale as positive, compared with 85 percent in 1973 (O'Rourke 2014). Increasingly, it is being recognized that what can be a deep divide between patient and physician, with correspondingly poor health outcomes and dissatisfaction on the part of the patient, as well as disillusionment and frustration on the part of the physician, may be addressed by training doctors not only in the physical and technical aspects of medical care, but also the emotional and psychological ones. Driven by an increased emphasis on patient-centric care, as well as insiders within the healthcare system who were encountering patients recounting "devastating" interactions with doctors that were not just "innocuous, but often experiences that were profound and deeply affected [their] lives" (Boodman 2015), a range of programs have been developed to train physicians (and other healthcare providers) in delivering medical care with empathy. Studies have linked empathy to greater patient trust in the physician, increased patient satisfaction, decreased physician burn-out, a lower risk of medical errors and malpractice suits, and demonstrably better health outcomes and medical efficacy (Boodman 2015). For instance, a study found that the rate of severe diabetes complications in patients of doctors who rated high on a standard empathy scale was 40 percent lower than in patients with low-empathy doctors, an effect comparable with the benefits seen as a result of the most intensive medical therapy for diabetes (O'Rourke 2014). As a result, starting in 2015, the Medical College Admission Test will contain questions about human behaviour and psychology, in recognition that being a good doctor "requires an understanding of people, not just science," according to the American Association of Medical Colleges (Boodman 2015).

Such training is just one illustration of how a cultural shift within an organization can have substantial benefits for multiple stakeholders, and yet result in relatively small costs. The need for such a philosophical shift is not an easy one to identify or to determine how to implement, but as accountability for healthcare metrics continues to focus on not only medical outcomes but also patient perceptions, such a cultural reorientation may be the best way to authentically connect with the true needs and values of multiple organizational stakeholders.

Organizational Metrics

Finally, the organization must be geared towards gathering key indicators that reflect the organization's performance in delivering value to patients and their families. Even patient advocates recognize that, to a certain extent, the measures of patient "satisfaction" currently in place are incomplete at best and deeply flawed at worst. Take, for instance, the patient satisfaction survey data collected by the U.S. Centers for Medicare & Medicaid Services. Consistent with the idea of managing to measurement, most hospitals have improved in the areas the surveys track, such as how clean and quiet their rooms are and how well doctors and nurses communicate, but the surveys have resulted in little shuffling in the rankings of high- versus low-performing hospitals (Rau 2015). In some cases, small variations in patient responses (which are well-recognized as being a normal part of using surveys as a research tool) can have drastic financial impacts; in determining how much to reimburse, the government only gives credit when patients say that they "always" got the care they wanted during their stay (such as their pain was "always" well-controlled). If a patient indicates that the hoped for level of care was "usually" provided, it doesn't count at all, and on a scale of 0 to 10 for rating a hospital stay, an organization must get a 9 or 10 in order for Medicare to fully reimburse them (Rau 2015). This approach to measurement fails to reflect or appreciate the complexities associated with self-report measures of any service experience, let alone a healthcare experience that takes place over an extended period of time, across multiple individuals, and which could reasonably be assumed to be affected by emotional and physical factors that may have little to do with the experience itself.

This approach also highlights a limitation of the assumption that only things that are quantitatively measureable are "real" and thus can be managed and controlled. That this perspective dominates within healthcare organizations and their assessors is not altogether surprising, given the typical "evidence-based" approach of traditional medicine. But many social science disciplines (including marketing, organizational behaviour, sociology, and anthropology) have demonstrated that there is much to be gained in true understanding by employing qualitative methodologies that yield "thick description" (McCracken 1988), making them better suited to fully exploring complex and ongoing interactions, such as those commonly observed in a typical "patient experience." Medical researchers could thus benefit from taking a cross-disciplinary approach that would better capture the occasionally intangible nature of the "patient experience" in order to truly embody the "outside-in" philosophy espoused by Day and Moorman (2010).

CONCLUSION

As primary stakeholders in the healthcare system, patients are becoming more empowered and more vocal about what they expect from healthcare providers and from the system itself. At the core of patient-centred care is the engagement of patients and their families in their own medical care. Engaging patients to ensure their satisfaction has the immediate effect of mitigating complaint behaviour, much of which will be behind the backs of healthcare providers. This complaint behaviour can come to embroil organizations in needless political battles. Furthermore, satisfied patients are more actively engaged in their own treatment which leads to better medical outcomes.

Engagement with, rather than refutation of, patient concerns enables the healthcare organization to be more attuned with broader societal trends. An important societal trend has been the legitimation of local knowledge in which individual patient experiences are at times more valued by societal stakeholders (such as governments) than is the "official" line of healthcare organizations. Embracing this societal context allows healthcare organizations to win broader societal support.

In order to attune themselves to these individual patient and broader societal trends, healthcare organizations must develop integrated and coordinated organizational structures, organizational cultures that are transparent and flexible, and incentive systems that reward organizational actors to attend to patient-centred care.

REFERENCES

Bardes, Charles L. 2012. "Defining 'Patient-Centered Medicine.'" *New England Journal of Medicine* 366(9): 782–83.

Beeson, Stephen C. 2006. *Practicing Excellence: A Physician's Manual to Exceptional Health Care*. Pensacola, FL: Fire Starter Publishing.

Boodman, Sandra G. 2015. "How to Teach Doctors Empathy." *The Atlantic Magazine*, March 15. http://www.theatlantic.com/health/archive/2015/03/how-to-teach-doctors-empathy/387784/

Day, George S., and Christine Moorman. 2010. *Strategy From The Outside-In: Profiting From Customer Value*. New York: McGraw Hill.

den Hond, Frank, and Frank G. A. de Bakker. 2007. "Ideologically Motivated Activism: How Activist Groups Influence Corporate Social Change Activities." *Academy of Management Review* 32(3): 901–24.

Epstein, Ronald M., and Richard L. Street, Jr. 2011. "The Values and Value of Patient-Centered Care." *Annals of Family Medicine* 9(2): 100–103.

Fligstein, Neil, and Doug McAdam. 2012. *A Theory of Fields*. Oxford: Oxford University Press.

Frampton, Susan, et al. 2008. *Patient-Centered Care Improvement Guide*. Planetree and Picker Institute. http://www.patient-centeredcare.org

Giese, Joan L., and Joseph A. Cote. 2000. "Defining Consumer Satisfaction." *Academy of Marketing Science Review* 1(2): 1–22.

Glickman, Lawrence B. 2009. *Buying Power: A History of Consumer Activism in America*. Chicago: University of Chicago Press.

McCracken, Grant. 1988. "The Long Interview." *Qualitative Research Methods* Series 13. Newbury Park: Sage Publications.

———. 2011. *Chief Culture Officer: How to Create a Living, Breathing Corporation*. New York: Basic Books.

McGraw, A. Peter, Caleb Warren, and Christina Khan. 2015. "Humorous Complaining." *Journal of Consumer Research* 41 (Feb): 1153–71.

O'Rourke, Meghan. 2014. "Doctors Tell All—and It's Bad." *The Atlantic Magazine*, October 14. http://www.theatlantic.com/magazine/archive/2014/11/doctors-tell-all-and-its-bad/380785/

Rau, Jordan. 2015. "Hundreds of Hospitals Struggle to Improve Patient Satisfaction." *Kaiser Health News*, March 10. http://kaiserhealthnews.org/news/hundreds-of-hospitals-struggle-to-improve-patient-satisfaction/

Tabler, Jennifer, Debra L. Scammon, Jaewhan Kim, Timothy Farrell, Andrada Tomoaia-Cotisel, and Michael K. Magill. 2014. "Patient Care Experiences and Perceptions of the Patient-Provider Relationship: A Mixed Methods Study." *Patient Experience Journal* 1(1), Article 13: 75–87.

Chapter 6

ENGAGING PATIENTS AND THE PUBLIC IN PLANNING FOR CARE AND DRIVING HEALTHCARE REFORMS

RÉJEAN HÉBERT

The aging of the population is dramatically changing the profile of diseases. From a preponderance of acute diseases in the last century, we are increasingly moving towards more chronic diseases (Hébert 2010a). This has many implications. First, the current hospital-centred healthcare system should move toward a community-centred system to support patients with chronic diseases who need long-term care in the community. Second, the relationship with health professionals has to shift from the dominant current model of the almighty physician who knows what is best for the patient to a model that features proactive, knowledgeable patients who are able to interact with many professionals from different disciplines—the "chronic care model" (Wagner et al. 2001). Third, healthcare managers and policymakers must also change their mindset: they need to stop thinking they know the best way to deliver high-quality, efficient care, but instead listen to the needs and will of the people.

In this chapter, patient and citizen engagement will be first defined and presented into a conceptual framework. We will then review patient engagement in direct care, and patient and public engagement in management, governance and setting public policy. The role of patients in professional training and research will then be summarized. We will finally discuss the limitations and pitfalls of patient and citizen engagement.

Managing a Canadian Healthcare Strategy, edited by A. Scott Carson and Kim Richard Nossal. Montreal and Kingston: McGill-Queen's University Press, Queen's Policy Studies Series. © 2016 The School of Policy Studies, Queen's University at Kingston. All rights reserved.

DEFINITION OF PATIENT ENGAGEMENT

Patient and public engagement represents a significant revolution in health-care (Richards et al. 2013). Coulter (2011) defines patient and public engagement as "the relationship between patients and healthcare providers as they work together to promote and support active patient and public involvement in health and healthcare and to strengthen their influence on healthcare decisions, at both the individual and collective levels." Patient engagement is rooted in support groups like Alcoholics Anonymous and AIDS support groups. These groups have developed close relationships with health professionals and health-care organizations to improve their responsiveness to patients' needs. Activist groups in mental health were also effective in sensitizing professionals and organizations to serve patients better and get them more deeply involved in the care process. The growing importance of chronic diseases and the role of the Internet in improving patient access to health information were significant factors in expanding patient engagement. Other related concepts such as shared decision making and patient-centered care were developed coincidently (Barry and Edgman-Levitan 2012; Légaré et al. 2012).

Patient engagement covers the entire spectrum of healthcare: from direct care to program management, governance of health organizations, public policy, and even training and research. Three levels in the continuum of engagement can be distinguished. Consultation with the patient is the primary level, where the patient or the public is informed and their opinion is sought by professionals, program managers or policymakers. Involvement is the second level, with the patient and public getting actively involved in the process. Partnership is the ultimate level, where patient and clinicians, citizens and managers or policymakers work closely together to co-build care, programs or policy (Carman et al. 2013). Table 6.1 summarizes the different levels of engagement for the different domains of healthcare.

Patient Engagement in Direct Care

In direct healthcare, Graffigna and Barello (2015) described in their conceptual framework that patients' engagement may go from awareness (they called it "arousal") to adhesion, and finally partnership with the multidisciplinary team of professionals. It should happen not only at the cognitive level but also at the emotional and behavioural levels. This sequence of thinking, feeling, and acting was where, in a real partnership, the disease is not just accepted but is finally integrated by the patient (they called this an "eudaimonic" state). The "Montreal model" is an interesting framework for developing patient and professional partnerships in healthcare (Pomey et al. 2015). It distinguishes four levels in the continuum of patient engagement: information, consultation, collaboration, and partnership. In the last stage, patient and professionals are co-constructing the care plan in a real partnership.

Many therapeutic education programs have been set up to foster patient engagement and self-management (Lawn and Schoo 2010). The best known is the

TABLE 6.1
Framework of Patient Engagement

Domain	Continuum of Engagement		
	Consultation	Involvement	Partnership
Direct care	Patients receive information	Patients are asked about preferences in treatment plan	Treatment decisions are made by the patient and professionals
Organizational design and governance	Patients are surveyed	Patients are involved in committees and councils	Patients are partners in decisions
Policy making	Consultations are held with the public and specific groups	Citizens and groups are involved in setting priorities and in making recommendations	Citizens and groups are partners in the decision-making process
Training professionals	Patients are consulted on program revisions and design	Patients are involved in committees and educational activities	Patients are partners in program design and activities
Health research	Patients' concerns and priorities are integrated into research	Patients sit on peer review and advisory committees	Patients are integrated into health research teams

Adapted from Carman et al. 2013.

Stanford program, a six-week group program led by lay people that inspired many other programs around the world (Newbould, Taylor, and Bury 2006). While the UK National Expert Patients Programme is based on the Stanford program, the groups are co-led by a patient and a healthcare professional (Taylor and Bury 2007). The Flinders Program developed in Australia is an individual program that includes capacity assessment, motivational interviews, the setting of priorities and defining of goals, and the negotiation of a health plan (Battersby et al. 2007). The American 5A Program (assess, advise, agree, assist, arrange) is also a well-known program implemented in various contexts (Fiore et al. 2000). Many tools for informing patients have been developed; the University of Ottawa has a comprehensive inventory of patient decision aids (https://decisionaid.ohri.ca/index.html).

Information technology may play a significant role in self-care. Internet portals are useful sources of information for patients about health problems. However, the quality of the information and its translation into lay vocabulary are critical for its usefulness. Tele-monitoring, tele-health and tele-medicine are also effective in improving patient self-care (Peeters, Wiegers, and Friele 2013).

Patient and Public Engagement in Management, Governance and Public Policy

In management and governance, patients and the public could be consulted using pools, satisfaction and priority surveys, or focus groups. Patients and citizens could also be involved in committees, not only to voice their opinions but also to involve them in making decisions. Ultimately, they can partner in the decision-making process for designing new programs and services or planning strategic orientations of health organizations. Deliberative methods require well-informed citizens discussing with policymakers to get to consensus (Abelson et al. 2003). This type of health democracy is rapidly expanding in health organizations.

According to Lomas (1997), there are three levels of public engagement in policy making. The macro level (government) relates to which services should be funded (health vs. other sectors). The meso-level relates to specific health services and programs (ministry). The micro-level relates to decisions about which classes of patient should receive services (local organizations).

Rowe and Frewer (2005) proposed a model for public engagement. They distinguished between communication (the sponsor informs the public), consultation (information is obtained from the public) and participation (exchange between the sponsor and the public). Public participation is defined as "the practice of involving members of the public in the agenda-setting, decision-making, and policy-forming activities of organizations/institutions responsible for policy development" (p. 253). Rowe and Frewer inventoried and classified the mechanisms and tools used to foster public participation. Communication could take the form of publicity, public hearing and meeting, Internet, or hotline. Many methods could be used for consultation: opinion pool or survey, referendum, consultation document, interactive website, focus group, open space or advisory panel. To foster public participation, citizens' juries, consensus conferences, task forces, deliberative panels, or town meetings with voting have all been proposed. The public could be defined according to three categories: individual citizens speaking on their own behalf, organized interest groups (advocates), or patients and consumers of services (Mitton et al. 2009). According to Contandriopoulos (2004), public representativeness could be formal (via election, designation, random selection); descriptive (in other words, where the representatives would be similar to the "average" member of the public); or symbolic (subjective perception of legitimacy).

In the United States, the Accountable Care Organizations (ACO) movement addressed the Triple Aim (better care for individuals, better health for populations, and lower cost) in setting standards for organizations, which include a focus on patient centredness promoted by the governing body and integrated into practice by leadership and management. Among the 33 performance standards, seven focus on patient-centred approaches such as communication with providers, health promotion and education, and shared decision making (Toussaint, Milstein and Shortell 2013).

Patients and citizens can be involved in setting clinical practice guidelines to incorporate patients' values and perspectives. This improves their relevance and effectiveness (Légaré et al. 2011). Patient and citizens could also be involved in health technology assessments. In England, the National Institute of Health and Care Excellence (NICE) involves specially trained lay people in all the processes of assessing the quality and relevance of health products. NICE also runs a Citizens Council to address moral and ethical issues.

In policy making, citizens are consulted on their priorities and preferences with respect to the healthcare system using pools and surveys. In some political parties, members are involved in designing the party's program, which could become the government's program if the party is elected. That kind of strategy was used in Quebec by the Parti Québécois (PQ) for incorporating prevention and a long-term care insurance plan in the party program and electoral platform, and then in the priorities of the PQ government of Pauline Marois in 2012 (Hébert 2015). Another example is the Public Consultation on Seniors' Living Conditions in Québec, which was co-chaired by an elderly women. The consultation process included forums in every region of Quebec to hear from older people, associations of older people, scientists, and stakeholders about what can be done to improve seniors' living conditions. However, the report from that consultation was not used immediately for setting public policy, except for support for the World Health Organization's Age-Friendly Cities program (Hébert 2010b). The application of this program in Quebec illustrates how the public could be involved in making policy using a community-building approach. The municipality forms a steering committee made up of older people and stakeholders from civil society, public administration, and political representatives. Then a social diagnosis of community resources and older adults' needs is carried out. The committee designs an action plan based on a logical model. Following formal approval by city council, the plan is implemented through intersectoral collaborations (Garon et al. 2014).

The Quebec Health and Welfare Commissioner holds public forums in the process of assessing the performance of the healthcare system. The National Seniors Council in Ottawa and the Senior Partners Committee in Quebec are examples of population representatives who advise governments on policies for older people.

Unfortunately, this type of public participation in public policy has become less popular; today, governments tend to focus on short-term political benefits by paying attention to citizens' opinions expressed in pools or focus groups. The introduction of social media does not necessarily support citizens' active participation. While this "socialnetworkcracy" is spreading fast, we should remember that social media does not reach a representative sample of society. Vulnerable people and patients are frequently excluded from this high-tech circle. In short, participatory democracy is still wishful thinking in most modern countries. We have to find new ways to involve the public in real partnerships for designing social and health policies that respond to the needs of the population.

Patient Engagement in Training and Research

Patient engagement is also important for training new generations of healthcare workers. Many medical schools are involving patients in programs and educational activities. The Uniformed Services University of the Health Sciences in Bethesda, Maryland, for example, developed concrete methods for fostering patient participation in medical training. The Université de Montréal medical school created a directorate for collaboration and partnership to support patient cooperation in the faculty (Pomey et al. 2015). These initiatives are critical in changing the culture of medical professionals towards greater patient involvement in healthcare. The hidden curriculum is often very effective in perpetuating the old culture of paternalistic clinician and passive patient (Anderson and Funnell 2005). Many training programs have been designed to support clinicians in fostering patient engagement by adopting a patient-centred approach. A recent systematic review from a Cochrane Collaboration Group concluded that such interventions are effective and that short-term training (10 hours or fewer) is as effective as longer training (Dwamena et al. 2012).

In research, the Canadian Institutes of Health Research held a workshop on patient involvement in January 2014. The aim of the Strategy for Patient-Oriented Research (SPOR) is to integrate patients better into the research process. Patients should be involved in the governance of health research organizations and teams, and should be part of the peer-review process. Patients should also be trained to participate in the research process. Mechanisms and tools for helping researchers to integrate patients were also identified (Canadian Institutes of Health Research 2014).

Limitations and Pitfalls of Patient and Public Engagement

Patient and public engagement has gained widespread traction because it is an idea that adapts well to the chronic care model, and because it seems compelling in an era when personal autonomy is so privileged. But is it scientifically sound? Following a systematic review of the literature, Coulter and Ellins (2007) found substantial evidence supporting patient engagement in healthcare for improving health literacy, clinical decision making, self-management, and patient safety. Many studies and reports stressed the impact of patient engagement on psychosocial variables (well-being, satisfaction, personal efficacy). Some studies showed a significant impact on biological variables, particularly in diabetes, on pain in arthritis, and on physiological parameters in lung diseases. Some studies included impact variables on healthcare utilization, but the results were not persuasive. There is thus an urgent need to document the impact of patient engagement, particularly on healthcare utilization and efficiency. Likewise, few studies have demonstrated the effect of patient engagement in management and governance (Conklin, Morris, and Nolte 2012). A clustered, randomized, controlled trial demonstrated that involving patients in a priority-setting process for a health organization increased agreement between patients' and professionals' priorities (Boivin et al. 2014).

The main criticism of patient engagement is patient selection. Patients involved in those programs are often more wealthy, better educated, and highly motivated to be involved in the care process. This approach does not reach out to vulnerable, older, illiterate, isolated, or migrant people. Those suffering from mental diseases are also frequently not involved (Lindsay and Vrijhoef 2009). This not only affects the external validity of scientific studies about patient engagement; it could also increase social inequities in healthcare. Patient engagement could be an additional barrier to accessing healthcare by people who are already marginalized.

At the policy-making level, patient engagement risks marginalizing scientific and organizational evidence. Public policy is based on three sets of evidence: scientific, organizational (feasibility), and political (Klein 2003). Public engagement could be a strong lever for increasing the role and weight of political evidence. Attention should then be paid to the scientific and organizational evidence to avoid implementing policies that are not scientifically sound or are impractical.

Also, mechanisms for the expression of public opinion should be structured so that they are as representative of the target population as possible, and thus as unbiased as possible. Vulnerable and marginalized people are often underrepresented in public forums and democratic processes. Public policies focusing on, or impacting, those people are particularly at risk. Also, while activist groups could be very effective in lobbying political representatives and governments, those groups may not be good representatives of the people targeted. Finally, there is a risk that private companies and other stakeholders could, directly or indirectly, unduly influence the process for their own benefit. Conflicts of interest are a major ethical issue in this context.

There are a number of potential obstacles to public engagement in healthcare policy. Some could be organizational, since public organizations may not have the human and financial resources to create appropriate mechanisms to involve the public. The timing of mechanisms for participation could also be incompatible with the policy-making timetable. There could also be community obstacles: citizens may be not interested in participating in these initiatives, or they may distrust government institutions. Political obstacles are also present, with policymakers being reluctant to engage the public in a participatory process and risk controversy. They could be concerned that such processes may be viewed by the public as an inability to set up projects, programs, or policies (Gauvin and Ross 2012).

To avoid those pitfalls, active strategies should be put in place to reach out specifically to vulnerable, marginalized, and underprivileged populations. Using a variety of strategies increases the probability of getting a good picture of the needs and priorities of the target population. Surveys, interviews, focus groups, and meetings should be designed to reach out to specific groups of people concerned by the program or policy. Although social media is a good way to reach many people, it should not be the only way. Training people and inviting them to sit on committees is another effective strategy put forward in the Montreal Model (Pomey et al. 2015). Training should focus on both the cognitive and emotional aspects to reduce inequities of patients' representatives involved in professional, managerial, and governance activities.

Formal mechanisms for getting patients and the public involved in the governance of healthcare organizations should be implemented and developed. In Quebec, elected representatives from the population used to sit on the boards of public health institutions. User committees were set up to inform users, improve quality, advocate for users' rights, and support users in the complaints process. Population forums were also created 10 years ago in every regional jurisdiction. However, these initiatives have been threatened by the last reform of the healthcare system in Québec by the Liberal government of Philippe Couillard. In February 2015, they passed Bill 10, which in a stroke dismantled local healthcare institutions and merged them into a single large regional organization. With this reform, board members are no longer elected but are appointed by the minister. Users' committees were merged into one large committee, much farther away from the local clinical situation. Importantly, the population forums will probably not survive this reform. Québec's step in the wrong direction should remind us that patient involvement in health policy is a fragile process that needs to be continuously nurtured.

CONCLUSION

Patient and public engagement is important in the context of the aging of the population and the pandemic of chronic diseases. It must be widely implemented in the healthcare system for direct care and in the management and governance of organizations. Public policy should also involve patients and the public in designing new programs and services to better meet the needs of the population.

Scientific evidence of the impact of patient engagement on the quality and efficiency of healthcare services should be supported. Strategies to reach out to vulnerable, illiterate, isolated, and marginalized populations should be used to mitigate the risk of increasing social inequities in health. Patient and public engagement should be balanced with scientific evidence and with organizational feasibility to get appropriate and effective public policies.

Patient and public engagement requires an important cultural shift for clinicians, managers and policymakers. Training is critical to foster this revolution. New governance methods and management structures should be developed to support patient engagement. Formal mechanisms should also be created to involve citizens in the political process and in creating new public policy.

Over the last decade, a democratic deficit has been growing in Canada. Once elected, governments no longer consult the public in creating new policies or ending important social programs. Electoral campaigns often fail to generate public debate on important issues. If governments do not introduce new formal ways of engaging people, the public will need to organize new ways to be heard. In history, bloody revolutions were the way populations made that happen. The "maple spring" in Quebec in 2012 was an example of how social media and demonstrations can be a new way to build peaceful revolutions. The Canadian healthcare system needs to be reformed; its performance lags far behind other western countries (Osborn et al. 2014). Public funding, accessibility and universality are challenged but they represent the pillars of the system. The public should be involved in reforming healthcare. We all need to stand up to show what we need to improve our health and well-being. If we do not, other people will decide, and not necessarily in our best interest.

REFERENCES

Abelson, J., P. G. Forest, J. Eyles, P. Smith, E. Martin, and F. P. Gauvin. 2003. "Deliberations About Deliberative Methods: Issues in the Design and Evaluation of Public Participation Processes." *Social Science & Medicine* 57: 239–251.

Anderson, R. M., and M. M. Funnell. 2005. "Patient Empowerment: Reflections on the Challenge of Fostering the Adoption of a New Paradigm." *Patient Education & Counseling* 57: 153–157.

Barry, M. J., and S. Edgman-Levitan. 2012. "Shared Decision Making—The Pinnacle of Patient-Centered Care." *New England Journal of Medicine* 366: 780–781.

Battersby, M., P. Harvey, P. D. Mills, E. Kalucy, R. G. Pols, P. A. Frith et al. 2007. "SA HealthPlus: A Controlled Trial of a Statewide Application of a Generic Model of Chronic Illness Care." *Milbank Quarterly* 85: 37–67.

Boivin, A., P. Lehoux, R. Lacombe, J. Burgers, and R. Grol. 2014. "Involving Patients in Setting Clinical Priorities for Healthcare Improvement: A Cluster Randomized Trial." *Implementation Science* 9: 2. doi:10.1186/1748-5908-9-24

Canadian Institutes of Health Research. 2014. *Strategy for Patient-Oriented Research: Putting Patients First*. Ottawa, ON: Government of Canada, http://www.cihr-irsc.gc.ca/e/documents/spor_framework-en.pdf

Carman, K. L., P. Dardess, M. Maurer, S. Sofaer, K. Adams, C. Bechtel, and J. Sweeney. 2013. "Patient and Family Engagement: A Framework for Understanding the Elements and Developing Interventions and Policies." *Health Affairs (Project Hope)* 32(2): 223–231. doi:10.1377/hlthaff.2012.1133

Conklin A., Z. Morris, and E. Nolte. 2012. "What is the Evidence Base for Public Involvement in Health-Care Policy?: Results of a Systematic Scoping Review." *Health Expectations* December. doi:10.1111/hex.12038

Contandriopoulos, D. 2004. "A Sociological Perspective on Public Participation in Health Care." *Social Science & Medicine* 58: 321–330.

Coulter, A. 2011. *Engaging Patients in Healthcare*. New York: McGraw-Hill Education.

Coulter, A., and J. Ellins. 2007. "Effectiveness of Strategies for Informing, Educating, and Involving Patients." *British Medical Journal* 335(7609): 24–27.

Dwamena, F., M. Holmes-Rovner, C. M. Gaulden, S. Jorgensen, G. Sadigh,

A. Sikoskskii, S. Lewin, R. C. Smith, J. Coffey, A. Olomu, and M. Beasley. 2012. "Interventions for Providers to Promote a Patient-Centred Approach in Clinical Consultations." *Cochrane Database of Systematic Reviews* 12:CD003267.

Fiore, M. C., W. C. Bailey, S. J. Cohen, S. F. Dorfman, M. G. Goldstein, E. R. Gritz et al. 2000. *Treating Tobacco Use and Dependence. Quick Reference Guide for Clinicians*. Rockville, MD: US Department of Health and Human Services.

Garon, S., M. Paris, M. Beaulieu, A. Veil, and A. Laliberté. 2014. "Collaborative Partnership in Age-Friendly Cities: Two Case Studies from Quebec, Canada." *Journal of Aging and Social Policy* 26(1-2): 73–87.

Gauvin F. P., and M. C. Ross. 2012. "Citizen Participation in Health Impact Assessment: Overview of Issues." *National Collaborating Center for Healthy Public Policy*. http://www.ncchpp.ca/docs/EIS-HIA_ParticipationOverview_En.pdf

Graffigna, G., and S. Barello. 2015. "Modelling Patient Engagement in Healthcare: Insight for Research and Practice. In *Patient-engagement: A consumer-centered model*. Berlin: De Gruyter.

Hébert, R. 2010a. "Home Care: From Adequate Funding to Integration of Services." *HealthcarePapers* 10(1): 58–69.

———. 2010b. "An Urgent Need to Improve Life Conditions of Seniors." *Journal of Nutrition, Health and Aging* 14(8): 711–714.

———. 2015. "Still-born Autonomy Insurance Plan in Quebec: Example of a Public Long-Term Care Insurance System in Canada." *HealthcarePapers* (in press).

Klein, R. 2003. "Evidence and Policy: Interpreting the Delphic Oracle." *Journal of the Royal Society of Medicine* 96(6): 429–431.

Lawn, S., and A. Schoo. 2010. "Supporting Self-Management of Chronic Health Conditions: Common Approaches." *Patient Education and Counseling* 80(2): 205–211. doi:10.1016/j.pec.2009.10.006

Légaré, F., A. Boivin, T. van der Weijden, C. Pakenham, J. Burgers, J. Légaré, S. St-Jacques, and S. Gagnon. 2011. "Patient and Public Involvement in Clinical Practice Guidelines: A Knowledge Synthesis of Existing Programs." *Medical Decision Making* 31: E45–74.

Légaré, F., S. Turcotte, D. Stacey, S. Ratté, J. Kryworuchko, and I. D. Graham. 2012. "Patients' Perceptions of Sharing in Decisions. A Systemic Review of Interventions to Enhance Shared Decision Making in Routine Clinical Practice." *Patient* 5(1): 1–19.

Lindsay, S., and H. J. M. Vrijhoef. 2009. "Introduction—A Sociological Focus on 'Expert Patients.'" *Health Sociology Review* 18(2): 139–144.

Lomas, J. 1997. "Reluctant Rationers: Public Input to Healthcare Priorities." *Journal of Health Services & Research Policy* 2: 103–111.

Mitton, C., N. Smith, S. Peacock, B. Evoy, and J. Abelson. 2009. "Public Participation in Health Care Priority Setting: A Scoping Review." *Health Policy* 91: 219–228.

Newbould, J., D. Taylor, and M. Bury. 2006. "Lay-Led Self-Management in Chronic Illness: A Review of the Evidence." *Chronic Illness* 2: 249–261.

Osborn, R., D. Moulds, D. Squires, M. M. Doty, and C. Anderson. 2014. "International Survey of Older Adults Finds Shortcomings in Access, Coordination, and Patient-Centered Care." *Health Affairs* 33(12): 2247–2255.

Peeters, J. M., T. A. Wiegers, and R. D. Friele. 2013. "How Technology in Care at Home Affects Patient Self-Care and Self-Management: A Scoping Review." *International Journal of Environmental Research and Public Health* 29; 10(11): 5541–5564. doi:10.3390/ijerph10115541

Pomey, M.-P., L. Flora, P. Karazivan, V. Dumez, P. Lebel, M.-C. Vanier, et E. Jouet. 2015. « Le modèle relationnel patient partenaire au profit des patients atteints de maladies chroniques: proposition d'une méthodologie de déploiement et d'appropriation. » *Revue de Santé Publique* 27(1 supp.): S41–50.

Richards, T., V. M. Montori, F. Godlee, P. Lapsley, and D. Paul. 2013. "Let the Patient Revolution Begin." *British Medical Journal* 346: f2614. doi:10.1136/bmj.f2614

Rowe, G., and L. J. Frewer. 2005. "A Typology of Public Engagement Mechanisms." *Science Technology Human Values* 30: 251–290.

Taylor, D., and M. Bury. 2007. "Chronic Illness, Expert Patients and Care Transition." *Sociology of Health and Illness* 29(1): 27–45.

Toussaint, J., A. Milstein, and S. Shortell. 2013. "How the Pioneer ACO Model Needs to Change: Lessons from its Best-Performing ACO." *Journal of the American Medical Association* 310(13): 1341–1342.

Wagner, E. H., B. T. Austin, C. Davis, M. Hindmarrrsh, J. Schaefer, and A. Bonomi. 2001. "Improving Chronic Illness Care: Translating Evidence into Action." *Health Affairs (Project Hope),* 20(6): 64–78.

Chapter 7

THE ROLE OF THE PRIVATE SECTOR IN CANADIAN HEALTHCARE: ACCOUNTABILITY, STRATEGIC ALLIANCES, AND GOVERNANCE

A. SCOTT CARSON

Canadian healthcare is very expensive compared to other developed countries. In 2014, total healthcare expenditures were forecast to be $214.9 billion, fully 10.9 percent of Canada's GDP, making it the seventh highest among Organisation for Economic Co-operation and Development (OECD) countries (CIHI 2014). On a per capita basis, Canada has the sixth costliest system, 36 percent higher than the OECD average (OECD 2013). Yet compared to OECD countries, Canada's performance is relatively mediocre across a wide range of quality measures (CIHI 2014). Indeed, in a 2014 Commonwealth Fund study of 11 developed countries, Canada ranked second-to-last overall in measures of quality, access, effectiveness, efficiency, and healthiness, ahead only of the United States.

Canadians generally approve of their healthcare system. And one of the main reasons why Canadians like their system is because they believe it is "public," by which is meant that it is universal and has a single government insurance payer. As Nik Nanos of Nanos Research puts it, "There are very few, if any, pillars of Canadian public policy of which Canadians approve as strongly as the principle of universal healthcare, which has been with us since it was first adopted by the Pearson government in the 1960s" (2009). This view is sustained in a poll commissioned by the *Globe and Mail* in 2012 (Cheadle, 2012), in which 94 percent of respondents called the Canadian universal system "an important source of collective pride." What lies behind the desire for universality is social justice. The social principles upon which Canadian healthcare is based are grounded in a sense of fairness. These are the principles that are reflected in the Canada Health Act, which declares the primary objective of Canadian healthcare policy to be "to protect, promote and restore the physical and mental well-being of residents of Canada and facilitate reasonable access to health services without financial or other barriers" (Sec. 3). This has been likewise articulated in various national healthcare reviews. For example, in his 2002 report, *Building on Values: The Future of Health Care in Canada*, Roy Romanow stated "Canadians have been clear that they still strongly support the core values on which our healthcare system is premised—equity, fairness and solidarity" (xvi).

In other words, despite the mismatch between cost and performance, what Canadians want is a healthcare system that meets certain crucial tests of social justice. The first criterion is financial security for patients and families. Universal, government-funded, and administered health insurance is seen to protect against financially ruinous hospital and physician costs, which are widely assumed to be what can happen when the healthcare system is "private." Second, universally available and government insured healthcare benefits need to meet the tests of both "fairness" in the form of universal "access," and "equity" in the availability to everyone of the same level of services. Again, Canadians widely believe that both access and equity would be at risk in a private system in which the service model is connected with private profit. A third consideration is "democratic control" in order to meet the responsibility for policy formation and accountability for outputs. Healthcare is seen to be a fundamental good and as such should be controlled, not by corporations and market forces, but by democratically elected governments.

What does this mean for the role of business in Canadian healthcare? Many proponents of a public system fear that if business plays a significant role in the system of healthcare, this would be tantamount to a private sector intrusion into the delivery of a Canadian public good. It would be, as Canadians often say, "like the American system." As such, many people think it would stand in opposition to the principles of social justice.

In this chapter, I will argue that there is much room in Canadian healthcare for the private sector that does not impede the goals of social justice or fairness, namely access and equity. In fact, the reverse is likely true: the involvement of the private sector in the right places in the system could readily promote access and equity—by adding financing, resource capacity, expertise, innovation, institutional learning, and reputation enhancement.

The main focus of my discussion will be on the third consideration—democratic control of the healthcare system. I will show that democratic policy making and system oversight are compatible with various forms of partnerships between the public and private sectors. The focus on the issue of system oversight and management is important because considerations one and two above, namely of personal financial security and system fairness (i.e., access and equity), fall within the purview of governments. So long as governments are not abdicating these responsibilities or ceding control of the healthcare system, they are not prevented by the private sector from living up to their responsibility to pursue the objectives of social justice. Instead, the private sector can be a valuable partner in meeting them.

I will consider, first, the role that the private sector plays in Canadian healthcare today. Second, different forms of partnership that are applicable to healthcare will be outlined, and I will explain how they can relate to each other. Third, I will propose a collaborative governance model that could provide oversight of public private partnerships that respects and promotes the democratic obligations of governments to exercise oversight in the healthcare system. Finally, I will argue that a case will be made for considering strategic alliances as a key form of partnership between the public and private sectors.

THE ROLE OF THE PRIVATE SECTOR IN CANADIAN HEALTHCARE TODAY

Whether making a case to support or to oppose participation by the private sector in Canadian healthcare, it is important to understand what is meant by the words "public" and "private," because in healthcare discussions there is much ambiguity, both in the meaning of these words, and the circumstances in which they are used. For example, Canadians widely believe they have a "public" healthcare system; most Canadians probably do not realize that some 30 percent of the system's expenditures are, in fact, private, not public. Greater clarity in terminology is thus needed.

First, consider how the Canadian system is funded. Public funding means coming from a government. For example, insurance coverage for payments to hospitals and physicians is provided by provincial/territorial governments, which in turn fund these payments from general tax revenues and (indirectly) from federal transfer payments. However, when we say that funding is private, such as payments made for prescription drugs, this can mean either funding by private sector corporations who provide insurance, or from the pockets of individuals. Opponents of private sector involvement in healthcare are more likely to be targeting corporations than private individuals, yet both are picked up by the word private.

Second, reference to the private sector can also be taken to be synonymous with "business," but there is also some ambiguity in this. Opponents of business participation in healthcare may be thinking of large corporations, such as multinational pharmaceutical or medical device manufacturers, but not a family-owned neighbourhood pharmacy or a biotech start-up. Both, however, are businesses—and businesses are part of the private sector, even though they are different from individual patients and families, who are also private payers for portions of their healthcare.

Third, when private is taken to be a proxy for business, the business being referred to may not pertain to funding but rather to a "business perspective." For instance, business schools teach their students the concepts, core principles, subject knowledge, and skills that not only generate competence in dealing with business problems but also a way of looking at problems—from a business perspective. Equally, someone who works in a business, whether in a multinational corporation, start-up venture, or small owner-operator company, is likely to develop a business perspective. This, too, can be what is meant by private, or by private sector.

Fourth, private sector can refer to "practices" that are commonly associated with what is found in businesses and what business schools research and teach. For example, the boards of directors of many large hospitals are structured and function in ways that are based on the theory and practice of corporate governance. Hospitals and other healthcare organizations have widely adopted, or adapted, these practices. Similarly, strategy processes such as the "balanced scorecard approach," which originated in business, are often used in hospitals and other healthcare institutions. Much the same can be said about financial systems, control and reporting, human resource theory, value creation processes such as the "lean" principles and techniques, and so on.

Taking all of this into account, when we talk about the private sector participating in healthcare, we have many possible ways in which that can occur. In the next section, I will be more specific about how much "participation" is in evidence in Canadian healthcare.

Funding of Healthcare

Think of private participation in healthcare in relation to how the healthcare system is funded. As indicated above, public sector expenditures are goods and services for which a government pays. As well as the operating costs of hospitals and patients' visits to physicians, this includes the cost of government health ministries and the funding of capital expenditures in hospitals, clinics, and entities in the other parts of the system. The private sector financing applies mainly to expenditures attributable to private insurance companies and out-of-pocket payments by patients.

Government Funding

A public/private split exists in most countries. Table 7.1 shows the relationship between public and private spending across OECD member countries. Mexico, Chile, and the United States have larger private sector funding percentages than the remainder of the 34 countries. Canada's private sector participation is the 12th highest, slightly higher than the OECD average, and higher as well than 22 other countries.

In absolute terms, Canada's private sector expenditures are $60.3 billion (CIHI 2014). By comparison with other developed countries, Canadian private expenditures are sizable. For instance, they are greater than the total public

TABLE 7.1
Expenditures on Health by Type of Financing, 2009 (or nearest year)

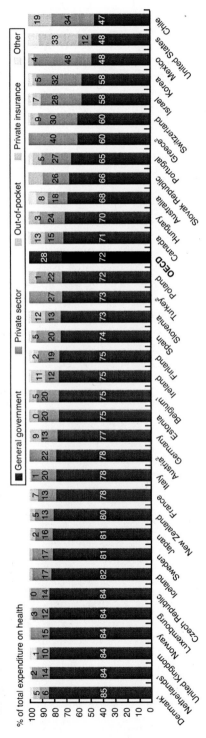

1. Current expenditure.
2. No breakdown of private financing available for latest year.
Source: Adapted from OECD Health Data 2011
StatLink: http://dx.doi.org/10.1787/888932526274

and private healthcare expenditures in both Sweden ($55.6 billion) and Austria ($49.3 billion; using data from The World Bank 2014). So it is clear that the private sector is currently playing a significant role in Canadian healthcare in funding terms.

Apart from the relative size of the private sector, it is useful to consider the roles that the private sector plays in healthcare delivery in other OECD countries. Canadians often focus on the US because of its size and proximity to Canada, but our comparators should be more broadly based. In the UK, for instance, specialists can practice simultaneously in both state funded and private clinics. The Australian and Swedish systems include both public and private hospitals. And the French system is a hybrid.

Healthcare Institutions

Hospitals are Canada's primary institutional service providers. They account for 29.6 percent, or $63.5 billion, of all healthcare expenditures, of which about $2.4 billion is paid by private insurance and out-of-pocket expenditures by households. However, outside the hospital, the private sector role has been growing either to provide new services or take over some hospital functions. There is private sector ownership of some specialized surgical hospitals (e.g., Shouldice Hospital), and a growing number of private clinics provide diagnostic imaging, laser eye surgery, optometry, and so on. In other healthcare fields such as dentistry, psychological counselling, chiropractic medicine, naturopathic medicine, and pharmacy (external to the hospital), entities are owned and operated variously by individuals, small practitioner groups, or corporations, and most offer their services on a private fee-for-service basis. Ownership of pharmacies ranges from owner operators, to large corporations, to food chains (e.g., Loblaws), to box stores (e.g., Walmart). Clearly, institutional healthcare delivery is dominated in financial terms by public hospitals, but in the scope of healthcare entities, the private sector is broadly represented and likely increasing.

Product and Service Providers

Ranging from small entrepreneurial entities to large corporations, businesses research, create, design, and manufacture medical technology, devices, and pharmaceuticals. In addition, private sector contractors design, build, finance, maintain, and operate hospitals; businesses provide services such as maintenance, janitorial, laundry, audit, legal, architectural, and purchasing; and consultants and lawyers provide advice: on everything from policy formation to risk management to organizational restructuring, to government policymakers, regional health authorities and hospital boards, and administrators.

Further, private clinics are increasingly providing diagnostic services such as MRIs. Optometrists/opticians, chiropractors, psychological counsellors, and other health service professionals provide services that lie outside of the Canadian health insurance system. Even physicians, physiotherapists, and pharmacists are, for the most part, in the private sector. For instance, of Canada's over

16,389 physiotherapists, 40.3 percent are in private professional practice (CIHI 2010). Also, of the 38,737 thousand pharmacists in Canada, 73 percent practice in the community or other non-hospital settings (National Association of Pharmacy Regulatory Authorities 2015). Within the domains of health policy, healthcare services, and healthcare institutional operations, the private sector is well represented. And of course, by private sector, we mean professionals who are practicing privately.

Business Perspectives

In hospitals, clinics, and community care centres, there is an important difference between the "care" of patients and their "operations." Consider the very considerable influence of business thinking that exists in the operational side of hospitals and other healthcare institutions. For instance, a hospital CEO's executive team includes not only the chiefs of medicine and nursing, but also those who are responsible for the hospital's finances, risk management, human resources, information technology and systems, and strategy and communications. The subject knowledge of these operational areas comes directly or is derived from business disciplines—i.e., finance, accounting, organizational behaviour, management information systems (MIS), and strategy. As well, the management processes employed in the hospital, such as strategic planning, balanced scorecards, lean processes, and so on, have their origins in business thinking and practice.

In addition, the executives, and many of their staff members, are often graduates of business schools or executive training programs, and many have private sector work experience. For example, both the vice president of finance and their reporting line staff may be graduates of commerce or business administration programs who have articled with a public accounting firm while completing the CPA designation. They may have worked in the private sector before moving into the healthcare sector. Similar cases would be found in MIS and human resources. Indeed, business schools anticipate the need for business-trained hospital and other healthcare leaders. For example, the MBA programs at Queen's University, the University of Toronto, York University, McGill University, Western University, and the University of British Columbia all have healthcare management specializations to prepare graduates for such positions.

Business perspectives are in evidence even beyond management. Boards of directors of hospitals (especially in Ontario's 151 hospitals) comprise both internal hospital members (ex officio and appointed) and externally elected members. A significant number of the elected members are from private sector firms—banks, consulting firms, manufacturing companies, and technology firms—and bring a business perspective to the governance of institutions. Table 7.2 shows the business and academic/professional backgrounds of external directors in 17 of Ontario's academic hospitals. Of 256 external directors, 70 percent have business experience and 75 percent have either business experience or a business degree/professional designation. At nine of the 17 hospitals, 80 percent or more of the directors have either business experience or a business

TABLE 7.2
Business Experience and Education of Elected Directors in Selected Ontario Academic Hospitals

Selected Academic Hospitals in Ontario (Hospitals with publicly available director bios)	Elected Directors	Ex Officio/ Appt. Directors	Total Directors	Elected with Business Experience (%)	Elected with Business Degree/ Professional Designation (%)	Elected with Combined Business Experience and Business Degree/ Prof. Designation (%)	Elected with Business Experience or Business Degree/ Prof. Designation
Hospital 1	17	6	23	15 (88)	8 (47)	7 (41)	15 (88)
Hospital 2	17	4	21	12 (71)	7 (41)	6 (35)	13 (76)
Hospital 3	16	6	22	8 (50)	5 (31)	4 (25)	9 (56)
Hospital 4	16	4	20	10 (63)	3 (19)	3 (19)	10 (63)
Hospital 5	12	5	17	8 (67)	5 (42)	4 (33)	9 (75)
Hospital 6	15	4	19	9 (60)	7 (47)	7 (47)	9 (60)
Hospital 7	18	6	24	17 (94)	9 (50)	9 (50)	17 (94)
Hospital 8	13	4	17	10 (77)	8 (62)	8 (62)	10 (83)
Hospital 9	11	6	17	3 (27)	4 (36)	3 (27)	4 (36)
Hospital 10	26	6	32	23 (88)	9 (35)	9 (35)	23 (88)
Hospital 11	12	5	17	9 (75)	4 (33)	5 (42)	10 (83)
Hospital 12	15	5	20	6 (40)	3 (20)	2 (13)	7 (47)
Hospital 13	15	3	18	9 (60)	7 (47)	4 (27)	12 (80)
Hospital 14	15	7	22	8 (53)	5 (33)	5 (33)	8 (53)
Hospital 15	7	11	18	7 (100)	2 (29)	2 (29)	7 (100)
Hospital 16	15	8	23	13 (87)	5 (33)	5 (33)	13 (87)
Hospital 17	16	9	25	13 (81)	9 (56)	8 (50)	15 (94)
TOTALS	256	99	355	180 (70)	100 (39)	91 (36)	191 (75)

degree/professional designation. Clearly, business thinking plays a significant role in hospital governance.

In addition, the board's processes, committee structures, self-assessment, and reporting frameworks are derived from private sector theory and practice. Equally, the governance of regional health structures, like the Local Health Integration Networks (LHINs) in Ontario, as well as their fundraising foundations, share these private sector characteristics. So private sector thinking, processes, and experience pervade healthcare institutions.

It should be noted that there is controversy in the field of management education regarding the extent to which the emphasis in business schools on profit and competitive advantage develops in students a worldview based on self-interest and lack of appreciation for broader social goals. This may overstate the importance that students attach to finance and strategy courses, and give insufficient recognition to the perceived value of course work in organizational behaviour and corporate social responsibility. But there can be little doubt that a corporate and commercial way of thinking does affect students. This, in turn, leads reasonably to the conclusion that business graduates are in general financially oriented, results-focused, and taught to think in terms of rational decision-making frameworks. It is in this way that leaders in healthcare institutions come to adopt a business perspective.

However, this perspective should not be confused with excessive attention to financial matters at the expense of patient health and safety. To do so would fly in the face of the principle of patient-centredness. Indeed, the restructuring of the NHS England in 2013 was strongly influenced by the results of a national investigative commission that linked unnecessary deaths and very poor patient safety in many hospitals to the over-concern of management and boards with budgetary matters at the expense of patients (Francis 2010).

While the patient care and operational aspects of healthcare institutions are "different," they are not "separate" from one another. Executives and their departments work together as a team in the enterprise of delivering healthcare to patients, families, and communities. Modern healthcare therefore blurs the dividing lines between public and private to deliver institutional healthcare.

Business Practices

Healthcare institutions today are strategic planners. The demands of accountability to governments, agencies, and the public require that hospitals and other institutions plan strategically. They must consider: (a) how they will function strategically in relation to the health system (e.g., LHINs) of which they are a part; (b) how they will be able to partner with community health and social services; (c) how to strategically focus and prioritize their medical services; (d) how to assess financial needs and sources of funding for operational and capital expenditures; (e) how to plan, prioritize, and fund research and teaching (for medical centres); (f) how to allocate health human resources, and address primary care; (g) how to establish plans for information and management technology; and (h) how to establish management processes, such as lean operations.

In each of these categories of practice, the theories, core concepts, processes, and practices are derived at least in part from management theory, research, and practice. Of course the implementation is adapted to healthcare, but the conceptual origins are traceable to business. At the provincial/territorial level, a similar connection to management can be seen. Of course, healthcare policy development is more traditionally the role of governments even if institutional application is business based. But even policy is influenced by business thinking when advisory commissions, councils, and consultations include private sector participants.

To conclude, private sector participation in Canadian healthcare can be thought of in terms of how the system and its components are funded, the infusion of business perspectives into the governance, management, and operations of the healthcare system, and the practices of managing and operating healthcare institutions that are derived or adapted from business. Looking at the delivery of Canadian healthcare today, it is not realistic to question whether business should be present in our "public" system. The question should be, where is the participation of business most likely to contribute to achieving the ideals and strategic objectives of our system?

In order to answer this, we need to understand the ways in which business and government are related to each other in Canadian healthcare. If the healthcare system requires democratic oversight in order to be in accord with social principles such as fairness, access, and equity, then we must understand why business should participate, and how business and government relate to each other in ways that make this oversight possible.

Why Should the Private Sector Participate in a Public System?

The benefits of private sector participation in healthcare should be assessed primarily on the basis of how well it promotes the interests of patients and their families. The overriding commitment should not be to the self-interests of professionals, organizational convenience of providers, pragmatic interests of politicians, or theoretical commitments of ideologues. It was said above that Canadians want healthcare to be guided by the principles of social justice—in particular fairness to patients and families in the form of access and equity. So the justification for private sector participation should be assessed on the basis of its contribution to the efficient and effective performance of the system that generates healthcare outcomes to meet the social principles.

While this will be addressed more fully below, it is useful to introduce the key points here. Figure 7.1 summarizes a framework that shows what a collaborative relationship can yield in terms of benefits. The framework sets out two categories of contribution: resources and growth. Within those categories are six drivers of beneficial outcomes. Those drivers (such as financing, capacity and expertise deriving from resources; and innovation, learning and reputation deriving from growth) work together to promote beneficial outcomes for the healthcare system, namely efficiency and effectiveness. In turn, these contribute to improved access and equity for patients.

Figure 7.1
Public and Private Sector Collaboration Framework

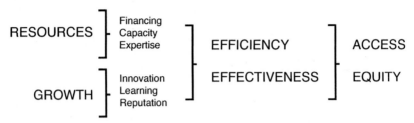

The framework categorizes the benefits of public and private entities working together; first, in terms of the resource contributions that derive from private sector strengths, and second, in the growth opportunities for the entity that constitute the relationship between the public and private sector. In more detail, the benefits are as follows.

The first is financing. The private sector partner often has access to financing for certain projects. If so, this not only adds financial resources to the project, but also it transfers financial risk from the government to the private sector partner. Collateral benefits to the government are both the freeing up of financial resources for spending on other programs, and the removal of the need for borrowing. The latter is important because adding debt to government balance sheets can affect bond ratings, which in turn can have a negative impact on future borrowing costs.

Second is capacity. Projects and other joint undertakings have non-financial resource requirements: human resources, technology, plant and equipment, business processes, and so on. Even limitations on time availability can be a capacity constraint. In some cases, a public sector partner may not possess the needed resources; even if they do have the resources, the government may need to deploy them elsewhere. Partnering with the private sector can offer a solution to capacity problems.

Third, a private partner may be able to contribute expertise. This could be in the form of unique experience in executing tasks required for the project to be successful. Or it could involve proprietary technologies or business processes, which are valuable to the project, rare in terms of availability, and difficult to imitate, or for which there are few viable substitutes.

The fourth enabler is innovation. Invention and discovery of feasible solutions to problems through new products and services is a classic strength of the private sector, especially when capacity is combined with expertise. To say that private and public sector entities working together will necessarily innovate is an overstatement. Innovation occurs when the conditions are favourable. However, the potential for innovation should be a consideration when evaluating private sector participation if, based on the best available evidence, innovation has a better chance of occurring when the public and private sectors work together than if they do not.

Institutional learning is the fifth benefit. In the process of working together, public and private sector individuals and institutions can learn much from each other. There is a human dimension of working together in which an individual learns the perspectives of the other as they develop a working rapport. Much was said about the business perspective above; for those whose careers have been in the public sector, the business orientation takes getting used to, and vice versa. In addition, new business processes can be learned—from the balanced scorecard approach to translating strategic objectives into measurable goals with targets, lean value enhancement processes, and so on. Finally, innovations and discoveries can be leveraged, extended, and transferred to other aspects of each partner's business (subject to contractual agreements).

Sixth, reputational enhancement is important to the ongoing work of both the public and private partners. For example, a research institute that has state-of-the-art facilities and technology because of a public private partnership enjoys numerous advantages. It makes recruitment of new high-quality researchers much easier. A reputation for leading-edge research follows naturally. And it improves the chances of success in applications for additional grants and other forms of research funding, completing the virtuous circle.

With these points in mind, we turn now to consider what forms participation between the private sector and public sector can take.

RELATIONSHIP BETWEEN PUBLIC AND PRIVATE SECTORS

In this section, I explore three ways in which the public sector, mainly governments, can relate to the private sector: regulation, ownership/control, and partnerships. I then set out a framework for assessing which forms of relationship are most suited to addressing healthcare issues.

Regulation

Public policy in healthcare is the purview of governments. In advancing a policy aim a government provides a regulatory framework within which the policies must be implemented. For instance, the Canadian government oversees the implementation of the Canada Health Act, and in doing so acts as a regulator for other governments (provincial and territorial) in terms of universal health insurance, and for private sector corporations with respect to pharmaceutical approvals. In turn, provinces and territories regulate medical device approvals. Regulatory frameworks in healthcare function in much the same way as they do in other areas of public policy. They ensure oversight while recognizing that other entities are better positioned to deliver products and services.

Ownership and Control

Canadians are familiar with crown corporations such as the Export Development Corporation and Canada Post Corporation. These are not-for-profit corporations, the shares of which are owned by the Crown, that compete with private sector counterparts. Agencies such as provincial securities commissions, gaming and lottery, and alcohol sales may have different legal structures (depending on the jurisdiction) in not having shares that are owned by the government. A government may prefer to own, rather than regulate, in order to implement its policies directly. Sometimes governments change their minds about ownership and divest their corporations. The Government of Canada divested itself of both Air Canada and the Canadian National Railway. Similarly, the Ontario government announced in October 2015 that it intends to sell part of its ownership of Hydro One, its electricity transmission system. Alternatively, governments sometimes transfer control of entities by means of long-term leases. The Canadian government did this in the 1990s when it leased major airports in Canadian cities to regional airport authorities.

Since governments still retain a public policy interest in many of their divested entities, they can continue their oversight by way of regulation as above. For example, the Ontario government constructed a toll highway (Hwy. 407) as a means of achieving a public policy objective, namely relieving traffic congestion on another major highway (Hwy. 401) in close proximity. Ontario subsequently sold the toll highway in 1999. Part of the sale involved a regulatory mechanism that tied future toll price increases to mandatory traffic volume targets. There were stiff financial penalties if the higher tolls resulted in reductions in the volume of traffic below a required threshold. As long as the toll road carried the required volume of traffic, it was deemed to be meeting the public policy objective of relieving traffic congestion on the other major highway. The regulatory structure was the government's tool for achieving this.

Regulation is an indirect way for governments to engage with the private sector. Except in cases where regulation is directly tied to a single company, the connection is usually impersonal because it is at an industry level. Ownership by contrast is more direct. But even here, the extent of direct involvement between owner and owned depends on the particular situation. A government can be more or less involved in the oversight and management of the entity it owns. Assessing whether either regulation or ownership is a desirable form of relationship in promoting public policy or programs by using the private sector requires us to think of the particular situation under consideration in relation to the four tests above: finance, capacity, expertise, and innovation.

Let us compare regulation and ownership with another important form of business and government relationship, namely partnerships.

Partnerships and Alliances

Contracting Out

At one end of the spectrum of partnerships is "contracting out" for goods and services. Governments enter into contracts with businesses to have them perform custodial and cleaning services in government buildings, highway snow removal, road construction, facilities maintenance, supply chain management for procurement, and so on. Hospitals contract out for laboratory services, linens, parking, legal and audit, and other services. The rationale for contracting out is often a matter of cost and expertise: it is less expensive to purchase the service, the service requires competency that does not exist in-house, there is insufficient capacity within the existing in-house resources, or the service required is not a core activity of the organization.

Characteristic of this form of partnership is that the relationship is: (a) established by the government partner; (b) contractually bound; (c) performance based; (d) limited in scope by the terms of the contract; and (e) time limited. In sum, governments pay for a service to be performed. Once the service has met the completion test established by the contract, the relationship ends, at least until it is renewed or reconstituted by a further contract.

Public Private Partnership

A partnership is created when two or more parties undertake some form of project or activity toward which each makes a contribution to establish the partnership and continue its operation. Contributions can be financial, real property, plant and equipment, expertise, or indeed anything of value that contributes to the venture. Often one partner takes the lead in managing the partnership. A partnership is not a defined legal entity such as a corporation; rather it gains legal status by virtue of legal agreements that the partners enter into between themselves. For example, lawyers and accountants establish partnerships to practice law or accounting together by sharing premises, administration, and business development expenses. Also, mining companies, even competitors, sometimes create a partnership to develop a mine where the cost would otherwise be prohibitive for either partner on its own; rival technology companies will also establish a jointly owned company to develop a new technology or application.

Another common form of partnership of importance to the healthcare discussion is a "public private partnership" ("P3"). This is a joint venture among partners, which, as the name implies, involves a government, either directly through a ministry, agency, or controlled entity, and at least one private sector partner. Each contributes to the establishment of the partnership.

A P3 shares certain features with contracting out, namely that the relationship is government established and led, it is contractual in nature, and it typically has a finite life that is usually coincident with the completion of a project for which the partnership has been formed. What makes it different from contracting out is that the undertaking in which the partners are venturing together is more complex than a simple contract—in some cases because multiple contracts are combined to achieve different but connected objectives.

In Canadian healthcare, a common form of P3s can be observed in hospital infrastructure projects. In a new or redeveloped hospital project, the government (or ministry) engages a partner, or partners, to design, finance, build, operate, or maintain a hospital. The partnership often involves a combination of some or all of these functions. Table 7.3 outlines some of the key P3s used for Canadian healthcare projects.

The rationale for P3s typically focuses on resources and expertise. The resource implications for governments are twofold. The first is financial. In contracting out, a government provides the funding to support the partner's performance of the contract. However, in a P3, the private sector partner often provides the financing for the partnership. Indeed, in all 84 healthcare projects summarized in Table 7.3, the private sector partner provides financing, in addition to design, build, and other functions. This relieves the government of either, or both, income statement or balance sheet pressure, which is to say that the government is thereby not required to use its own operating or capital funds for the project and it does not need to add debt to its balance sheet through borrowing. The second implication is that governments may not have the resource capacity—e.g., workforce, equipment, technology—to take on a large construction or other project. Since the private sector partners are in business to perform these roles, it makes sense for their resources to be utilized by government.

Table 7.3
Public Private Partnership Projects in Healthcare Sector Across Canada

Models/ Provinces	Design-Build-Finance-Maintain-Operate	Design-Build-Finance-Maintain	Design-Build-Finance-Operate	Design-Build-Finance	Build-Finance-Maintain	Build-Finance	Totals
British Columbia	1	11	1				13
Alberta			1				1
Saskatchewan		2					2
Ontario	1	16	1	4	3	31	56
Quebec	5	3		1			9
New Brunswick		2					2
Northwest Territories		1					1
Totals	7	35	3	5	3	31	84

Note: Canadian healthcare P3 projects at Request for Proposal stage, under construction or recently completed, as at June 2015.
Source: Prepared from The Canadian Council for Public and Private Partnerships (Canadian PPP Project Database, June 2015); http://projects.pppcouncil.ca/ccppp/src/public/searchproject?pageid=3d067bedfe2f4677470dd6ccf64d05ed

Expertise does not always reside within government, but it can sometimes be sourced from the private sector. Project design, construction, and management are the specific expertise of some companies, which can be leveraged by governments through industry partnerships.

A key factor for the determination of the viability of a P3 is whether it, or a potential private sector partner, has greater expertise in the evaluation of the risks and benefits of a given project, and who is in the best position to manage those risks once identified. Matched with the question of expertise is the matter of resource capability and capacity. Granted, not all projects should be P3s. Each case needs to be evaluated on its own merits. However, where there is a stronger argument for partnering based on resource and expertise considerations, P3s should be seriously considered as an option.

As a further note, we must keep in mind that it is in the nature of "partners" in any undertaking to have aspirations, objectives, and motives that differ from each other. A partnership must accommodate these differences in a way that "corporations" do not. The latter can remove dissonances that inhibit the corporate purpose. They can fire recalcitrant executives, refuse to accept divisional strategies and plans that do not align with the corporate objectives, and harmonize the corporate culture to promote conformity of purpose and perspective. However, partnerships must accommodate differences. Successful partnerships achieve this accommodation whereas unsuccessful partnerships fail and dissolve.

In the realm of healthcare P3s, then, it is to be expected that the private sector partners will have commercial objectives and the government partners will want to achieve public policy ends. Successful P3s are those that accommodate both because doing so allows each partner to achieve outcomes that promote its own objectives, while together partners achieve outcomes that fulfill collective goals. In sum, partners learn to work together, rather than one subsuming the other.

Strategic Alliances

Strategic alliances are a form of joint venture partnership. Often the terminology of joint venture and strategic alliance is used interchangeably. However, as I use the term here, a strategic alliance refers to a partnership that is more open-ended. Alliance partners have a purpose in going beyond existing projects (Carson 2015a). They come together in order to explore opportunities for the future that are in pursuit of broader strategic goals (Doz and Hamel 1998). The Canadian Partnership Against Cancer is an example: It is funded by the federal government to promote cancer control by bringing together cancer experts, charitable organizations, governments, cancer agencies, national health organizations, patients, survivors, and other groups, to implement a Canada-wide cancer control strategy. Its main functions span a continuum encompassing prevention through healthy communities and lifestyle, cancer screening, system performance and quality guidelines, treatment, and follow-up and survivorship (Canadian Partnership Against Cancer 2015).

A project can be an undertaking of such a relationship, but the purpose of the alliance itself is to pursue business opportunities that go beyond simply a project to include ventures that explore new processes, technologies, or products that may not yet have been identified. An illustration from the technology industry is an alliance that formed in the 1960s between Fuji and Xerox to compete against Canon and Ricoh in the paper copier market. That partnership later grew to include a new partnership that formed between Xerox and Rank Organization and many smaller companies. Collectively they were able to pursue new technological innovations, even though they individually had their separate corporate objectives (Gomez-Casseres 1996).

Some alliances are called "pooling" alliances. They bring together organizations that have similar resources, for example a purchasing alliance that involves a group of hospitals and preferred device suppliers. A "trading" alliance comprises organizations with different resources. An example is the alliance formed in 2011 between General Electric's healthcare unit and M+W Group to produce biopharmaceuticals such as vaccines, insulin, and biosimilars for emerging nations. GE brought its technical expertise to the partnership, and M+W contributed its global engineering, construction, and project management (General Electric Company 2011). Indeed, the Premier Healthcare Alliance in the United States includes 2,300 hospitals and $33 billion in purchases (Zajac et al. 2011). Figure 7.2 compares in summary form the three main forms of partnership.

The P3 model, which is common in healthcare, especially with respect to infrastructure development, tends to have many of the features of a strategic alliance. Yet the strategic alliance may hold a special promise for Canadian healthcare because it brings partners together around shared strategic priorities. Could governments in Canada feasibly pursue strategic alliances in healthcare with business? The opportunities that could be explored are considerable insofar as the private sector is able to contribute resources and expertise to the alliance. The public sector contributions would include public policy, strategic objectives, and alliance leadership. Let us consider this more fully.

Public Private Strategic Alliances

In what parts of the healthcare system would strategic alliances be most appropriate? How should strategic alliances be structured in order to ensure that governments retain their public policy and accountability roles and responsibilities?

There are many areas where strategic alliances are appropriate in the healthcare system. For example, in the United States, General Electric, Siemens, and Philips have developed strategic alliances with academic medical centres, hospital systems, and physician groups. In a Canadian example, a group of hospitals in southeastern Ontario have established a supply chain company to purchase and deliver medical supplies to achieve cost synergies. A possibility also exists for a cluster of hospitals to partner with a device manufacturer or technology company to leverage resources and to explore new clinical practice models. Finally, there are possibilities for strategic alliances in which the private sector provides financing and management expertise to build laboratories and the hospitals provide research programs and resources. None of these are radical or untried, but they are not as well developed or far-reaching as they

Figure 7.2
Partnership Form Comparison

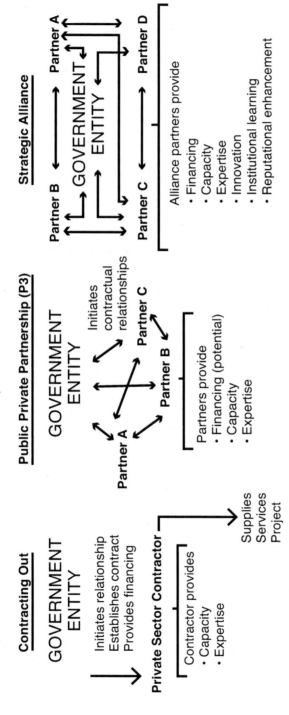

Contracting Out

GOVERNMENT
ENTITY

Initiates relationship
Establishes contract
Provides financing

Private Sector Contractor

Contractor provides
· Capacity
· Expertise

Supplies
Services
Project

Public Private Partnership (P3)

GOVERNMENT
ENTITY

Initiates
contractual
relationships

Partner C

Partner B

Partner A

Partners provide
· Financing (potential)
· Capacity
· Expertise

Strategic Alliance

Partner A

Partner B

GOVERNMENT
ENTITY

Partner C

Partner D

Alliance partners provide
· Financing
· Capacity
· Expertise
· Innovation
· Institutional learning
· Reputational enhancement

could be. In short, alliances can form between "suppliers" such as pharmaceutical and biotech firms for drug development and commercialization, or medical device and information technology firms for such things as remote monitors; "suppliers and providers" as in the case of hospital researchers and medical imaging firms; "clusters of providers" such as pharmacies and retail stores; "buyers and providers" such as a manufacturing company establishing on-site clinics for employees; and "buyers and other buyers" such as a medical device manufacturer, which, as an employer, forms an alliance with a health insurance group (Zajac et al. 2011).

Alliances are not a panacea. Conditions may not be conducive to success. The macro environment—political, economic, technological, and social conditions—needs to provide support for the strategic objectives of the alliance. And the strategic priorities of the partners must align, or success will be difficult to achieve. Further, the alliance partners need to be able to establish a management and governance structure that enables them to work together collaboratively. Finally, the behavioural characteristics of the alliance partners need to be compatible with working together. Some partners are better at working cooperatively than others. Indeed, there is a gradation in the degree of cooperativeness: fully cooperative, to quasi-cooperative, to indifferent, to competitive, to vengeful (Zajac et al. 2011). At some stage, cooperativeness can fade to the point where the alliance is untenable. Finding and maintaining a collaborative relationship is difficult but potentially valuable if it can be sustained. Still, even successful alliances have limitations to their life.

Of course, conflicts of interest and other problems can arise in strategic alliances. However, this does not provide an argument against alliances per se, but rather points to areas where management of the relationship requires attention. As the public and private sectors gain more knowledge of each other's perspectives through the infusion of business thinking in healthcare, and the expansion of private sector service delivery across the continuum of care, the ability to resolve issues and problems increases.

Strategic alliances are a powerful form of partnership, and they can help to promote social justice objectives. This does not mean that all projects and undertakings need to involve this or any other form of business and government partnerships. Rather, it is certain specific undertakings that should be considered, such as projects, strategic research and development, product research and development, service delivery innovations, system integration prototypes and experiments, and so on.

The challenge for a government in a strategic alliance relationship is that it is a "partner" in a strategic venture rather than being in "control" as in a P3. Even though a P3 does not always allow for the immediacy of control that exists in the contracting out relationship, there are, nevertheless, levers of control. These levers are less available in a strategic alliance—a partnership of equals. The question then is, how does government build into the relationship a control feature that allows it to exercise its democratic policy and accountability oversight?

The answer, I suggest, is at the governance level. I propose a bicameral governance structure in the context of a collaborative governance model.

BICAMERAL COLLABORATIVE GOVERNANCE

Collaborative governance is emerging as a powerful oversight model in multi-stakeholder undertakings, which involve a government and two or more non-government partners. The non-government partners may not include a private sector partner, but for present purposes these collaborations of interest will involve a private sector partner. In a collaborative governance entity the partnership is initiated by the government partner. The government's objective is to create a multiparty entity that will implement a policy or program. While the government is the originator of the collaborative entity, it may or may not be active in its operations. The new Ontario Health Links are an example of such an entity: the government seeks to achieve certain of its local healthcare integration policies through entities that link multiple health providers, such as hospitals, nursing homes, community social services, medical teams, and so on. The governance of such a collaborative entity is a body that is representative of the collaborators. Their relationship to each other may be contractual, but is more likely determined by informal agreements in reference to the government's policies, mandate assignments, and regulations. Typically, collaborative governance functions by discussion and consensus, rather than legal authorities and performance deliverables (Ansell and Gish 2008).

The collaborative governance model has broader application than entities such as Health Links. It could apply to strategic alliances that address major strategic challenges such as health system transformation, in which the collaborators could involve different private sector companies. If so, one of the weaknesses of the collaborative governance model should be easy to see. With such a reliance on discussion and consensus, collaborative governance is most compatible with entities that are closely aligned in terms of overarching objectives, purpose, and values. Corporations have commercial objectives such as growth, profitability, and enhancement of shareholder value. This does not always align with patient-centred and broader social goals. How then could a collaborative governance model effectively address conflicts and contrasting objectives? The answer is that in order for governments to be satisfied that they have a mechanism for asserting some form of control over the entity, something must be added to the governance model.

It can be suggested that the best alternative is a bicameral governance structure, which contains a dual oversight component (Carson 2015b). The board of directors of the collaborative entity—the Operating Board—would be mandated to oversee the management and operations of the collaborative to ensure the achievement of its objectives. To ensure that clarity exists between the Operating Board and management, there must be an "operating agreement," which would govern the day-to-day functioning of management and provide the control feature of management oversight. The ongoing operations of the alliance would be the responsibility of management. The Operating Board would provide the same governance role as any corporate board exercises with respect to management.

The second component of the bicameral structure is what we might call the Policy Council. This is a board whose members would include representatives of the government and the private sector. Its role would be to ensure that the collaboration continued to serve the policy purpose for which it was formed. The Policy Council would also be the means by which the government was able to ensure that its policy authority and accountability requirements were met. It is not the role of the Policy Council to concern itself with day-to-day operations, or to intervene in the sphere of the Operating Board's responsibility.

The Canadian Blood Services provides an excellent illustration of the bicameral structure. As an operating entity, the corporation and its management are overseen by a board of directors. The board's responsibility is to ensure that management is acting in the best interests of the corporation in accordance with its mandate. In our terminology this is the Operating Board. But the Canadian Blood Services has a second component to its governance structure. The corporation's activities are funded by the provinces (except Quebec), so each province has an interest in ensuring that its objectives are being met overall. The Canadian Blood Services version of what we would call the Policy Council is the entity that reviews the corporation from this overarching point of view. There is a council that is composed of government officials who review the broad functioning of the corporation in relation to its purpose for being. This is not its operational role. In this way the corporation's bicameral governance structure provides two types of oversight (Sher 2015).

It is important to distinguish between a "bicameral model" and what we might call a "two-tier model" in which one board provides oversight to the other. In the latter model, the upper level board is more "senior" than the lower-level board. In a bicameral structure, by contrast, the boards have different purposes and roles.

It is true that the Policy Council would have a more senior level standing than the Operating Board, for the Policy Council has the power to end the relationship between the government and its alliance partners. But its senior position does not imply a duty of oversight or a duplication of its role in supervising the senior management of the organization. Figure 7.3 summarizes the structural difference between a two-tier governance model and a bicameral model.

STRATEGIC ALLIANCES IN CANADA

What is being proposed here is a non-politicized approach to advancing Canadian healthcare in spheres that can best benefit by organizations and individuals from both public and private sectors working together in collaboration. This is not the place to outline in detail where specific opportunities might lie. However, the six-point framework outlined above (i.e., financial, capacity, expertise, innovation, institutional learning, and reputational enhancement) is a

Figure 7.3
Two-Tier and Bicameral Governance

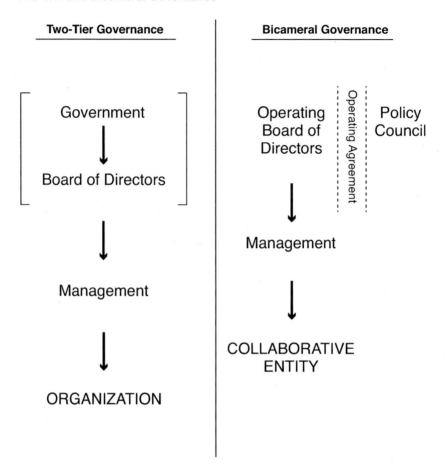

useful evaluative tool, both for assessing the viability of an alliance candidate and for seeking out and prioritizing new opportunities.

In challenging times of resource constraint, many public sector healthcare institutions focus on the first three components of the framework—financial, capacity, and expertise—as a way of bolstering what might be absent or in short supply. As an illustration, the Council of Academic Hospitals of Ontario (CAHO) expresses a deep concern about funding for the research enterprise in its 2013–14 Annual Report. Referring to its own study of funding pressures it says:

> These findings by the CAHO community provide the basis for
> an informed discussion with investment partners in government,
> industry and the philanthropic community. CAHO will continue to

work to develop a model for sustainable, long-term investment in
health research...

In this statement, CAHO is recognizing the importance of public private collaboration, but the focus is placed on resource constraint. This is not a criticism
of CAHO because this was the purpose of their study. Still, it draws attention
to the importance of looking for strategic opportunities beyond the financial
aspects.

The opportunities in Canadian healthcare are numerous and varied. Many
involve connecting entrepreneurs or corporations who have developed a new
technology with providers and patients. For instance, the Ontario Telemedicine
Network is a world leader in telemedicine that links technology, specialists,
primary care professionals, and patients. For example, a patient in a remote
location can send a photograph of a mole on her arm to a dermatologist who
responds with a diagnosis in days, rather than the patient waiting weeks or
months for an in-person consultation. Or, a patient wearing a remote monitoring device can be monitored by a practitioner who interprets the data for early
intervention at the local level, rather than in the emergency room of a hospital.
Alliances such as these achieve not just cost savings, capacity, and expertise,
but also innovation, new learning, and reputational enhancement.

Some alliances form because the partners conceive of an innovative solution
to a problem coming from the application of an existing technology. In other
cases, the alliance partners begin with a problem and together design an original solution that itself can give rise to future applications. Both alliances bring
value that goes beyond other forms of partnership with respect to innovation.
The latter, though, has the potential to generate more learning and reputation
than the former. When thinking of the continuum of partnerships discussed
above in relation to Canadian healthcare, all are valuable, but the strategic alliance has the most to offer.

As a summary of partnership structures, Table 7.4 sets out the considerations
for selecting the most appropriate form of partnership for the objectives to be
met.

Choosing the most appropriate form of partnership should be based on a
clear understanding of the risks and benefits to be derived. Contracting out for
services or supplies is a government-driven relationship that can result in cost
savings, capacity enhancement, expertise availability, and reduction of risk by
transferring it to a contractor. Alternatively, P3s enable government-led partnerships to provide opportunities of revenue generation or alternative financing
availability, resource capacity expansion, expertise availability for each of the
partners, and risk reduction or sharing. Further, the strategic alliance provides
virtually all of the benefits of a P3, but it adds something very important, namely the capacity of the partners to innovate—to explore new opportunities for research, and system or technology transformation—to learn and grow, and to develop an enhanced reputation for excellence that leads to further opportunities.

Table 7.4
Partnership Summary

Forms	Contracting Out	Public Private Partnerships	Strategic Alliances
Roles	Services: Maintenance, professional (accounting, audit, IT) Supplies: Hospital medical, technical, devices, equipment	Projects: Hospital, clinical, and other infrastructure design, build, finance, operate, maintain. Services: Pooling of resources to achieve shared objectives.	Strategic system change processes Research and development Strategic technology transformation: At either system or institutional levels: strategy, planning, management
Relationship	Government strategy, management Government funded	Government as policy and strategic lead Private sector responsible for management and execution of project Funding: government or private sector	Government and private sector as co-leads Private sector responsible for management and execution of venture Funding: government or private sector
Value Contributions	Cost saving Resource efficiency Expertise availability	Revenue generation/financing availability, risk reduction Cost saving Capacity expansion Expertise	Revenue generation, cost saving, risk transfer Capacity expansion Expertise Innovation Institutional learning Reputation enhancement
Risk to Democratic Accountability	Minimal: Government establishes contract details. Service and supply providers tender.	Medium: Governments are partners. Contracts often contain flexibility for private sector. Potential to extend outside government control.	High: Governments are equal partners in the venture. Dispute mechanism and exit arrangements are essential for both parties.
Control Feature	Legal contractual control	Partnership influence, legal remedies, cancellation of partnership	Bicameral collaborative governance

CONCLUSION

In the Canadian healthcare system, the public and private sectors have increasingly been coming together. The private sector is participating ever more broadly as the role of healthcare providers expands beyond hospitals and across the continuum of care. As well, the influence of business theory and practice is found throughout the governance and management of institutional delivery of care. This convergence of purpose and thinking presents valuable opportunities for partnerships and alliances.

Public private partnerships have the potential to contribute much to the development of infrastructure and other capacity in Canadian healthcare systems. But in pushing the boundaries of partnership structures, strategic alliances have the capability to bring in further resources and expertise to achieve certain public policy objectives. They represent a special type of partnership in which both the government and the private sector partners can have an alignment of strategic objectives and pursue their objectives more successfully by working together rather than apart.

A strategic alliance shares many of the features of a public private partnership, but the essential difference is in the coming together of strategic priorities between the government and the corporation. A public private partnership may be a very effective way of achieving an overall public policy goal, but this is often achieved despite the fact that the private sector party's goals are more commercial than public policy related. Strategic alliances are different than public private partnerships precisely because they represent an opportunity for business and government to come together in a joint undertaking where both have strategic objectives that do in fact align. It is this alignment that creates the exceptionally strong capability of the partners working together—both want substantially the same things because each has found a way to integrate its individual goals with those of the alliance.

Of course, strategic partners still have their differences. The private sector, after all, has profit-related goals that it cannot ignore. However, the bicameral governance structure provides a mechanism for drawing together both the public and private sector partners in a way that enables both to achieve common strategic objectives while ensuring they meet their obligations to their stakeholders. Through well structured and governed strategic alliances, the principles of social justice that underpin our public health system can not only be protected, but also the performance of our Canadian healthcare system could be significantly improved.

REFERENCES

Ansell, C., and A. Gish. 2008. "Collaborative Governance in Theory and Practice." *Journal of Public Administration and Research* 18: 543–71.

CAHO (Council of Academic Hospitals of Ontario). 2015. *2013–2014 Annual Report.* http://caho-hospitals.com/wp-content/uploads/2013/09/CAHO-Annual-Report-2013-2014-final2.pdf.

Canada Health Act. R.S.C. 1985, c. C-6. Ottawa: Government of Canada. http://laws-lois.justice.gc.ca/PDF/C-6.pdf.

Canadian Partnership Against Cancer. 2015, http://www.partnershipagainstcancer.ca/about/who-we-are/partnershipoverview/.

Carson, A. S. 2015a. "Why Canadians Need a System-Wide Healthcare Strategy." In *Toward a Healthcare Strategy for Canadians*, edited by A. S. Carson, J. Dixon, and K. R. Nossal, 11–37. Montreal and Kingston: McGill-Queen's University Press.

———. 2015b. "If Canada Had a Healthcare Strategy, What Form Could It Take?" In *Toward a Healthcare Strategy for Canadians*, edited by A. S. Carson, J. Dixon, and K. R. Nossal, 255–76. Montreal and Kingston: McGill-Queen's University Press.

Cheadle, Bruce. 2012. "Universal Health Care Much Loved among Canadians, Monarchy Less Important: Poll." *Globe and Mail*, November 25, http://www.theglobeandmail.com/news/national/universalhealth-care-much-loved-among-canadians-monarchy-less-importantpoll/article5640454/.

CIHI (Canadian Institute for Health Information). 2010. *Physiotherapists in Canada, 2009.* http://www.cptbc.org/pdf/CIHIReport.PTinCanada.2009.pdf.

———. 2014. National Health Expenditure Trends, 1975 to 2014 (National health indicator database). Ottawa: CIHI, http://www.cihi.ca/web/resource/en/nhex_2014_report_en.pdf.

Doz, Y. L., and G. Hamel. 1998. *Alliance Advantage: The Art of Creating Value through Partnering.* Boston: Harvard Business School Press.

Francis, R. 2010. *Independent Inquiry into Care Provided by Mid Staffordshire NHS Trust: January 2005–March 2009.* Vol. 1. UK: The Stationary Office.

General Electric Company (GE). 2011. "GE Healthcare and M+W Group Form Strategic Alliance in Vaccines, Insulin and Biopharmaceuticals." News release, 13 December, http://www3.gehealthcare.com/en/news_center/press_kits/ge_healthcare_and_mw_group_strategic_alliance.

Gomez-Casseres, B. 1996. *The Alliance Revolution: The New Shape of Business Rivalry.* Cambridge, MA: Harvard University Press.

Nanos, N. 2009. "Canadians Overwhelmingly Support Universal Healthcare; Think Obama is on Right Track in United States." *Policy Options* (November). http://policyoptions.irpp.org/issues/health-care/canadians-overwhelmingly-support-universal-health-care-think-obamais-on-right-track-in-united-states/.

National Association of Pharmacy Regulatory Authorities (NAPRA). 2015. National Statistics, http://napra.ca/pages/Practice_Resources/National_Statistics.aspx?id=2103.

OECD (Organisation for Economic Co-operation and Development). 2011. *Health at a Glance 2011: OECD Indicators.* Paris: OECD Publishing, http://dx.doi.org/10.1787/health_glance-2011-en.

———. 2013. *Health Care Quality Indicators.* (Health Policies and Data). Paris: OECD Publishing, http://www.oecd.org/els/health-systems/healthcarequalityindicators.htm.

Romanow, R. 2002. "Building on Values: The Future of Health Care in Canada—Final Report." Commission on the Future of Health Care in Canada. Ottawa: Government of Canada, http://www.sfu.ca/uploads/page/28/Romanow_Report.pdf.

Sher, G. D. 2015. "Canadian Blood Services as an Example of a Canadian Healthcare Strategy." In *Toward a Healthcare Strategy for Canadians*, edited by A. S. Carson, J. Dixon, and K. R. Nossal, 39–62. Montreal and Kingston: McGill-Queen's University Press.

World Bank, The. 2014. "Health Expenditure, Total (% of GDP)." http://data.worldbank.org/indicator/SH.XPD.TOTL.ZS.

Zajac, E. J., T. A. D'Aunno, and L. R. Burns. 2011. "Managing Strategic Alliances." In Shortell and Kaluzny's *Health Care Management: Organization Design and Behavior*, edited by L. R. Burns, E. H. Bradley, and B. J. Weiner, 321–46.

Chapter 8

HEALTHCARE PROFESSIONALS AS AGENTS OF CHANGE

CHRISTOPHER S. SIMPSON, KARIMA A. VELJI, LISA ASHLEY, AND OWEN ADAMS

Among the key agents of change in reshaping the national health policy agenda are healthcare professionals themselves, and in particular their national organizations, such as the Canadian Nurses Association (CNA) and the Canadian Medical Association (CMA). In this chapter, we examine the efforts of the CNA and the CMA to advocate for a national health policy agenda. We argue that these associations should have an important role in reshaping the health policy agenda. We demonstrate the importance of creating an environment for change that results from building networks and relationships, bringing credible evidence to the table, collapsing power differentials, and showcasing diversities. Approaches for healthcare professionals to move forward in mobilizing change on key healthcare issues are presented including creating collaborative visions and building shared agreements.

MODELLING CHANGE

The CMA and the CNA have long contributed to health policy capacity and advocacy in Canada since being established in 1867 and 1908 respectively, well before the federal Department of Health in 1919.

Advocacy for the health and well-being of Canadians was foundational to the reason why both associations were established and why we continue to exist today. Like most national health organizations, the CMA and CNA have a two-fold mission of representing both the interests of our members and the Canadian population. The CMA's vision includes being "the national voice for the highest standards for health and healthcare" (2015a), and the CNA's objects and goals include: "to advocate in the public interest for a publicly funded, not-for-profit health system" and "to shape and advocate for healthy public policy provincially/territorially, nationally and internationally" (2015). This capacity has become more important in the past few decades as the federal government has increasingly disengaged from the health policy arena, starting in the late 1970s when the original 50:50 cost-sharing for Medicare was replaced by the combination of tax points and per capita cash grants with the Established Programs Financing (EPF) Act of 1977.

The dynamics of federal/provincial/territorial relations on healthcare since the 1990s have provided challenges and opportunities both to us and to other health stakeholders. We have certainly learned the value of collaboration between our organizations and in working with others. While the CNA and CMA have had some common objectives since the beginning, bilateral collaboration did not start until 1991, when we became two of seven charter members of the Health Action Lobby (HEAL).[1]

HEAL was established following the 1991 federal budget, which provided that the health and social transfers would be frozen in per capita terms through 1994–95, after which they would grow at a rate of GNP growth minus three percentage points (Department of Finance Canada 1991). HEAL was concerned that the federal freeze in EPF transfers would have a destabilizing effect on Medicare. One of HEAL's first activities was to commission a report on the EPF program. The report demonstrated that the changes to EPF would result in $30 billion in healthcare funding reductions from 1986 to 1996, and that as a result of the growth in the value of the tax point transfer, the cash component was on track to disappear over the next decade (Thomson 1991). HEAL was concerned that this would eliminate the ability of the federal government to enforce the Canada Health Act (CHA). Early in its activities, HEAL established ten guiding principles (Table 8.1; 1991).

TABLE 8.1
HEAL's Guiding Principles for Health and Healthcare

1. Health goals (national and provincial)
2. Continuum of care
3. Shared responsibility for safeguarding Canada's health system
4. Consumer participation in healthcare decision making
5. Individual rights

---

[1] Seven charter members were Canadian Hospital Association, Canadian Long Term Care Association, Canadian Medical Association, Canadian Nurses Association, Canadian Psychological Association, Canadian Public Health Association, and Consumers Association of Canada.

6. Cooperation (interdisciplinary, inter-sector, intergovernmental)
7. Stability of funding
8. Efficient and effective management
9. Voluntarism
10. Professional self-regulation and licensure

In its early years, there was frequent interaction among HEAL members. This fostered trust in working together that has facilitated other collaborations. Another lesson from HEAL was the value in bringing credible evidence to the table. The initial report on EPF was followed by other commissioned expert reports. Today HEAL continues its activities and includes some 40 members.

One of the challenges of collaboration at a national level is trying to raise awareness and support among provincial/territorial constitutional associations and the grassroots membership. Indeed, just one year after HEAL was formed, a motion was put forward at the CMA General Council in 1992 that called for CMA to disassociate itself from HEAL. The motion was defeated. At one point there was discussion of creating HEAL organizations at the provincial level. An attempt by Manitoba to create such an organization was short-lived and was not pursued in other jurisdictions.

The stage for continued collaboration between CNA and CMA was set with the 1995 federal budget, which announced the consolidation of health and social transfers in the Canada Health and Social Transfer (CHST). The CHST was set to take effect on 1 April 1996, at which time the federal government reduced the cash transfer by $6 billion over two years. This was on the heels of restraint from the recession of the early 1990s that saw a small decline in real per capita public spending on healthcare from 1993 to 1996. As a result, the issue of long wait times for tests and procedures began to rise steadily as a concern among both the public and providers.

In 2004 CNA-CMA released a joint discussion paper, "The Taming of the Queue: Toward a Cure for Health Care Wait Times," (CNA-CMA 2004) based on roundtable deliberations informed by CMA's commissioned international research among key stakeholders in Australia, New Zealand, and Europe. The CNA-CMA paper set out a 10-point plan for the measurement and management of wait times (Table 8.2).

TABLE 8.2
10-Point Action Plan for Managing Wait Times

1. Set priorities through broad consultation
2. Address patient/public expectations through transparent communications
3. Address immediate gaps in health human resources and system capacity
4. Improve data collection through investments in information systems
5. Develop wait-time benchmarks through clinical and public consensus
6. Strengthen accountability by way of public reporting
7. Maximize efficiencies by aligning incentives properly
8. Address upstream and downstream pressures by investing in the continuum of care
9. Expand inter-jurisdictional care options by enhancing portability provisions
10. Commit to adoption of best practices

The discussion paper was followed by a telephone survey of both physicians and nurses in 2004. The results showed that physicians and nurses were very much on the same page in terms of experiences with wait times and the impact on patients. Access to family physicians topped both of their lists of access problems. Both groups shared the same view on declining access for services of specialists, nursing care in hospitals, emergency room services, and surgery. Large majorities of each group agreed that Canada needs a national system that measures waiting times for health services and diagnosis (Ipsos Reid 2004).

The "Taming of the Queue" discussion paper and poll results were released on the eve of the First Ministers' conference that was convened by Prime Minister Paul Martin on 13–16 September 2004. The CMA and CNA, along with senior representatives of the Canadian Healthcare Association and the Canadian Pharmacists Association, were present at the meetings. The premiers had the discussion paper—during the meetings, Newfoundland and Labrador premier Danny Williams waved it in the air to make a point—and it was clear that the combined advocacy effort of the premiers and the stakeholders had an effect on the federal government's position. Going into the meeting, the federal government circulated a proposal with an offer of $24.9 billion in additional health funding over a 10-year period (Canada 2004); by the end of the meeting, however, the federal government had increased its commitment to $41.3 billion, including a $5.5 billion Wait Times Reduction Fund (Canadian Intergovernmental Conference Secretariat 2004).

Another key commitment of the 2004 Health Accord was an agreement by governments to increase the supply of health professionals, and to make their action plans public by 31 December 2005. This commitment inspired a new collaboration between the CMA and CNA to develop a set of core principles and strategic directions for a pan-Canadian health human resources plan, something that, separately, we had both advocated for a long time. The resulting green paper contained 10 core principles, each of which had strategic directions identified (Table 8.3). The report (CNA-CMA 2005) was released jointly by the CMA and CNA at a special session at the CMA General Council in August 2005.

Table 8.3
Core Principles for a Pan-Canadian Health Human Resources Plan

1. Needs-based planning
2. Collaboration among disciplines
3. The health workforce is a national resource
4. Greater self-sufficiency
5. Recognize the global environment
6. Inclusive policy planning and decision-making processes
7. Competitive human resource policies
8. Healthy workplaces
9. Balance between personal and professional life
10. Lifelong learning

This was followed soon after by the release in September of A Framework for Collaborative Pan-Canadian Health Human Resource Planning by the Federal/Provincial/Territorial Advisory Committee on Health Delivery and Human Resources, and there is significant commonality between the two reports (ACH-DHR 2007).

FEDERAL GOVERNMENT LEADERSHIP

In our view, policy analysts have been too quick to discount the leadership role of the federal government in promoting health reform in a pan-Canadian context. The $800 million Primary Health Care Transition Fund (PHCTF), for example, was a federal government commitment under the First Ministers' 2000 Health Accord that resulted in a series of national and provincial/territorial projects that were directed at five common objectives to promote and enhance the delivery of multidisciplinary primary care (Health Canada 2007). The CMA and CNA collaborated with eight other health professional organizations on an initiative funded under the PHCTF to develop a set of principles and a framework to enhance interdisciplinary collaboration in primary healthcare (EICP). In the course of this project all collaborating organizations reached out to engage both our grassroots members and our leadership. During one large leadership gathering, it became evident that one of the barriers to effective collaboration was a lack of awareness about the role and function of the different providers. This initiative resulted in six principles and seven framework elements (Table 8.4; EICP 2006a).

TABLE 8.4
Enhancing Interdisciplinary Collaboration in Primary Health Care: Framework and Principles

Framework Elements	Principles
Patient/client engagement	Health human resources
Population health approach	Funding
Best possible care and services	Liability
Access	Regulation
Trust and respect	Information/communications technology
Effective communication	Management and leadership
	Planning and evaluation

During the course of this project, one positive development was the release of a joint statement, in 2005, by the Canadian Medical Protective Association and the Canadian Nurses Protective Society, on liability for nurse practitioners and physicians in collaborative practice (2013). This statement identified the liability risks in collaborative practice and set out seven stops to decrease those risks.

At the conclusion of the project, the EICP principles and framework were endorsed by all participating organizations. While it is difficult to judge the direct impact that the project has had on the ground, there is little doubt that it influenced other stakeholders at the national and provincial/territorial levels. Indeed, 39 organizations, including professional associations, regulatory bodies, and health regions, signed on as supporters of the final document (EICP 2006b). Importantly, the intense and continuous collaboration over its course has also continued to foster trust among the participating organizations that paved the way for further joint efforts.

In addition to collaborative endeavours, both our organizations have undertaken major efforts to outline a path forward for transformational change in healthcare. While we have carried these out independently, they are highly congruent in embracing the Institute for Healthcare Improvement's (IHI) Triple Aim approach (2015). In developing the Triple Aim, IHI has taken the approach that optimal health system performance can only be achieved through the simultaneous pursuit of three dimensions:

- improving the experience of care (including quality and satisfaction);
- improving the health of populations; and
- reducing the per capita cost of care.

CMA—HEALTHCARE TRANSFORMATION

In 2008, the CMA General Council adopted a resolution calling for the development of "a blueprint and timeline for transformational change in Canadian health care to bring about patient-focused care." The first phase of the Health Care Transformation (HCT) initiative was an international study tour: CMA President Dr. Robert Ouellet and two staff members interviewed 75 people from 36 organizations and groups in five European countries that were selected on the basis of having introduced significant change in their health systems (Canadian Medical Association 2009a). The focus of the interviews was on both the "what" and the "how" of transformational change, and was modelled loosely on John Kotter's eight-stage process of change, beginning with establishing a sense of urgency through to institutionalizing new approaches (Kotter 1996).

The findings of this study served as the foundation for a discussion paper that was examined at the 2009 General Council, and then refined into a policy document in 2010 (Canadian Medical Association 2009b; 2010). The policy document set out a framework for transformation that is based on five pillars:

- building a culture of patient-centred care;
- providing incentives to enhance access and improve quality of care;
- enhancing patient access along the continuum of care;
- helping providers help patients; and
- building accountability and responsibilities at all levels.

This was followed in early 2011 by a series of six public town hall meetings held across Canada, conducted in partnership with *Maclean's* magazine, in which members of the public were engaged on issues of value in healthcare, the responsibility that patients and their families have for their health, and the expansion of the CHA (Canadian Medical Association 2011). Further external engagements have included the striking of an expert Advisory Panel on Resourcing Options for Sustainable Health Care in Canada in 2011 and a second cross-national series of town hall meetings on social determinants of health in 2013.

CNA NATIONAL EXPERT COMMISSION

In 2011, the CNA established an independent National Expert Commission (NEC), comprising 10 leaders from the fields of nursing, medicine, law, academia, economics, and healthcare policy. The NEC was organized around the Triple Aim framework and it carried out extensive stakeholder and public consultation, including:

- 19 public roundtables carried out in partnership with YMCA Canada;
- stakeholder meetings;
- public polling;
- a call for submissions that resulted in almost 50 individual submissions from nurses, the public, and other health professionals, and eight organizational submissions; and
- three commissioned research syntheses on each of the Triple Aim elements of better care, better health, and better value (National Expert Commission 2015).

The NEC's final report (National Expert Commission 2012) was published in June 2012, and it contained a nine-point action plan (Table 8.5).

TABLE 8.5
National Expert Commission: Nine-Point Action Plan

1. Challenge all Canadians to rank in top five nations for five key health outcomes by 2017
2. Set pan-Canadian goals through local solutions
3. Implement primary care for all by 2017
4. Invest in social determinants of health
5. Identify the health and healthcare needs of vulnerable and marginalized people
6. Governments should integrate health in all policies
7. Use best evidence to promote safety and quality
8. Train providers to match system transformation
9. Use technology to its fullest

Following the release of the report, the CNA engaged Drs. Adalsteinn Brown and Terrence Sullivan to conduct an interactive, evidence-based process to select the top five indicators (2013). The final five indicators are shown in Table 8.6.

Table 8.6
CNA Top 5 in 5 Indicators for 2017

1. Increase the percentage of primary care practices offering after-hours care
2. Increase chronic disease case management and navigational capacity in primary care
3. Increase Canadians' access to electronic health information and services
4. Decrease hospital admissions for uncontrolled diabetes-related conditions
5. Decrease the prevalence of childhood obesity

Through our respective transformation initiatives the CMA and CNA have come to fully embrace the Triple Aim framework and its three elements, which we have termed better care, better health, and better value. In 2011, we developed guiding principles for healthcare transformation that build on the foundational principles of the Canada Health Act (CMA-CNA 2011). These consist of six principles that are organized under the Triple Aim framework (Table 8.7).

Table 8.7
CMA-CNA Guiding Principles for Healthcare Transformation

Better Care
• Patient-centred care that is seamless along the continuum of care
• Quality services appropriate for patient needs

Better Health
• Health promotion and illness prevention
• Equitable access to care and multi-sectoral policies to address the social determinants of health

Better Value
• Sustainability based on universal access to quality health services
• Accountability by stakeholders—the public/patients/families, providers and funders—for ensuring the system is effective

Upon the release of the principles in July 2011, we began to solicit endorsements from national and provincial/territorial organizations starting with our own bodies. They have since been endorsed by all of the provincial/territorial medical and nursing organizations, and in total by more than 130 organizations.

The healthcare transformation initiatives of the CNA and CMA, as well as those of other organizations, were motivated in significant measure by the anticipated negotiations around the renegotiation of the 2004 First Ministers' Health Accord that was set to expire in March 2014. Based on the precedents of the 2000, 2003, and 2004 Accords, there was every reason to believe that this would be the case.

However, it was not to be. At a meeting of federal/provincial/territorial (FPT) finance ministers on 19 December 2011, finance minister James Flaherty made the announcement that the 6 percent escalator in the CHT would be extended through 2016–17, and thereafter lowered to 3 percent or the rate of nominal GDP growth through 2023–24, and would be reviewed in 2024 (Department of Finance Canada 2011).

At their January 2012 meeting, the premiers announced the formation of the Health Care Innovation Working Group (HCIWG) that would consult with healthcare providers in carrying out this work. The CNA, CMA, and Health Action Lobby were invited to participate in working groups to address the following:

- Scope of practice (team-based models): examining the scope of practice of healthcare providers and teams in order to better meet patient and population needs in a safe, competent and cost effective manner.
- Human resources management: address health human resource challenges and explore more coordinated management to address competition across health systems.
- Clinical practice guidelines: accelerating the development and adoption of best clinical and surgical practice guidelines so that all Canadians benefit from up-to-date practices (Council of the Federation 2012).

Prior to getting involved with the HCIWG, in early 2012, the Canadian Nurses Association invited the CMA to co-host a Health Stakeholder Summit (CNA-CMA 2012) focused on primary health care (PHC) to provide Health Canada with recommendations for future policy directions, by identifying and prioritizing key opportunities and mechanisms to support the integration and implementation of PHC across Canada. With funding support from Health Canada, the Summit was designed as a facilitated policy dialogue that

- explored fresh perspectives, promising practices, and key enablers to advancing PHC;
- identified policies and mechanisms to increase access to quality PHC for Canadians; and
- identified how PHC can be fully integrated into the Canadian healthcare system.

The Summit was attended by 30 participants from six jurisdictions, and a wide variety of professional backgrounds was represented, including a patient representative. The participants identified the barriers to advancing primary healthcare and reached consensus on seven strategies to move forward, including a call to support the development of innovative integrated delivery models for PHC through interprofessional teams designed to meet the needs of the patient populations served. The Summit built on previous collaborations of the CMA and CNA and other health organizations, and we were well positioned to contribute to the HCIWG's team-based models initiative.

The team-based models working group adopted principles and criteria developed by CNA and CMA built on the Triple Aim to identify models that promote optimal collaborative and inter-professional care. The principles are shown in Table 8.8 (Health Care Innovation Working Group 2012b).

TABLE 8.8
Principles for Selection of Team-Based Models of Care

1. Patient-centred
2. Enhances the integration of care
3. Increases equitable access to care
4. Evidence-informed
5. Supports health promotion and illness prevention
6. Sustainable
7. Incorporates innovations
8. Optimizes skills and scope of practice

Similarly, the CMA and CNA had experience in the area of CPGs to contribute. As part of the development of the HCIWG CPG initiative, our organizations developed a paper to guide the selection of the initial topics (CMA, CNA 2012).

The HCIWG's first report was tabled at the premiers' summer meeting in Halifax. It contained 12 recommendations. In the area of CPGs, it was recommended that ministers work with clinical communities to adopt the C-Change Guidelines for Heart Disease and the Registered Nurses' Association of Ontario Guidelines for the Assessment and Management of Foot Ulcers for People with Diabetes. In the area of team-based models, eight models were identified to address needs in the following areas:

- access to primary care;
- access to emergency services in rural communities; and
- access to enhanced home care (Health Care Innovation Working Group 2012a).

One year later, the HCIWG reported that success was being achieved in lowering the price for both generic and brand name drugs. The premiers asked the HCIWG group to look at appropriateness of care and seniors' care, and directed the team-based models working group to identify opportunities to increase the role that paramedics and pharmacists play in the delivery of front line services.

One of the challenges of the HCIWG is that it has not been provided with the resources to put a secretariat in place, although at their September 2014 meeting the provincial and territorial health ministers announced that Ontario would establish an office for the Pan-Canadian Pharmaceutical Alliance (Canadian Intergovernmental Conference Secretariat 2014). The senior government officials and the CNA/CMA/HEAL staff who have contributed have been doing so with limited financial and human resources.

On 18 February 2015, a summit was convened to review 10 models that featured the roles of pharmacists and paramedics. This meeting finalized the HCIWG's work on team-based models. The focus of this phase was on collaborative models in which pharmacists and paramedics play enhanced roles in the provision of team-based front line services. A task force that consisted of representatives from FPT governments and health provider groups selected examples. Local professionals presented 10 innovative models with an emphasis on the needs identified by the team, the tools and resources developed, and barriers, enablers, and impact of the model on patients and providers. There was also discussion around the nature of innovation, which is based on local population health needs, emphasizing the importance of creating conditions to support change. Research and evaluation of models should seek to find those that are best for the patient, cost effective, and that support quality of care. The outcomes of this meeting will be part of a final report on the work on team-based models that will be submitted to deputy ministers, ministers, and premiers for further consideration.

At their summer 2014 meeting, the premiers announced the formation of a task force for the purpose of launching a dialogue with Canadians and stakeholders on the issue of population aging, and to examine the impact of the aging population on Canada's social and economic future (Council of the Federation 2014). The issue of seniors and their health and healthcare is of longstanding interest to both the CMA and CNA. It is not clear when or how the task force is proceeding and no update was released at the premiers' 2015 summer meeting. Immediately prior to the premiers' meeting on 30 January 2015, we wrote to the co-chairs to urge them to place the future mandate of the working group on seniors' care on the agenda. We were pleased to see that this was discussed, and in their communiqué the premiers called on the federal government to provide funding in support of services that enhance the well-being of Canada's seniors (Council of the Federation 2015). At the conclusion of their July 2015 meeting, the premiers wrote to each of the five federal party leaders challenging them to address the needs of the aging population, including increasing the level of the Canada Health Transfer to at least 25 percent of provincial/territorial health spending (Council of the Federation 2015b).

CNA/CMA/HEAL SUMMITS ON INTEGRATED CARE

Starting in 2012, the CNA and the CMA, in partnership with HEAL, initiated a summit process that brought provider groups, governments, and patients together to introduce and define new and existing evidence to support the transition to a fully and functionally integrated person- and family-centred health system that offers the right provider, at the right time, for the right care. A central dimension to this shift called for the enhancement of access along the full continuum of care and a strong focus on not only ensuring smooth transitions as people navigate their journey through the system, but also on addressing social and environmental determinants of health. It was clear that governments alone would not be successful in achieving the necessary change, but that physicians, nurses, pharmacists, and other health providers must also provide leadership.

Within a rapidly changing context, and with the imperative of bringing expert advice to guide health system transformation in Canada, the CNA and the CMA conducted a three-phase summit process in 2012–2013, which was grounded in two sources: The Principles to Guide Health Care Transformation in Canada, and the Triple Aim framework. This was an important opportunity for health providers to explore the core elements and design of a functionally integrated health system that enhances access across the full continuum of care.

The purpose of the first phase of the summit process involved a national workshop focused on mapping out the continuum of care using a chronic disease prevention and management framework in three high impact areas, to be selected from hypertension, cardiovascular disease, stroke, diabetes, colorectal cancer, and chronic obstructive pulmonary disease. After identifying the characteristics of an ideal continuum, workshop participants created seven functionally integrated continuums of care that resulted in visual concepts of what an ideal continuum might look like. The Phase II national workshop built upon Phase I from the perspective of individuals' needs. It further considered seamless healthcare pathways (along and within the continuum of care) that account for the factors that determine and maintain health and have an impact on how well we deliver the right care, to the right person, at the right time, and in the right place (CNA-CMA 2013).

As a result of the summit workshops, it became clear that a strong foundation in primary health care principles, as well as collaboration and communication within and between different health professionals, was essential for achieving functionally integrated care. The third phase of the summit involved the dissemination of survey results from the HEAL membership and patients about patient and provider expectations. The expectations for the five foundations of integrated care that had been identified were confirmed by summit participants: (1) patient access; (2) patient-centred care; (3) informational continuity of care; (4) management of continuity of care; and (5) relational continuity of care. Expectations for each of the five foundations were created using five scenarios: aboriginals with diabetes, adults with COPD, children with obesity, seniors with dementia, and youth with mental health concerns (Vogel and Ashley 2014). When the expectations that follow are in place to support these five foundations of integrated care, the result will be better health, better care, and better value for Canadians.

After wide stakeholder consultation, HEAL (2014) released a consensus statement in December 2014 that called on all levels of government, and the federal government in particular, to commit to a renewed and sustained working relationship to improve Canada's health system. The document proposes the following vision statement for the federal government in health and healthcare: "To advance the health and health care of Canadians, working collaboratively with the provinces and territories, health care providers and the public to ensure the promotion and delivery of appropriate, integrated, cost-effective and accessible health services and supports."

It calls for a framework for performance improvement and innovation modelled on the Triple Aim and underscores the need to promote fiscal fairness with respect to the CHT in light of the changes since 2011. The statement identifies three areas where there is a significant leadership opportunity for the federal government, including the aging population, prescription drugs, and fostering innovation. It recommends a National Health Innovation Fund that focuses on three priority areas:

- Primary healthcare
- Mental health and addictions
- A national health human resources organization to promote coordinated planning efforts across disciplines and jurisdictions

SEVEN SUCCESS FACTORS TO MOBILIZE CHANGE

Building capacity among healthcare professionals to mobilize change on key issues often means stepping outside of one's comfort zone, collapsing power differentials, and addressing common concerns while often having competing interests. It is about working with others to create an emotional connection to an issue and tell a story (Bevan and Fairman 2014).

First, it is essential to build upon evidence-based opportunities and strategic challenges in a manner that convey the imperative for change. A common concern of many healthcare professionals is the belief that current Canadian healthcare systems are not sustainable. Canada does not have a high-performing health system, currently ranked 10th out of 11 countries on the Commonwealth Fund's most recent international study (Commonwealth Fund 2014). A second concern is the patchwork quilt across the country of access to home and community care and prescription drugs.

Second, it is critical to build networks and relationships of trust through frequent and ongoing communication to build shared agreement on the burning-issue platform. While the CMA and the CNA have been fairly successful among providers and patient organizations, there is room for improvement in creating a synergistic environment for change. The CNA, the CMA and other national healthcare, home care and seniors organizations recognize that achieving better health, better care and better value for all Canadians requires the engagement of all stakeholders: governments, health providers, organizations, the private sector, and Canadians. We share concerns about the sustainability of health expenditures and recognize that improving system performance should reduce the growth rate of expenditures.

Third, greater focus is needed to address common concerns. The numerous provincial and federal reports of the past two decades have most typically put forward numerous recommendations that cover the waterfront of health system reform; but little change has resulted. A shared focus with clear system and health targets would systematically transform Canada's health system to achieve improved health outcomes.

Fourth, patience and perseverance are crucial. The experience of making sustainable change is in recognizing and acknowledging diversities. The examples in this chapter took place over years. It is not easy to sustain interest and momentum within and among stakeholders—if you can define and agree on what success will look like upfront, and chart some quick wins, that will help. For example, our concerted effort on wait times and access began in early 2004; we have made progress but the problem has by no means been solved.

Fifth, creating collaborative visions is essential. The CNA and the CMA, together with other healthcare organizations, have agreed upon and adopted a principle-based approach to any of our collaborations. That greatly facilitates the continuous process of monitoring and challenging ourselves along the way.

Sixth, all stakeholders have to assume responsibility and accountability for their role in bringing about change. Most of the levers for change lie within the provider community and we need to acknowledge that. It is about not laying blame, but by creating an emotional connection through storytelling.

Finally, and most important, change needs to occur by putting the patient at the centre. This involves healthcare professionals stepping aside and collapsing power differentials. Citizen participation must inform decisions related to the development, funding and delivery of healthcare in Canada. Collaborative strategies should emphasize the principles of social justice and health equity, and realize the significant role of the social and environmental determinants in shaping health at the individual, community, and population levels.

MOVING FORWARD

The CMA and the CNA have invested considerable resources in complementary initiatives to advance the health of Canadians and the transformation of healthcare on the national policy agenda. As we move forward, our advocacy efforts are also taking a "health in all policies" approach—to ensure that all levels of government understand the consequences of their decisions on the health of Canadians. Broad sectors of public policy and legislation such as education, transportation, environment, communication, natural resources, income security and foreign trade are being developed with little or no consideration for their implication on population health.

This is being exemplified through our work on advancing care for seniors 65+ who represent one in six (15 percent) of Canadians and account for fully just under half (47 percent) of provincial/territorial government health spending. By 2036, these figures are projected to increase to one in four (25 percent) and just under two-thirds (62 percent; assuming that the 2012 age-sex pattern of per capita health spending remains unchanged). While most provinces have initiated some form of seniors' strategy, there is wide variability among them and there has been no concerted national policy discussion about the prospects of seniors beyond retirement income security.

For its part, the CNA is focusing on issues of healthy aging, improved access to community-based care, and support for family caregivers. This call is strongly supported by the results of a national Nanos poll of the public:

- 93 percent agreed on the importance of having the ability to age at home with access to home care;
- 89 percent supported improving financial support to family caregivers; and
- 90 percent supported an enhanced role for nurses in providing home care to seniors and helping them navigate the health system (Nanos Research 2014a).

The CMA is focusing on the need for a national seniors' strategy also strongly supported by a Nanos poll that was conducted in ridings that were won by 3 percent or less in the 2011 election:

- 86 percent of those polled agreed that federal parties should make seniors' care a top priority in their political platform for the next election; and
- 87 percent supported the position of Canada's doctors and nurses in calling for a pan-Canadian strategy on seniors' care (Nanos Research 2014b).

As the CNA and the CMA move forward on this policy agenda, the focus will be on building capacity among our members across the country to advocate for seniors care and healthy aging. Tools have been created by both associations that assist members to develop skills, to get informed, and to get politically active. The CMA and CNA will continue to call on all levels of government to address seniors' issues through broad stakeholder consultations. The approach we have taken reflect our key learning that effective advocacy must engage the full range of stakeholders, including patients, clients, the public, providers, and payers at the front-end of any initiatives and innovations.

CONCLUSION

Over the past two decades, the CMA and the CNA and other national healthcare organizations have come to subscribe to the African proverb, "if you want to go fast, go alone; if you want to go far, go together." Aside from the collaborations discussed above, we trade notes in advance of every opportunity to advocate to the federal government, including federal elections, pre-budget consultations, and presentations to various parliamentary committees. We believe that this on-going collaboration enhances both our collective and individual effectiveness.

Assessing our activities since 1991, we believe that the CMA and the CNA have had a positive influence in maintaining the engagement of the federal government in the healthcare system and preserving the publicly funded character of the Medicare program. However, the job is far from complete. Wait times for non-emergency services remain too long, and access to health services beyond those provided by doctors and in hospitals remains unaffordable to many Canadians, and can also depend on where they live. While we and other health organizations and governments subscribe to patient and family-centred care, the reality falls short. Consider the following list of indicators set out by Leatt, Pink, and Guerriere in 2000, by which patients will be able to tell when an integrated health system exists (Table 8.9).

TABLE 8.9
How Patients Will Know When an Integrated Healthcare System Exists

It exists when they
- do not have to repeat their health history for each provider they encounter;
- do not have to undergo the same test multiple times for different providers;
- are not the medium for informing their physician that they have been hospitalized or treated by another provider;

- do not have to wait at one level of care because of incapacity at another level of care;
- have 24-hour access to a primary care provider;
- have easy-to-understand information about quality of care and outcomes in order to make informed choices about providers and treatments;
- can make an appointment for a visit to a clinician, a diagnostic test, or a treatment with one phone call;
- have a wide choice of primary care providers who are able to give them the time they need; and
- with chronic disease, are routinely contacted to have tests to identify problems before they occur, and are provided with education and support to maximize their autonomy.

Source: Adapted from Leatt, Pink, and Guerriere, 2000

We venture that very few, if any, Canadians would be able to check off all nine indicators. This speculation is certainly borne out in the recent findings of the Commonwealth Fund's 2014 International Survey of Older Adults, on which Canada ranks poorly among the 11 countries surveyed (Osborn et al. 2014). If we are going to move the yardsticks on indicators such as these, we are going to have to build on the good work we have done on public and member engagement, and continue to build capacity among healthcare professionals as change agents. We must redouble our outreach efforts to our members to provide them with tools and information to enable them to engage in health system transformation.

REFERENCES

ACHDHR (Advisory Committee on Health Delivery and Human Resources). 2007. *Framework for Collaborative Pan-Canadian Health Human Resources Planning*. Revised edition. Ottawa: Federal/Provincial/Territorial Advisory Committee on Health Delivery and Health Human Resources.

Bevan H., and S. Fairman. 2014. *The new era of thinking and practice in change and transformation: A call to action for leaders of health and care.* NHS Improving Quality. http://media.nhsiq.nhs.uk/whitepaper/index.html

Brown A. D., and T. Sullivan. 2013. *Canada's Top 5 in 5: Building National Consensus on Priority Health-Improvement Indicators.* Ottawa: Canadian Nurses Association. http://www.cna-aiic.ca/~/media/cna/files/en/nec_top5_final_report_e.pdf?la=en

Canada. 2004. *Improved Access and Reduced Wait Times: A Summary of The Federal Proposal.* Ottawa. September.

Canadian Intergovernmental Conference Secretariat. 2004. *A 10-Year Plan to Strengthen Health Care.* Accessed 20 April 2015. http://www.scics.gc.ca/CMFiles/800042005_e1JXB-342011-6611.pdf

———. 2014. "Provinces and Territories Talk Health Care." Press release, 30 September. http://www.scics.gc.ca/english/conferences.asp?a=viewdocument&id=2217

Canadian Medical Association (CMA). 2009a. *Appendix 2. What We Heard: A Review of Five European Health Systems. A background report for CMA's transformational change project.* April. http://www.facturation.net/multimedia/CMA/Content_Images/Inside_cma/Advocacy/HCT/Appendix-2-WhatWeHeard_en.pdf

————. 2009b. "Toward a Blueprint for Health Care Transformation." Discussion paper prepared for the 143rd meeting of the Canadian Medical Association General Council. August. http://resident.cma.ca/multimedia/CMA/Content_Images/Inside_cma/Advocacy/HCT/Blueprint-HCT_en.pdf

————. 2010. *Health Care Transformation in Canada. Change That Works. Care That Lasts.* http://policybase.cma.ca/dbtw-wpd/PolicyPDF/PD10-05.PDF

————. 2011. *Voices Into Action: Report on the National Dialogue on Health Care Transformation.* https://www.cma.ca/Assets/assets-library/document/en/advocacy/HCT_townhalls-e.pdf

————. 2015a. "History, Mission, Vision and Values." https://www.cma.ca/En/Pages/history-mission-vision.aspx

Canadian Medical Association–Canadian Nurses Association (CMA-CNA). 2011. *Principles to Guide Health Care Transformation in Canada.* https://www.cma.ca/Assets/assets-library/document/en/advocacy/2593%20Principles%20to%20Guide%20HCT-e.pdf

————. 2012. "Selecting Initial Topics for Share Clinical Practice Guidelines. Advice in Response to a Request from the Health Care Innovation Working Group." February.

Canadian Medical Protective Association and Canadian Nurses Protective Society. [2005] 2013. "CMPA/CNPS Joint Statement On Liability Protection For Nurse Practitioners And Physicians In Collaborative Practice." http://www.cnps.ca/upload-files/pdf_english/CMPA_CNPS_Joint_Statement_Nov_2013.pdf

Canadian Nurses Association (CNA). 2015. "About CNA." http://www.cna-aiic.ca/en/aboutcna

Canadian Nurses Association (CNA), Canadian Medical Association (CMA). 2004. *The Taming of the Queue: Toward a Cure for Health Care Wait Times.* Ottawa.

————. 2005. *Toward a Pan-Canadian Planning Framework for Health Human Resources: A Green Paper.* Ottawa.

————. 2012. *Primary Health Care Summit Summary Report.* http://www.cna-aiic.ca/~/media/cna/page-content/pdf-en/primary_health_care_report_e.pdf

————. 2013. *Integration: A New Direction for Canadian Health Care. A Report on the Health Provider Summit Process.* November. http://www.cna-aiic.ca/~/media/cna/files/en/cna_cma_heal_provider_summit_transformation_to_integrated_care_e.pdf?la=en

Commonwealth Fund. 2014. *Mirror, Mirror on the Wall, 2014 Update: How the U.S. Health Care System Compares Internationally.* http://www.commonwealthfund.org/publications/fund-reports/2014/jun/mirror-mirror

Council of the Federation. 2012. "Premiers Announce Health Care Innovation Working Group." http://canadaspremiers.ca/phocadownload/news-
room-2012/communique_task%20force_jan_17.pdf
———. 2014. "Premiers' Task Force to Support Chair's Initiative on Aging."
28 August. http://canadaspremiers.ca/phocadownload/newsroom_2014/
news_release_aging_aug28-final.pdf
———. 2015a. "Canada's Premiers Collaborate on the Economy and Call
for a Better Partnership with the Federal Government." 30 January. http://
canadaspremiers.ca/phocadownload/newsroom-2015/communique-
jan_30_2015.pdf
_____. 2015b. "Canada's Premiers engage federal party leaders." http://
www.canadaspremiers.ca/phocadownload/newsroom-2015/election_let-
ters_communique-final2.pdf
Department of Finance Canada. 1991. *The Budget 1991*. Ottawa: Department
of Finance Canada. http://www.budget.gc.ca/pdfarch/1991-plan-eng.pdf
_____. 2011. "Backgrounder on Major Transfer Renewal." Archived. Otta-
wa. Modified 19 December 2011. http://www.fin.gc.ca/n11/data/11-141_1-
eng.asp
EICP (Enhancing Interdisciplinary Collaboration in Primary Health Care).
2006a. *The Principles and Framework for Interdisciplinary Collaboration
in Primary Health Care*. March. http://www.eicp.ca/en/principles/march/
eicp-principles-and-framework-march.pdf
———. 2006b. "List of Supporters." http://www.eicp.ca/en/principles/list.asp
Health Action Lobby (HEAL). 1991. *Medicare: A Value Worth Keeping*. http://
www.healthactionlobby.ca/images/stories/publications/1991/MedicareVal-
ueWorthKeeping.pdf
———. 2014. *The Canadian Way: Accelerating Innovation and Improving
Health System Performance. A Consensus Statement by the Health Action Lobby*. December. http://healthactionlobby.ca/images/stories/publica-
tions/2014/HEAL_TheCanadianWay_EN_NoEmbargo.pdf
Health Canada. 2007. *Primary Health Care Transition Fund*. http://www.hc-sc.
gc.ca/hcs-sss/prim/phctf-fassp/index-eng.php
Health Care Innovation Working Group. 2012a *From Innovation to Action:
The First Report of the Health Care Innovation Working Group*. http://cana-
daspremiers.ca/phocadownload/publications/health_innovation_report-e-
web.pdf
———. 2012b. "Scope of Practice Models. Principles and Criteria for Selec-
tion of Models."
Institute for Healthcare Improvement (IHI). 2015. "IHI Triple Aim Initiative."
http://www.ihi.org/Engage/Initiatives/TripleAim/pages/default.aspx
Ipsos Reid. 2004. "Health Care Professionals Views on Access to Health Care."
Research report submitted to Canadian Medical Association and Canadian
Nurses Association.
Kotter J. 1996. *Leading change*. Boston: Harvard Business Review Press.
Leatt P., G. H. Pink, and M. Guerriere. 2000. "Towards a Canadian Model of

Integrated Healthcare." *Healthcare Papers* 1(2): 13–35.

Nanos Research. 2014a. "CNA Hill Day Project Summary." November. http://www.cna-aiic.ca/~/media/cna/page-content/pdf-en/nanos-research-report-for-cna-hill-day-2014_e.pdf?la=en

———. 2014b. "Project Summary—Canadian Medical Association." April. http://www.nanosresearch.com/library/polls/POLNAT-W14-T601.pdf

National Expert Commission. 2012. *A Nursing Call to Action: The Health of Our Nation, the Future of Our Health System.* http://www.cna-aiic.ca/~/media/cna/files/en/nec_report_e.pdf?la=en

———. 2015. "How the Commission Proceeded With its Work." http://www.cna-aiic.ca/~/media/cna/files/en/how_the_commission_proceeded_e.pdf?la=en

Osborn R., D. Moulds, D. Squires, M. Doty, and C. Anderson. 2014. "International Survey of Older Adults Finds Shortcomings in Access, Coordination and Patient-Centred Care." *Health Affairs* 33(12): 2247–55.

Thomson A. 1991. *Federal Support for Health Care: A Background Paper.* Health Action Lobby. http://healthactionlobby.ca/images/stories/publications/1991/FedSupportHealthCare.pdf

Vogel M. and L. Ashley. 2014. "Integration: A New Direction for Canadian Health Care." Presentation to the Health Action Lobby, June.

Part 3

MOVING HEALTHCARE REFORM FORWARD

Chapter 9

CLEARING THE WAY: BEYOND THE ROADBLOCKS TO HEALTHCARE REFORM

NEALE SMITH AND HARVEY LAZAR

This chapter focuses on factors and conditions that have the potential to facilitate or block pan-Canadian healthcare reform. It draws from the lessons of the past about the nature and extent of health-care policy reform, and speculates as to how these factors may play out over the coming years, and what this implies for strategic efforts to advance system change. It is mainly focused on the future prospects for enhancements to universal publicly funded healthcare and the instruments in the federal government and federal-provincial toolkits that are germane to that purpose.

Development of the current healthcare system has involved federal, provincial, and intergovernmental actions. These, we argue, occurred in two distinct periods: a period of innovation up to 1984, when the basic configuration was debated and ultimately established, and a period of consolidation after 1984, when consensus on the features of Canadian Medicare was enshrined in the Canada Health Act. Since that time, no further system building or transformation initiatives have been launched.

In the section "Building Medicare," we will analyze what enabled the creation of these institutions up to 1984. A powerful set of ideas about equity, set among conditions of political competition and relative economic prosperity, allowed for the construction of a set of arrangements for universal and compre-

Managing a Canadian Healthcare Strategy, edited by A. Scott Carson and Kim Richard Nossal. Montreal and Kingston: McGill-Queen's University Press, Queen's Policy Studies Series. © 2016 The School of Policy Studies, Queen's University at Kingston. All rights reserved.

hensive hospital and physician insurance for Canadians. Where the health sector was relatively undeveloped, and entrenched interests were few, advantage went to the first governments to act. We continue then to consider why change has been so difficult to come by in the post-1984 era. We update recent research (Lazar et al. 2013a) showing that in key health policy domains, progress is incremental at best. Given Canada's federal system, which leaves control over administration of healthcare in the provincial sphere, money has been the main driver of reform. Compared to the earlier era, however, strong federal leadership has been lacking, and spending constraints stronger. With the support of entrenched interests that now benefit from Medicare's arrangement, change is limited to the search for greater efficiencies.

In the following section, "Possible Futures," we consider the effect of alternative scenarios on the future of Canadian healthcare. The focus of these alternative scenarios is not on the specifics of policy options to mitigate the risks or seize the opportunities inherent in them. Rather, it is on considering the likely adequacy of our system of governance and institutional framework for anticipating and responding to potential political, social, economic, and technological developments. In the final section, we draw out the implications of this analysis to suggest where those who want to advance health reform efforts might find leverage points.

BUILDING MEDICARE: PHASE ONE REFORM (1945–1984)

Events immediately following World War II set the stage for the agenda of healthcare policy reform that created the modern Canadian welfare state. This story has been detailed extensively elsewhere (e.g., Maioni 1998; Taylor 1978; Tuohy 1999); we recap the main events here, through the lens of an analytic framework of factors enabling or constraining reform.

Several pressures for implementing reform existed. There was a desire to give back to Canadians who had endured the Depression and fought the war; that they might in peacetime return to a better country than they had left. For the existing federal and provincial governments, there was also a growing political threat from the political left: domestic social democrats inspired by policy ideas emanating from intellectuals in the UK and Western Europe. The Co-operative Commonwealth Federation (CCF), forerunner of today's New Democratic Party (NDP), was topping some national opinion polls for a period in 1943 and was elected to power in Saskatchewan in 1944. At the same time, there were barriers to reform. Canada's federal constitution limited Ottawa's law-making authority in what was considered a provincial jurisdiction. Reform was perceived to require significant spending, and some Canadians and governments found the idea of a bigger state ideologically unacceptable, running counter to their values of personal self-reliance and limiting public spending to only the "deserving" poor.

If there ever was a time to assert a strong Ottawa-centric view of the federation, this was it. The Dominion government was the order of government that had prosecuted and won the war; its prestige in 1945 was high. This Ottawa-centric view was found in the federal government's positions on macro-economic stabilization policy, revenue-sharing with provinces, and for our purposes, its 1945 proposals to the Dominion-Provincial First Ministers' Conference on Reconstruction. Importantly, the health field was essentially a blank policy slate as there had been little to no previous governmental activity in this sphere. In setting an agenda for discussion of healthcare reform, then, the federal government was the *first mover*. Its substantial and detailed proposals included:

- large improvements in provincial healthcare planning, funded by Ottawa;
- a more systematic approach to public health, with federal financial support;
- large supply side growth—more hospitals, beds, physicians, nurses and other caregivers with federal sharing in capital costs; and
- government-funded services to address the demand side (first dollar universal comprehensive Canada-wide healthcare insurance). These were proposed to include hospital care, primary care, (i.e., doctors), visiting nurses, dental care, medical specialists' services and prescription drugs. The programs were to be administered by provinces or not-for-profit bodies appointed by provinces. The Dominion government was to pay for a fixed share of the costs on an ongoing basis (60 percent was the percentage first proposed but with caps).

In a nutshell, money would be the lever to secure policy reforms.

The main competitor to a universal comprehensive publicly funded Medicare program was a voluntary privately funded program. This alternative was put on the table by some provincial premiers (i.e., Ontario, Quebec,[1] and Alberta), who objected both to publicly funded healthcare on a mandatory basis and to the idea that the federal government had a role to play in whatever arrangements were reached. No consensus on health insurance proposals was achieved in 1945, and what followed was a two-decade long struggle to achieve reform. This pitted Ottawa and some provincial supporters (especially Saskatchewan) against those provinces advocating the privately funded programmatic approach, who fronted shifting coalitions of interests and institutions centred on provincial medical associations supported by the Canadian Medical Association (CMA), and the life insurance industry.

In the case of hospital insurance reform, the Canadian Hospital Association and the affiliated Catholic Hospital Conference and their provincial counterparts were also nominally among those resistant to universal public insurance, but they were not nearly as politically powerful as medical associations (especially outside of central Canada)—and not nearly as committed (Taylor 1978).

---

[1] While the stance of the Quebec government in federal-provincial negotiations coincides from time to time with that of other provinces, because its overarching political imperatives are to protect the French language and culture, and to seek greater autonomy (or outright sovereignty), its position on all issues must always be interpreted with this distinction in mind.

The hospital associations were made up overwhelmingly of privately owned, not-for-profit (NFP) corporations: mainly religious orders, other charitable organizations, and municipalities, incorporated under provincial NFP companies' law. With some exceptions these hospital corporations were financially weak and many looked to a national publicly funded healthcare program with relief as much as regret. Publicly funded hospital insurance would not leave them with unpaid bills and accumulating debt. This part of the debate terminated with the passage in 1957 of the federal Hospital Insurance and Diagnostic Services Act (HIDSA).

In the case of medical insurance, the resistance to the universal/mandatory government-funded approach was much better organized and more determined. The leadership came from those who thought they would lose from a publicly funded medical care policy. Private commercial insurance companies were first among these losers. They had developed a market for private health insurance; by 1965 commercial private insurers were providing some degree of coverage to almost five million Canadians (Taylor 1978), out of a total population of about 20 million, and were unwilling to abandon this market easily. At the same time, provincial medical associations had established or approved of not-for-profit, pre-paid, private insurance plans in their jurisdictions—a strategy that the CMA encouraged. Each plan was based on a fee-for-service (FFS) schedule that the physicians had designed or supported. These initiatives helped the profession maintain control over both the delivery and pricing of services.

In the end, the supporters of universal publicly funded healthcare won. Those provinces that had already introduced legislation based on the voluntary model—Ontario, Alberta and British Columbia—lost. When the federal Medical Care Act (MCA) was passed in 1966, it put considerable federal money on the table. Few provinces were prepared, or could afford, to forego this—it would have been too big a sacrifice for their taxpayers. Whatever political view a province held prior to the federal legislation, it could not afford to wait too long and have its federal taxpayers subsidize federal taxpayers in other provinces.

The federal MCA left most design decisions to the provinces. Each province acted independently. Each chose to adopt the tariff schedule which the physician-sponsored, or physician-approved, not-for-profit plans had been using or planning to use. In this way, provincial governments more or less assured themselves of physician cooperation in the design and delivery of medical insurance. They chose not to impose the inevitably heavy hand of government in areas where the medical profession was accustomed to self-governance. While provincial medical associations "lost" on the issue of mandatory public versus voluntary private coverage, the public system was made dependent on physician influence in many ways. Bilateral forums involving provincial health ministries and provincial medical associations have sought to jointly manage efforts to improve the efficiency and effectiveness of existing healthcare programs, largely working out of public sight.

Arenas and Instruments

Intergovernmental conferences were key venues for debating options for healthcare policy reform. The first ministers' federal-provincial conference was the main institutional arena. Owing to the sheer financial magnitude of the healthcare programs, they were bound to have a profound influence on the fiscal framework of all jurisdictions. It thus followed that the federal and provincial finance ministers were the principal advisers to their first ministers on the broad parameters of the programs. The Federal-Provincial Health Ministers' Conference (and their deputy ministers' committee) was a relatively small actor (admittedly on a vast agenda) during these years, and its agenda was technical most of the time (O'Reilly 2001).

Absence of formal decision rules for federal/provincial ministerial conferences enabled Ottawa to structure incentives to buy provincial support/acquiescence, one by one. For example, the specifics of the federal matching grant proposals for hospital and subsequently medical insurance were such that provinces that received equalization payments from Ottawa would have more than 50 percent of their eligible costs covered and the non-equalization-receiving provinces would receive less than 50 percent. The federal government thus ensured that the Atlantic provinces would buy in. Another example is in the 1966 federal legislation under which the federal government offered provinces the opportunity to opt out of the federal hospital insurance program and receive tax points rather than transfer payments, as long as provinces that took up the offer established an equivalent program complying with the principles of HIDSA. The federal offer was such that the net fiscal effect was nil for all provinces. This was really an offer meant to meet Quebec's political needs, which was the only province to take it up.

Yet another example is that different prime ministers established different thresholds for how many provinces would need to "sign on" before a joint program would proceed. In the case of hospital insurance, Louis St. Laurent's position evolved over time and he eventually proposed six provinces (a majority) in the 1957 HIDSA. That meant that the law would come into force when six provinces had enacted the appropriate parallel hospital insurance legislation. The following year the new Progressive Conservative government under John G. Diefenbaker reduced the minimum number of provinces to five as this ensured that the legislation would come into force quickly. Almost a decade later, the Pearson government proceeded with its medical care insurance legislation without any minimum number of provinces (Taylor 1978; Kent 1988).

Federal spending power was the key lever to health reform; conditional federal grants to provinces were the instruments. This also delimited the extent of reform: the costs of achieving the first steps—hospital and medical insurance—were substantial enough that the federal government was unwilling to consider more expansive coverage. Once in place however, the amounts offered by the federal government were influential enough that Ottawa was able to unilaterally alter the terms of its grants several times during phase one without leading to provincial withdrawal. Most notably, in the late 1970s, the federal government changed its financing commitment from an open-ended one to a capped one, through Established Programs Financing (EPF). EPF severed the link between provincial expenditures on health and federal contributions, and presumably gave provinces greater incentive to rein in their own spending. This change was substantively propelled by the federal finance department but politically involved first ministers. Provinces were unified in rejecting the idea of a cap on the federal matching grant contribution, but Ottawa eventually secured it after the health programs were established and provinces could not politically abandon them.

Looking back at the agenda of the 1945 Dominion-Provincial First Ministers' Conference on Reconstruction, we can see that phase one policy reforms transformed Canadian healthcare, most particularly in public health, the supply side, and part of the demand side. Other big reforms proposals were excluded, however. The blank policy slate at the outset of the period effectively meant existing interests had few long-established or deeply cherished positions to defend. But there was no shortage of ideas. On one side was the Keynesianism and "welfare state" thinking that permeated Western Europe and to a lesser degree the rest of the developed world. In opposition to it was the more conservative approach reflected in classical economics and the idea of personal responsibility. The status quo favoured the latter schools of thought.

With the benefit of hindsight, it is apparent that Ottawa's 1945 proposals shaped the policy agenda for many decades into the future. First-mover status mattered: the agenda was set by the Dominion government in 1945, and the subsequent evolution of this agenda was governed by political promises, electoral considerations, and political strength, on the one hand, and fiscal factors communicated through federalism's structures on the other. Politically, elected leaders responded both to external competition and internal diversity of opinion. While CCF strength in the late-1940s was an early incentive for the federal Liberal government to act, this pressure abated in the 1950s. It was replaced by meaningful competition for power between the Liberals and Progressive Conservatives between the mid-1950s and mid-1960s (as seen in the election of several minority governments following almost 20 uninterrupted years of Liberal dominance). While Liberals attempted to stake a claim as the Medicare party, internal positions within both parties were somewhat in flux. The Liberal prime minister, Louis St. Laurent, for instance, was wary of the implications of universal healthcare programs, while Conservative leader Diefenbaker would express a more open position than his party had historically been prepared to espouse (Taylor 1978).

The fiscal context was at first relatively favourable, with the 1950s and 1960s being a period of sustained economic growth. Conditions worsened subsequently (the 1970s brought stagflation and wage/price controls, and in the early 1980s, recession). These changing circumstances helped push the federal government to limit its exposure to escalating healthcare costs through the EPF arrangements. The only public arena available was intergovernmental; federal-provincial grants were the instrument of the moment. The bargain with physicians ensured short-term peace, but left the system with what many felt to be a flawed incentive structure. Since money was the incentive to encourage reform, more attention was given to money than the content of health policy itself.

BUILDING MEDICARE: PHASE TWO REFORM (1985–PRESENT)

The passage of the Canada Health Act (CHA) was a symbolic capstone to the first era of reform. Where we characterize the first four decades after the Second World War as an era of big reform, the years since 1985 represent incremental and often ineffectual change at best. Policy making no longer has a blank slate, but must build from the existing "facts-on-the-ground," that is, broad support among both the public and political classes for the CHA and the publicly funded hospital and physician services which it covers. This consensus has endured at all levels through changes of government. Parties on the right have emphasized cost control and greater use of market mechanisms, but have been unwilling to broach any fundamental change to the status quo; parties on the left meanwhile have called for expansions to the system, but in practice have taken a mostly defensive position and have been unwilling to open up the CHA for extensive debate out of fear of losing what has been obtained in the past.

Debate continues about unfinished elements from phase one (for example, how, if at all, to establish a national pharmacare program). However, much of the attention, especially at the provincial level, has been about how best to manage a "mature" system in order to maximize the effectiveness and efficiency of program spending. Canada's healthcare system is one of the costliest among OECD nations, with relatively poorer health outcomes than those achieved by comparator countries (Carson 2015). Canada's total public sector health expenditures grew from 6.4 percent to 8.0 percent of total GDP between 1995 and 2010, a 25 percent jump (Marchildon 2013); when added to the private share, Canada is thus in "the top quartile of spenders in the OECD with regard to total health expenditure per capita" (CIHI 2014, 85).

In the provinces, health accounts for a projected 37.7 percent of total government program expenditures, as of 2013 (CIHI 2014). The largest amounts go to hospitals (29.6 percent), physician services (15.5 percent), and pharmaceuticals (15.8 per cent; CIHI 2014). The first two are covered by the Canada Health Act, giving provinces an incentive to design systems heavily reliant upon these. Nonetheless, the proportion dedicated to hospitals has fallen since 1995, down from 40 percent at that time. Pharmaceutical costs first surpassed those of physician services in 1997 (CIHI 2014). Regarding health outcomes and satisfaction, Canada sits, at best, in the middle of the pack of OECD countries (Marchildon 2013; Mossialos et al. 2015). We rate near the bottom in the safety of care, and absolute last on the list in respect to timeliness of care (Mossialos). And Canada ranks second to last among 15 countries in the number of people who say the health system works well (Mossialos 2015).

Not surprisingly, given the above, the health sector is among one of the largest economic fields in Canada, more than twice the size of the energy sector (even before the huge decline in oil prices). It employs 1.4 million Canadians, 9 percent of all jobs in the country. It has been estimated that health spending (as of 2011) is responsible for almost $120 billion in direct contributions to the economy, with additional benefits in the upstream supply chain of $44 billion and 500,000 jobs (Bounajm 2013). The size of the health sector means that any efforts to address Canada's internationally dismal health reform performance record will be scrutinized by many eyes for their potentially adverse effects on jobs and profits.

There has never been any shortage in phase two of proposals for a reform agenda, to parts or the entirety of the system (Mhatre and Deber 1998; Lazar et al. 2013a). The Conference Board of Canada (Prada and Brown 2012) for instance identified 18 major reports released between 1997 and 2011, at both the federal (e.g., National Forum on Health, Commission on the Future of Health Care in Canada [Romanow], Standing Senate Committee [Kirby]) and provincial levels (e.g., Mazankowski, Fyke, Clair, TD Bank [Drummond, 2010]), as well as under the aegis of professional groups in medicine and nursing. According to the Conference Board review, these reports collectively produced 432 recommendations for action across seven themes. System management approaches and funding models were most commonly addressed, with considerable attention also to quality and value for money; health human resources; health promotion and disease prevention; innovation and technology; and access to care. Collectively, these reports provide a widely shared understanding of what kinds of changes to the Canadian healthcare system might be pursued in order to advance success around common goals, objectives, and values (Lazar et al. 2013a, Annex 1).

In June 2014, the Conservative government of Stephen Harper commissioned David Naylor, president emeritus at the University of Toronto, to report on promising areas of health innovation that could control costs while leading to improved quality and accessibility of care. Naylor's report, the Advisory Panel on Healthcare Innovation (2015), called for new federal leadership around patient engagement, systems integration, technological transformation, better approaches to procurement and reimbursement, and efforts to spur health innovation as a potentially powerful economic driver for the future. Like many of its predecessors, the report raised challenges which political leaders seemed unwilling to take on (Simpson 2015). When it comes to actual health system reform in Canada, phase two has produced much more talk than action.

In *Paradigm Freeze* (Lazar et al. 2013a), we argued that healthcare reform efforts from the early 1990s onward resulted in meager results even in the areas of greatest focus (See text box, *Paradign Freeze*). Have there been any instances of substantive reform in the years since that would challenge the assessment reached in that book? We think not. In the following section, we review developments in each of the six *Paradigm Freeze* policy areas which have been observed in the last half-decade, in order to support this conclusion. Note that our analysis in this chapter speaks to events that have occurred, but does not attempt to render judgments of magnitude in the same structured fashion.

Paradigm Freeze

Paradigm Freeze (Lazar et al. 2013a) was a program of research which looked at six policy areas, representing four conceptually distinctive types of policy (Lavis et al. 2002) across five provinces, from the early 1990s to 2010:

- Regionalization of health service delivery, representing the domain of governance arrangements (i.e., who holds policy, organizational, commercial and professional authority to make which kinds of decisions, including the role of stakeholders, patients and the public)
- Needs based funding formulas for health regions, and alternative payment plans for physicians, representing the policy domain of financial arrangements (i.e., how revenue is raised, spending disbursed, and healthcare users incentivized)
- For profit delivery of medically necessary services, and waiting list management, examples of the policy domain of delivery arrangements (i.e., how care is provided, where and by whom)
- Prescription drug plans, representing the program content domain (i.e., what goods and services are provided via the public financing)

The *Paradigm Freeze* research program offered some explanations from 30 province-issue case combinations for why health reform in Canada is so difficult to achieve. Chances of successful reform were shown to be influenced by exogenous factors (such as changes in government, fiscal crisis, public opinion, and technological change), exogenous/endogenous factors (such as ideologies and institutional features like intergovernmental relationships) and endogenous factors (such as the influence of healthcare provider interests; Lazar and Church 2013).

Reform was defined as policy choices that moved toward implementation of the consensus of directions proposed by health care commission reports from the 1980s through 2003. These represent closely considered ideas repeatedly endorsed after expert, and often public, scrutiny. Comprehensive reform would involve full implementation of all directions, with "significant," "moderate," and "limited" reforms indicating less action. The conclusion of "meagre" (Lazar et al. 2013b) is based on observation that eight cases produced no reform at all, and another eight only the barest change to account for limited progress.

While this research only looked in detail at five provinces, they were purposefully chosen to represent a range of factors, e.g., population, economy, and political history, which should make their experiences generalizable to the Canadian context as a whole.

Regionalization

Between 1989 and 1997, nine of 10 provinces established—or, in the case of Quebec, substantially overhauled—some form of regional health authority (RHA), which we can define as geographically based entities which consolidate responsibility for both provision and purchasing of health services across a range of functions, from public health and community care, to acute care hospitals, to long-term and continuing care (Lewis and Kouri 2004). The scope of services included in regions varies somewhat from province to province, but most significantly, always excludes physician services and out-of-hospital drug coverage. Ontario, the holdout province, subsequently created Local Health Integration Networks (LHINs), which are similar to regions in some ways, but serve strictly as purchasing and coordinating bodies, without direct service delivery.

Since this flurry of activity, the main trend has been to consolidate the number of regions: British Columbia, Alberta, Saskatchewan, Manitoba, and New Brunswick all took this route in the early years of the 21st century. In two provinces, Alberta and Prince Edward Island, there is one single healthcare "region" that covers the province as a whole; however, these units still operate as a region distinct from the provincial ministry of health. In 2015 Nova Scotia consolidated its nine regions into one, to operate alongside an independent tertiary care hospital with Maritime-wide responsibilities, following the election of a new Liberal government. Quebec's Liberal government also consolidated health organizations in spring 2015. In Ontario's 2014 provincial election, the opposition Conservative party campaigned on a platform to abolish the LHINs. Though the Liberal government was re-elected, it now proposes to reorganize the system by combining LHINs with the Community Care Access Centres, thereby adding continuing and long-term care to their existing responsibilities (M.R. Cohn 2015).

Several provinces (e.g., British Columbia, Saskatchewan, and Newfoundland and Labrador) have initiated the development of "shared services organizations," meant to create efficiencies by allowing for regional authorities to jointly carry out purchasing and other administrative functions (CADTH 2011)[2].

In only one province, British Columbia, has a new authority been created: the First Nations Health Authority (http://www.fnha.ca/). This unique entity arose in 2013 from devolution of federal programs to a province-wide, aboriginal-controlled authority as part of tripartite negotiations. It delivers mostly environmental health, community-based health promotion, wellness and addictions services.

As Boychuk (2009, 356) put it, "Regionalization appears to have taken its place in the historical evolution of Medicare as an enduring, yet ambiguous and contested institution." Recent years have seen on-going tinkering with organi-

---

[2] See http://www.3shealth.ca/; http://www.hssbc.ca/default.htm; http://www.releases.gov.nl.ca/releases/2015/health/0806n02.aspx.

zational structures for the administration of health services delivery, such that "continued evolution in system governance across and within jurisdictions has made it difficult to assess the outcomes of these reforms" (Prada and Brown 2012: 16).

Needs-based Funding for Healthcare Institutions

The creation of RHAs was generally accompanied by the adoption of population-based funding formulas, typically with adjustments meant to account for various facets of "need" (McIntosh et al. 2010). This is a relatively straightforward approach to health system funding that allows for reallocation across spending priorities. But in itself, this approach creates limited incentive to provider institutions to become more efficient or to act on any other policy goals which the funder may desire. Thus, some provinces have begun to test alternative health funding models such as pay-for performance (P4P) or activity-based funding (ABF); these can be seen as complements to the needs-based model (Sutherland 2011). Pay-for-performance typically involves additional payments offered to providers for achieving certain targets. Activity-based funding provides money for each treatment provided; i.e., it rewards volume of care. P4P has been implemented in Ontario (Li et al. 2014; Kiran et al. 2014) and British Columbia (Cheng and Sullivan 2013), as well as Manitoba and Nova Scotia (Wranik and Katz 2015), while ABF has been deployed in Ontario, British Columbia, Alberta, and Saskatchewan (Prada and Brown 2012).

These funding models have been promoted as a way of incentivizing delivery of desired treatments (e.g., primary prevention activities), to clear away backlogs, and to encourage more efficient use of available resources. However, it is unclear if major impacts can be expected. A systematic review of ABF found no evidence that it was better or worse than other forms of funding in relation to key patient outcomes (Palmer et al. 2014); similarly, reviews of P4P schemes have found the impacts to be relatively modest at best (Petersen et al. 2006; Gillam, Siriwardena, and Stell 2012).

For-Profit Delivery of Healthcare Services

Increasing the role of private for-profit firms in the delivery of health services in Canada has been one of the more contentious reforms considered. While *Paradigm Freeze* (Lazar et al. 2013a) identified some provincial premiers as vocal proponents of such efforts (e.g., Ralph Klein in Alberta and Mike Harris in Ontario), on-the-ground change was actually quite limited. This remains the case. The 2005 Supreme Court of Canada ruling on Chaouilli v. Quebec (*Chaoulli v. Quebec (AG)* [2005] 1 S.C.R. 791, 2005 SCC 35) was touted as a major shaping event that could force open doors towards private delivery (Forget 2005). However, little seems to have come to pass. Labrie—a proponent of market forces in healthcare—suggests that the Quebec government's response has been "timid" (2015); Daniel Cohn (2015) has argued that despite the opening of such a policy window, there has been no major change to health policy in

Canada's provinces in this regard "because neither politicians nor the major insurance companies could benefit from embracing the change on offer" (11–12). However, others argue that the Chaouilli decision has had major adverse effects upon Quebec's adherence to the CHA principles (Brouselle and Contandriopoulos 2015). These are seen in the contentious Bill 20, passed by the Couillard government in November 2015 (Derfel 2015) which appears to accept and will regularize by regulation the "accessory" fees to be charged to patients who receive publicly funded services in for-profit clinics (Forbes 2015; Meili and Martin 2015). Such fees have not been subject to CHA enforcement (Brouselle and Contandriopoulos 2015); since 2007–2008 only British Columbia has been subject to consistent and continuing deduction from its federal transfers due to violation of CHA principles (Health Canada 2014).

Some other court challenges around CHA and provincial legislation relating to private payment for health services continue to slowly work their way through the legal system. In 2016, for instance, British Columbia courts will hear a case against that province's Medicare Protection Act spearheaded by Dr. Brian Day, a leading operator of private healthcare clinics in the province and former president of the Canadian Medical Association (Labrie 2015).

Alternative Payment Plans

Physicians have long seen fee-for-service (FFS) payment as a right, and replacing it with an alternative such as capitation or salary as an attack on the freedom of physicians to practice medicine as self-governed professionals. However, much research over a long period of time establishes that FFS produces undesirable incentives. Efforts to change this proceed haltingly. In terms of physician remuneration, phase two has seen the continuation of a slow trend toward greater use of alternative payment plans. The National Physician Survey (2013) reported that the majority of doctors in Canada were now paid by mixed or blended forms, rather than strictly fee-for-service: "In 2004, 51% of respondents were paid predominantly by fee-for-service. This number fell to 42% in 2010, and to 38% in 2013." Changing attitudes among younger physician cohorts have been reported (CHSRF 2010), and this may have led to greater willingness of medical associations to bargain such schemes with their provincial ministries as part of physician master agreements. The use of alternative payment plan models for physician payment varies considerably across the different provinces, however, much as it did while the *Paradigm Freeze* (Lazar et al. 2013a) research was conducted.

Prescription Drug Plans

As noted earlier, pharmaceuticals account for approximately 15 percent of health expenditures in Canada. Governments have worked to manage these costs through a variety of means, such as establishing formularies to determine which drugs will be paid for by provincial plans (e.g., via the Common Drug Review or the pan-Canadian Oncology Drug Review) or requiring substitution of generic for brand name prescriptions when comparable products are available. In 2012, the provinces (excepting Quebec) worked together through the Council of the Federation to establish bulk purchasing (Taber, 2012). This is known as the pan-Canadian Pharmaceutical Alliance (pCPA). Munson (2015) suggests that as of March 2015, "The pCPA has [saved] patients \$315 million per year on prescriptions by negotiating prices for 49 new, brand name drugs. The group, which is run through the provinces' and territories' Council of the Federation secretariat, currently has another 20 negotiations on the go." Further savings might be expected to be obtained if the federal government joins this group, as Prime Minister Justin Trudeau has proposed to do. However, such savings could be easily overwhelmed by the arrival on the scene of some vastly expensive new therapies, and price hikes for existing drugs. Access to pharmaceuticals for those not currently insured remains an issue, and so national pharmacare continues to be mooted by many (e.g., Morgan et al. 2015).

Wait Times

This is a specific instance of questions about performance measurement and management in the health system. Addressing wait times was a major concern of the 2003 and 2004 Health Accords. In these, first ministers committed to publication of comparable health indicators for several procedures of public interest, to allow comparison of waits across jurisdictions. The Health Council of Canada (HCC) was created to monitor progress toward system goals agreed in the Accords. All provinces now post online wait-time data for public review, though the HCC was shut down by the Harper government in 2014. Individual provinces have worked on their own with special medicine sectors, (such as the Cardiac Care Network of Ontario, or the Alberta Bone and Joint Initiative), to further address wait issues. For instance, the ABJI collects and compiles surgical data from the province's orthopods; it is reported confidentially to each surgeon and in aggregate for different provincial zones (Dick and Woodhouse 2014). Centralized intake offers patients the chance to wait for a preferred provider, or to seek a shorter wait elsewhere. CIHI data (2015) suggest that wait times have stabilized across the country, while larger numbers of patients are being seen and procedures delivered; about 80 percent of services are delivered within benchmarked times.

Nationally, the Canadian Medical Association endorses the "Choosing Wisely" campaign, based on a US model, which should help to manage waits by reducing efforts spent on low value, non-evidence based or improper treatments. Annual events such as the Taming of the Queue conferences (CFHI 2015) and the release of report cards by groups such as the Wait Time Alliance (http://www.waittimealliance.ca) or the Fraser Institute (2015; also Globerman 2013) continue to keep wait time issues visible and draw attention to governments' perceived progress, or lack thereof, in addressing these.

In short, it appears that governments have largely exhausted structural change such as re- or de-regionalization. There appear to be few prominent advocates of privatization or alternative payment plans, and there are vocal advocates for national pharmacare, but apparently little obvious governmental leadership, willingness, or commitment. Physicians have retained privileged standing though all phases of reform debates on some issues: for instance their insistence that there be compulsory arbitration if provinces paid them too little, their control over distribution of compensation, and their rejection of physician budgets being handed to the regional level. Where there is ongoing activity, such as funding formulas or wait time measurement, this consists mostly of tinkering with established programs. Overall, the fact that limited reforms have occurred shows continuity with the preceding period (the post-1984 Canada Health Act era). It suggests that, barring change in any baseline conditions, we should expect reform to remain difficult to achieve. But the focus of this current book is about how proponents might successfully advance strategies for reform, so we will turn our attention to that.

HEALTHCARE IN CANADA—POSSIBLE FUTURES

To help us get a handle on how to advance strategy, we turn to scenario techniques; these have long been considered to fit well together (http://patimes.org/rethinking-strategy-public-agencies/). This "futures" approach was developed in the mid-1960s, and has been adopted from its corporate sector origins for use in healthcare planning and research purposes (Vollmar, Ostermann, and Redaelli 2015), including a consideration of the overall direction which healthcare policy and the health system might take. Some Canadian examples include Mendelson and Divinsky's work (2002), which described four scenarios with an emphasis upon the effects of globalization, and Maxwell, Rosell, and Forest's work (2003) with the Romanow Commission (2002), which sought public input for possible alternative healthcare futures: increased public investment in traditional Medicare, a major restructuring of service delivery in the public system, increased private payment, and the creation of an entirely parallel private system. This kind of scenario work is our model for what follows.

Scenario development, briefly, consists of identifying key driving forces and constructing alternative narratives which show how these drivers lead to different possible circumstances. They create outlines or sketches, rather than comprehensive portrayals (Vollmar et al. 2015). Scenarios are not predictions; they must be plausible, but not necessarily equally probable (Wilkinson and Kupers 2013). The scenarios here depict what would be considered to be desirable or less desirable outcomes, which point at least implicitly to possible policy recommendations. However, they are the product of discussion among the authors, using a qualitative and intuitive approach (Van Notten et al. 2003), and readers should bear this informality in mind.

The general *continuation of the status quo* is one scenario; it presumes that Canadian healthcare's legislative foundations, governance, financing and policy will continue to evolve slowly, much as they have done in the years since 1984. Based on our assessment of health system configurations over this period, we can define today's "status quo" as a situation where:

- The healthcare system is publicly funded for hospital care and physician services, per the Canada Health Act, i.e., a bio-medical model. Coverage is "narrow and deep" (Marchildon 2014).
- The federal government plays a role in financing, via transfers, while provinces have main administrative responsibility including control over organization, regulation, and delivery of services. Federal leadership has been transactional rather than visionary or transformative.
- Professional interests, especially organized medicine, have a considerable degree of influence.
- This existing model maintains strong public support as a visible symbol of Canadian identity and values.
- Within what are perceived to be ongoing financial constraints on healthcare spending, Canadian governments seek ways to pursue efficiencies and manage trade-offs. Spending decisions are informed to some degree by the work of the Canadian Agency for Drugs and Technologies in Health and other health technology assessment bodies.
- International flows of goods and services have been protected through a range of free-trade agreements negotiated and approved by Canadian governments over the last 30 years, but the public nature of Canada's system has also been protected.

Numerous issues may compete for some attention on governments' agendas. Projecting from what has been observed to date, governments have been receptive to calls for spending on the elderly population (Kershaw 2015). Analyses (e.g., Robson 2001) have contended that the aging of Canada's population will increase demand upon the healthcare system, though other research disputes this (e.g., Barer, Evans, and Hertzman 1995). Nonetheless, clamour for such spending recurs regularly when federal/provincial/territorial fiscal relations are discussed. This suggests that a status quo scenario will see increased spending on seniors' health issues. As a result, pressures around other issues, such as increasing inequities in access to pharmaceuticals due to lack of universal coverage, or the deplorable state of health in aboriginal communities, will mount but the barriers which have prevented action on these issues in the past will remain largely in place.

This scenario projects no substantial change in the proportion of government spending devoted to healthcare, or the current balance between public and private healthcare expenditures (approximately 70–30 percent). Healthcare will remain the largest of governments' expenditure programs, as it has been for the last four and more decades. Likewise, the long-standing intimate relations between provinces and medical associations will remain intact. The medical profession will maintain insider status on all issues that have the potential to influence compensation.

The Harper Conservative government (2006–2015)—to an exceptional extent for post-Second World War Canadian experience—downplayed any federal role or FPT collaboration in the healthcare sphere. For instance, the FPT Conference of Health Ministers did not operate; the federal government made unilateral decisions regarding the amount of federal transfers to provinces; a number of independent think tanks or arm's length bodies lost funding, or were wound down, such as the Health Council of Canada.

On such matters, a return to the status quo ante is likely. While the Liberal government of Justin Trudeau and its successors may be relatively more open to intergovernmental discussions in coming years, and while provinces may be expected to continue pushing for bigger transfers, no dramatic changes to FPT fiscal relations are likely. Independent institutions and think tanks may be re-established, though it will take time for them to achieve credibility and influence. One such body is dubbed the Health Observatory—it could facilitate "knowledge exchange throughout the country and beyond on leading practices" (Royal College of Physicians and Surgeons 2010).

The remaining scenarios should be conceived of as going beyond this baseline, to deliver meaningful and substantive change; in other words, they "bend the curve" rather than project current trends linearly into the future.

We have labelled the second scenario *Medicare plus*. The parameters are similar to those of the status quo: improvements to the public healthcare system can be achieved through collaboration and negotiation among governments and key provider interests. While such change may be described as gradual and incremental, it nonetheless is the product of near countless hours of intergovernmental meetings and repeated refinement and exchange of policy proposals. The occurrence of this scenario would likely be due to a more activist federal government willing to take the lead along with greater provincial willingness to commit to shared goals. There will be continued unwillingness to reopen the CHA for limited reforms due to fears that there will be no way to manage the scope of public debate once this genie is out of the bottle. Despite this constraint, the *Medicare plus* scenario posits the achievement of a number of not-insignificant enhancements to the Medicare package. In addition to seniors' health and well-being, we might expect to see greater federal transfers earmarked for primary healthcare and mental health, First Nations and Inuit health, and some form of coverage for catastrophic drug costs. Even in good economic times, there is little perceived financial scope to expand healthcare, so we might expect to see the emergence, or increased use, of alternative policy instruments, such as refundable income tax credits. Their use, of course, is complicated in the Canadian federal context where federal and provincial revenues tend to be linked through a shared tax collection infrastructure: changes which decrease taxable federal incomes will decrease provincial returns as well.

A third scenario reflects more dramatic movement toward greater government action and expansion in healthcare protections. The driver of change in this case would be the election of a federal government with a strong platform and policy commitment to reforming healthcare in a more *egalitarianism* direction—a victory for interests which have consistently promoted a fairness agenda and defended the original vision of Medicare. This scenario would include most, or all, of the *Medicare plus* enhancements, but would guarantee them through entrenchment within universal publicly funded programs. This additional coverage could be through amendments to the CHA or entirely new legislation—a politically important decision which would be the subject of considerable contestation. An additional part of the reform package would be new or amended legislation to prevent and even reverse trends to more unequal access to medically necessary services. To make funds available for these expansions, the federal government and provinces would need to make more use of cost-control mechanisms such as health technology assessment (where funding would be contingent upon new products and services demonstrating cost- and outcome-superiority over existing counterparts). A more substantive structural change propelled by the fairness agenda of this scenario would be implementation of bilateral or trilateral agreements with aboriginal communities for the transfer of dollars and control over programs to First Nations and indigenous authorities. The First Nations Health Authority in British Columbia may be an early model for this.

Our fourth scenario, *technology-driven reform*, would see the healthcare policy agenda driven substantially by government efforts to both react to, and anticipate, rapid developments in medical science and technology. While many types of technological change are possible, one of the most anticipated is in genomics and personalized medicine. Personalized medicine, sometimes referred to as precision medicine, is an approach to disease prevention and treatment that tailors medical decisions and practices by taking account of differences in people's genetics and lifestyles. Knowledge from diagnostic tests is used to determine how individuals are likely to respond to treatment, for instance, if a particular class of drugs is more likely to lead to adverse effects for some. This is an exemplar of fast developing technologies with potential wide effect which we can use to illustrate the impacts of this scenario. Personalized medicine offers significant individual health benefits, potentially leading to a marked increase in healthy years of life. Physicians and the public—including both genuine patient advocacy groups and "astro turf" groups, which are supported by large corporate interests for the sole purpose of lobbying in favour of their products (Appolliono and Bero 2007)—will push strenuously for the rapid inclusion of such services in the Medicare bundle. Given the importance of the health sector as an economic driver, there will be many ears receptive to these arguments. While the federal government has considerable constitutional power here as a result of its authority for food and drug safety, there is uncertainty as to whether regulatory institutions will be able to keep pace with demand, particularly if personalized medicine becomes rapidly available in the US or other jurisdictions. As a result, debate over the potential benefits and costs of expanded private financing of care will be reopened to a degree unlike that of the other scenarios. It is likely that there will be greater acceptance of growing inequality and of the idea that patients should be able to spend out-of-pocket on healthcare goods and services. Individual rights will take precedence over the "social rights of citizenship" (Bhatia 2010).

TABLE 9.1
Possible Effects of the Health Policy Status Quo and of Alternative Scenarios on Canada's Healthcare Future

Scenario	Direction, Speed, Timing, Magnitude, and Drivers of Reform	Who Benefits Most? Who Benefits Least?	Role of Government vs. Private Provision in Funding Healthcare	Impact on Public Finances	Adequacy of Institutions/Availability of Tools	Governance Arenas and Arrangements
Status quo [SQ]	DIRECTION: Baseline case. SPEED AND TIMING: Any changes will occur slowly and incrementally, likely following lengthy periods of discussion and negotiation. MAGNITUDE: Meagre for healthcare policy writ large. DRIVERS: Endogenous and exogeneous factors (e.g., population aging).	Those who benefit most from status quo include: Provincial Medical Associations; Big Pharma; Union members (who have coverage for most health services not covered by CHA). Those who benefit least include the poor and those who go without prescribed drugs.	No significant change in funding. Some for-profit privatization but mainly as contractors to provincial health services that are short of specific services in specific regions. Public programs generally pay for for-profit facilities no more than not-for-profit facilities.	Small reforms in health context may loom large in public finance due to sheer size of health expenditure programs.	Assumes continuation of current laws and practices, and F/P/T funding commitments. Assumes ongoing F/P/T efforts, at a technical level, to improve efficiency and cost effectiveness of health sector programs	Overlapping of F/P/T responsibilities favours collaborative federalism. Healthcare discussions and setting of broad system parameters continue at first ministers' and health ministers' tables, along with continued leading role played by finance ministries. Continued privileging of provincial medical associations in their relationships with provincial health ministries.

... continued

TABLE 9.1, continued

Scenario	Direction, Speed, Timing, Magnitude, and Drivers of Reform	Who Benefits Most? Who Benefits Least?	Role of Government vs. Private Provision in Funding Healthcare	Impact on Public Finances	Adequacy of Institutions/ Availability of Tools	Governance Arenas and Arrangements
Medicare Plus This scenario would see ad hoc efforts to address a number of perceived gaps, e.g., drug coverage, seniors' care, home and community care, primary and mental health care, aboriginal health.	DIRECTION: Slightly more proactive government activity in healthcare policy field SPEED AND TIMING: Any changes will occur slowly and incrementally. MAGNITUDE: Modest impact overall. Reforms may be significant for targeted populations DRIVERS: Endogenous and exogeneous factors (e.g., population aging).	Relatively small differences compared to status quo. Provincial Medical Associations, Big Pharma, union members benefit as under SQ. Should impact targeted groups and thus improve status of least advantaged relative to SQ	Mixed effects on government role relative to SQ. For instance, some private insurance will be displaced from drug coverage policies. However, increases in assisted living, home care and other seniors' supports likely to be delivered through existing private insurance and provider models.	Large enough to make a measurable dent in current resource allocation. Will add to federal deficit and debt through both increased direct spending and tax incentives. Will require more public funding to create new physical and human capital paid for through a mix of sources.	Vertical fiscal imbalance suggests that federal prescription drug coverage will be the most feasible way to address catastrophic costs. New federal transfers to P/Ts will be notionally targeted for mental health and other priority areas. Demand for additional healthcare spending may require exploration of new fiscal tools alongside tax increases: e.g., deductibles and co-payments, using the amounts generated to widen coverage. New financial tools may be employed to deal with aging population. For example, Income Tax Act provisions to encourage private care including respite for caregivers.	Political leadership from a more activist federal government initiates a re-activation of F/P/T Conferences. A strong focus on government response to aging population may lead to pressures for creation of freestanding seniors' ministries.

... continued

TABLE 9.1, continued

Scenario	Direction, Speed, Timing, Magnitude, and Drivers of Reform	Who Benefits Most? Who Benefits Least?	Role of Government vs. Private Provision in Funding Healthcare	Impact on Public Finances	Adequacy of Institutions/ Availability of Tools	Governance Arenas and Arrangements
Egalitarianism. This scenario would widen universal healthcare in ways that more fully address gaps and policy areas described in the Medicare Plus scenario. New government-to-government relationships with First Nations will be established.	DIRECTION: This scenario privileges the state. SPEED AND TIMING: Unpredictable but if it occurs, key developments will be relatively rapid. For this scenario to come to fruition, economic times likely must be good. MAGNITUDE: Greater than anything so far in the post-1984 years. DRIVERS: Changes are largely idea-driven (i.e., via political commitment) and therefore endogenous.	The less advantaged benefit most. Those with excellent coverage benefit least as they will pay more tax for current services. Spreading the benefits more widely may also mean increased use of non-physician human resources which may be contentious and lead to clashes between governments and organized medicine.	Policies driven by a strong fairness agenda will contain, and possibly in some spheres reduce, the private sector role in favour of public provision. Governments will be (uncharacteristically) more willing to take on entrenched corporate interests.	Should be expected to lead to considerable increases in public healthcare spending. Provinces have differing fiscal abilities to serve urban Aboriginal populations	The high cost of delivering expensive technologies on an egalitarian basis is an ongoing tension. This can be tackled through stricter use of health technology assessment processes and generic drug purchasing policies to control pharmaceutical costs. The Health Observatory offers a way to promote evidence-based policies. Efforts at Aboriginal reconciliation likely will take the form of bilateral and tripartite intergovernmental agreements with First Nations. These may raise questions of accountability.	The strong political commitments which bring this scenario into being suggest that it will be highly dominated by a reinvigorated first ministers' process with strong backup by finance ministries and health ministries. Compared to the SQ, the influence of finance ministries is weaker as pledge for greater spending seen as something that must be delivered upon. Greater attention to social determinants of health leads to increased cross-ministerial collaboration and the adoption of health-in-all-policies approaches.

... continued

TABLE 9.1, continued

Scenario	Direction, Speed, Timing, Magnitude, and Drivers of Reform	Who Benefits Most? Who Benefits Least?	Role of Government vs. Private Provision in Funding Healthcare	Impact on Public Finances	Adequacy of Institutions/ Availability of Tools	Governance Arenas and Arrangements
TECHNOLO-GY-DRIVEN REFORM: This scenario is driven by growth in personalized medicine emerging from fast growing genomics sciences.	DIRECTION: Governments react to developments largely generated in the private sector. SPEED AND TIMING: Timing is unpredictable; speed may be very rapid. MAGNITUDE: Over decades it may be massive. DRIVERS: Exogenous (scientific change).	The focus on genomic science as a means to improve wellness and diagnose and treat patients individually will amplify the influence of the medical profession. Effects will depend on who owns new processes, technologies, and drug formulations. Where private ownership prevails, price will shape who benefits most and least. Most	Government strives to "get out of the way" of healthcare entrepreneurs who are perceived as more nimble and better able to respond to challenges such as population aging. Probable large increase in federal regulatory role in verifying drug and procedure safety.	Governments are likely to be cautious in including treatments within the Medicare core. Private insurers, at least in the early stages, are also likely to be cautious in assuming uncertain risks—thus individuals may be the main payer.	Existing legislation enables the federal government to regulate the safety of foods, drugs, and controlled substances. To the extent that treatment entails risks, the federal Patented Medications Prices Review Board may be an appropriate instrument.	Existing legislation enables the federal government to regulate the safety of foods, drugs, and controlled substances. To the extent that treatment entails risks, the federal Patented Medications Prices Review Board may be an appropriate instrument. Questions of access will be discussed foremost in the political realm. Food and drug safety and other technical issues will normally be discussed within specialized forums. Key decisions will be guided by pressures from international trade

... continued

TABLE 9.1, continued

Scenario	Direction, Speed, Timing, Magnitude, and Drivers of Reform	Who Benefits Most? Who Benefits Least?	Role of Government vs. Private Provision in Funding Healthcare	Impact on Public Finances	Adequacy of Institutions/ Availability of Tools	Governance Arenas and Arrangements
		likely, momentum will emanate from the US and tend to increase inequality of access.				and economic development arenas. (Canadian residents as importers of products, or medical tourists; and Canadian providers as exporters are interests that will compete to be heard and influence policy).
Public health emergency In this scenario, a rapid series of public health emergency and climate change impacts will push traditional	DIRECTION: Strengthens the federal government's role in managing events or threats that (broadly conceived) endanger all Canadians. TIMING AND SPEED: Unpredictable,	Effective public health measures benefit the Canadian population as a whole. There is some potential for negative impacts on individual rights (e.g., quarantine regulations or international travel restrictions.)	Public health will remain a core function of government; there is unlikely to be any increase in the private sector's roles.	In themselves, this scenario's drivers do not increase healthcare costs significantly. However, there may be pressure on health budgets as governments	Assignment of public health response responsibility is based on legal mandates; however, given the ease with which emerging vectors travel, current law is much outdated. A series of federal-provincial bilateral agreements have to be signed. Needed is increased federal authority to manage contagious diseases by	Many of the required decisions and actions are technical in nature, and required institutions already exist in the form of public health agencies with appropriate mandates. Issues are largely addressed by health ministries. There may be some involvement of public safety and customs/

... continued

TABLE 9.1, continued

Scenario	Direction, Speed, Timing, Magnitude, and Drivers of Reform	Who Benefits Most? Who Benefits Least?	Role of Government vs. Private Provision in Funding Healthcare	Impact on Public Finances	Adequacy of Institutions/ Availability of Tools	Governance Arenas and Arrangements
healthcare policy issues away from the centre of the agenda.	though climate change projections suggest that there may be increases in exposure to disease vectors as the range of tropical insects grows. MAGNITUDE: The larger the effects of global climate change that are observed, the more traditional healthcare policy debates will be displaced. Impacts will vary dramatically by region. DRIVERS: Largely exogenous factors.			increase spending on climate change mitigation and adaptation. The costs of responding to actual emergencies should, in principle, be lower due to enhanced efficiency.	eliminating the requirement that disease must be found in at least two provinces before PHAC can take charge. Public health and hospital infrastructure services and protocols may demand upgrading to deal with contagious diseases and multi-drug resistant "super bugs."	immigration functions. There may be efforts to shift some questions to legal forums having to do with civil rights issues.

The final scenario, *public health emergency*, also offers governments a chance to be either proactive—to plan for public health challenges that can readily cross national and internal borders—or to react when confronted by crisis. Healthcare policy—and public policy generally—will be dominated by the need to respond to global climate change. The spread of disease-transmitting insects into new ranges, as well as the emergence of multi-drug resistant "superbugs" will increase the likelihood and frequency of communicable disease threats such as Ebola, Zika, or others as yet unknown. Similar to the 2003 SARS crisis, the inadequacy of hospital infrastructures and containment protocols will be revealed. Despite popular concern over the perceived magnitude of the danger, healthcare budgets will be constrained due to the need to invest heavily in climate change mitigation and adaptation strategies across policy sectors. While effective public health measures benefit the Canadian population as a whole, this scenario will see some negative impacts on individual rights (e.g., via quarantine requirements or international travel restrictions).

Table 9.1 provides a more structured summary of the highlights of, and provides additional details about, each of these five scenarios.

CONCLUSION—OR WHY IT IS SO HARD TO REFORM HEALTHCARE POLICY IN CANADA REDUX

What would a continuation of the status quo mean? Likely, no change in the core services funded by Medicare, with only small and variable reforms made incrementally at federal or provincial levels. There will continue to be interprovincial differences in wealth, and in political cultures/dominant ideas; over time, these may lead to further gradual divergence among provinces in access to and quality of care.

In our view, continuation of the status quo is not at all unlikely. However, the aim of the current analysis is to offer suggestions about the "leverage points" where advocates of health reform might focus attention if they want to bring about strategic change in the healthcare system. What might we conclude from this analysis?

At the federal level, dollars are still the main policy instrument available. If their use is accompanied by leadership and moral authority, as exercised in phase one and, to a lesser extent, parts of phase two, this might be a catalyst for health system reform (see Gardner, Fierlbeck, and Levy 2015 on this point; also see Forest, 2015, who in contrast downplays the necessity for federal leadership). Change in government is likely to be a time when windows for policy change open (Lazar et al. 2013a). The October 2015 transition to a federal Liberal government may signal new willingness to reengage with provinces, and to promote the Medicare plus scenario. The Liberals may return us to a period of increased deficit financing. However, if other policy instruments are considered, such as changes to the tax system, this might require additional sets of skills and knowledge, and additional and atypical partnerships to be cultivated by those who wish to influence healthcare policy changes.

Ideas change slowly for the most part, but there is evolution sometimes due to the introduction of new knowledge and evidence into the system (such as the growth of neo-liberal ideas and new public management-style approaches). Arm's length bodies, such as the former Health Council of Canada or the proposed Health Observatory, can be effective at bringing evidence to bear on policies. Egalitarian ideas have remained strong throughout the history of Medicare and are a powerful foundation for building and mobilizing support. We can envision changes among the balance of interests; pressures could see new ones arise and old ones lose in relative influence. Under some scenarios the finance bureaucracy or health bureaucracy will hold sway, while in other circumstances inter-departmental models like "health-in-all-policies" (Stahl et al. 2006) will allow new access points. The privileged position of organized medicine is likely to continue, especially in a future where we are unprepared for disruptive technologies. Changes in the basic institutions of healthcare and health policy are unlikely, but could radically reset the game. Greater power to sovereign First Nations governments may be one example.

Some external shocks are relatively predictable, others less so, but they tend to be reacted to rather than proactively anticipated. Climate change, potential disease-related vectors arising from this, and economic disruption seem most likely to have major impacts on the political, policy, and health systems. Thus we might hope that the worst effects of a public health emergency scenario could be averted with vigourous government preparation now; similarly, work on the regulatory infrastructure for drug safety might allow governments to get ahead of the impacts of new disruptive technologies that might otherwise create pressures that work against the solidaristic values of Medicare.

In short, reflecting on the history of healthcare reform in Canada, and on scenarios of its possible evolution, helps us to identify and assess factors that may enable more effective strategies for advancing policy change to be pursued by health system stakeholders and advocates in the public, the professions, and academia.

REFERENCES

Advisory Panel on Healthcare Innovation. 2015. *Unleashing Innovation: Excellent Healthcare for Canada* (Naylor Report).

Apolliono, D. E., and L.A. Bero. 2007. "The Creation of Industry Front Groups: The Tobacco Industry and 'Get Government Off Our Back.'" *American Journal of Public Health*, 97: 419–427.

Barer, M. L., R. G. Evans, and C. Hertzman. 1995. "Avalanche or glacier? Health Care and the Demographic Rhetoric." *Canadian Journal on Aging* 14(2): 193–224.

Bhatia, V. 2010. "Social Rights, Civil Rights, and Health Reform in Canada." *Governance: An International Journal of Policy, Administration, and Institutions*; 23(1): 37–58.

Bounajm F. 2013. "Health Care in Canada: An Economic Growth Engine."

Briefing 1—The Economic Footprint of Health Care Delivery in Canada.
Ottawa ON: Conference Board of Canada.

Boychuk, T. 2009. "After Medicare: Regionalization and Canadian Health Care Reform." *Canadian Bulletin of Medica History* 26(2): 353–378.

Broussele, Astrid, and Damien Contadriopoulos. 2015. "Why Trudeau Must Save Medicare in Quebec." *Toronto Star,* 5 November.

CADTH (Canadian Agency for Drugs and Technologies in Health). 2011. *Shared Services in Health Care*; Environmental Scan.

CFHI (Canadian Foundation for Healthcare Improvement). 2015. "Taming of the Queue, 2015." http://www.cfhi-fcass.ca/NewsAndEvents/Events/Taming_of_the_Queue.aspx

CHSRF (Canadian Health Services Research Foundation). 2010. "Mythbusters website." Now archived at http://www.cfhi-fcass.ca/Migrated/PDF/Mythbusters/mythbusters_APN_en_FINAL.pdf

CIHI (Canadian Institute for Health Information). 2014. *National Health Expenditure Trends, 1975–2014.*

———. 2015. *Wait Times for Priority Procedures in Canada, 2015.*

Carson, A. S. 2015. "Why Canadians Need a System-Wide Healthcare Strategy." In *Toward a Healthcare Strategy for Canadians*, edited by A. S. Carson, J. Dixon, and K. R. Nossal, 11–37. Montreal and Kingston: McGill-Queen's University Press.

Cheng, A. H., and J. M. Sutherland. 2013. "British Columbia's Pay-for-Performance Experiment: Part of the Solution to Reduce Emergency Department Crowding?" *Health Policy* 113(1-2): 86–92.

Cohn, D. 2015. "Chaouilli Ten Years On: Still About Nothing?" Paper presented at the 2015 Canadian Political Science Association conference, Ottawa ON.

Cohn, M. R. 2015. "The Plan to Reboot Health Care, Home Care in Ontario." *Toronto Star,* 17 December. http://www.thestar.com/news/queenspark/2015/12/17/the-plan-to-reboot-health-care-home-care-in-ontario-cohn.html

Commission d'étude sur les services de santé et les services sociaux (Clair Report for Quebec). Emerging Solutions. 2001. http://publications.msss.gouv.qc.ca/acrobat/f/documentation/2001/01-109-01a.pdf

Commission on Medicare (Fyke Report for Saskatchewan). 2001. *Caring for Medicare—Sustaining a Quality System.*

Commission on the Future of Health Care in Canada (Romanow Commission Interim and Final Reports).2002. "Shape the Future of Health Care." February. http://www.publications.gc.ca/collections/Collection/CP32-76-2002E.pdf

Derfel, Aaron. 2015. "Bill 20: IVF No Longer Covered Under Medicare, Private-Clinic Fees Soon to be Regulated." *Montreal Gazette,* 10 November. http://montrealgazette.com/news/local-news/bill-20-ivf-no-longer-covered-under-medicare-private-clinic-fees-soon-to-be-regulated

Dick, Don, and Linda Woodhouse. 2014. "Take a Look at Alberta Before Fretting Over Hospital Wait Times." *Globe and Mail.* 19 June. http://www.

theglobeandmail.com/opinion/take-a-look-at-alberta-before-fretting-over-hospital-wait-times/article19236516/

Drummond, Don. 2010. "Charting a Path to Sustainable Health Care in Ontario." TD Bank. http://lin.ca/resource-details/17316

Forbes, Cindy. 2015. "Statement." 4 October. https://www.cma.ca/En/Lists/Medias/2015-oct04-cma-statement-bill20-e.pdf

Forest, P-G. 2015. "A Case of Severe Withdrawal Syndrome." *Healthcare Papers* 14(3): 39–44.

Forget, C. E. 2005. "Promises, Promises—Setting Boundaries Between Public and Private." In *Access to Care, Access to Justice: The Legal Debate Over Private Health Insurance in Canada*, edited by C. M. Flood, K. Roach, and L. Sossin, 393-412. Toronto: University of Toronto Press.

Fraser Institute. 2015. "Waiting Your Turn: Wait Times for Health Care in Canada," 2015 Report. 8 December. https://www.fraserinstitute.org/studies/waiting-your-turn-wait-times-for-health-care-in-canada-2015-report

Gardner, W., K. Fierlbeck, and A. Levy. 2015. "Breaking the Deadlock: Towards a New Intergovernmental Relationship in Canadian Healthcare." *Healthcare Papers* 14(3): 7–15.

Gillam, S. J., A. N. Siriwardena, and N. Steel. 2012. "Pay-For-Performance in the United Kingdom: Impact of the Quality and Outcomes Framework—A Systematic Review." *Annals of Family Medicine* 10(5): 461–468.

Globerman, S. (editor). 2013. *Reducing Wait Times for Health Care: What Canada Can Learn From Theory and International Experience*. Vancouver BC: The Fraser Institute.

Health Canada. 2014. *Canada Health Act: Annual Report, 2013–2014*, http://www.hc-sc.gc.ca/hcs-sss/alt_formats/pdf/pubs/cha-ics/2014-cha-lcs-ar-ra-eng

Kershaw, P. 2015. *Measuring the Age Gap in Canadian Social Spending*. Vancouver, BC: Generation Squeeze (UBC Human Early Learning Partnership).

Kent, T. 1988. *A Public Purpose*. Montreal: McGill-Queen's University Press.

Kiran, T., A. S. Wilton, R. Moineddin, L. Paszat, and R. H. Glazier. 2014. "Effect of Payment Incentives on Cancer Screening in Ontario Primary Care." *Annals of Family Medicine* 12(4): 317–323.

Labrie, Y. 2015. *The Public Health Care Monopoly on Trial: The Legal Challenges Aiming to Chance Canada's Health Care Policies*. Montreal, QC: Montreal Economic Institute.

Lavis, J. N., S. E. Ross, J. E. Hurley, J. M. Hohenadel, G. L. Stoddart, C. A. Woodward, and J. Abelson. 2002. "Examining the Role of Health Services Research in Public Policymaking." *Milbank Quarterly* 80(1): 125–154.

Lazar, H, and J. Church. 2013. "Patterns in the Factors That Explain Health-Care Policy Reform." In *Paradigm Freeze: Why It Is So Hard to Reform Health Care in Canada, edited by* H. Lazar, P-G. Forest, J. N. Lavis, and J. Church, 219-252. Montreal/Kingston: McGill-Queen's University Press.

Lazar, H., P-G. Forest, J. N. Lavis, and J. Church (editors). 2013a. *Paradigm Freeze: Why It Is So Hard to Reform Health Care in Canada*. Montreal/

Kingston: McGill-Queen's University Press.

Lazar, H., P-G. Forest, J. N. Lavis, and J. Church. 2013b. *"Canadian Health-Care Reform: What Kind? How Much? Why?"* In *Paradigm Freeze: Why It Is So Hard to Reform Health Care in Canada*, edited by H. Lazar, P-G. Forest, J. N. Lavis, and J. Church, 219-252. Montreal/Kingston: McGill-Queen's University Press.

Lewis, S., and D. Kouri. 2004. "Regionalization: Making Sense of the Canadian Experience." *Healthcare Papers* 5(1): 12–31.

Li, J., J. Hurley, P. DeCicca, and G. Buckley. 2014. "Physician Response to Pay-For-Performance: Evidence From a Natural Experiment." *Health Economics* 23(8): 962–78.

Maioni, A. 1998. *Parting at the Crossroads: The Emergence of Health Insurance in the United States and Canada*. Princeton, NJ: Princeton University Press.

Marchildon, G. 2013. "Canada: Health System Review." *Health Systems in Transition* 15:1. Geneva: WHO Europe.

————. 2014. "The Three Dimensions of Universal Medicare in Canada." *Canadian Public Administration* 57(3): 362–82.

Meili, Ryan, and Danielle Martin. 2015. "Federal Politicians Should be Denouncing Quebec's New Move on Health-Care Fees." *Montreal Gazette*. 13 October.   http://montrealgazette.com/news/quebec/opinion-federal-politicians-should-be-denouncing-quebecs-new-move-on-health-care-fees

Maxwell, J., S. Rosell, and P-G. Forest. 2003. "Giving Citizens a Voice in Healthcare Policy in Canada." *BMJ* 326: 1031–33.

McIntosh, T., M. Ducie, M. Burka-Charles, J. Church, J. Lavis, M-P. Pomey, N. Smith, and S. Tomblin. 2010. "Population Health and Health System Reform: Needs-Based Funding for Health Services in Five Provinces." *Canadian Political Science Review*, 4(1): 42-61. doi:http://ojs.unbc.ca/index.php/cpsr/article/view/130/278

Mendelson, M., and P. Divinsky. 2002. *Canada 2015: Globalization and the Future of Canada's Health and Health Care*. Caledon Institute of Social Policy.

Mhatre, S. L., and R. B. Deber. 1998. "From Equal Access to Health Care to Equitable Access to Health: A Review of Canadian Provincial Health Commissions and Reports." In *Health and Canadian Society: Sociological Perspectives*, 3rd edition, edited by D. Coburn, C. D'Arcy, and G. M. Torrance, 459-484. Toronto: University of Toronto Press.

Morgan, S. G., M. Law, J. R. Daw, L. Abraham, and D. Martin. 2015. "Estimated Cost of Universal Public Coverage of Prescription Drugs in Canada." *Canadian Medical Association Journal*. doi:10.1503/cmaj.141564

Mossialos, E., M. Wenzel, R. Osborne, and C. Anderson. 2015. *International Profiles of Health Care Systems*. New York, NY: The Commonwealth Fund.

Munson, James. 2015. "Pharmacare Deferred: What Happens After Ottawa Starts Buying Drugs in Bulk?" *iPolitics*. 26 March. http://ipolitics.ca/2015/03/26/pharmacare-deferred-what-happens-after-ottawa-starts-buy-

ing-drugs-in-bulk/
National Forum on Health. 1997. "Canada Health Action: Building on the Legacy." www.hc-sc.gc.ca/hcs-sss/pubs/renewal-renouv/1997-nfoh-fnss-v1/ index-eng.php
National Physician Survey. 2013. *National Physician Survey 2013 Backgrounder.* http://nationalphysiciansurvey.ca/wp-content/uploads/2013/10/ OFFICIAL-RELEASE_NPS-2013-Backgrounder_EN.pdf
O'Reilly P. 2001. "The Federal/Provincial/Territorial Health Conference System." In *Federalism, Democracy and Health Policy in Canada*, edited by D. Adams, 107–30. Montreal-Kingston: McGill-Queen's University Press.
Palmer, K. S., T. Agoritsas, D. Martin et al. 2014. "Activity-Based Funding of Hospitals and Its Impact on Mortality, Readmission, Discharge Destination, Severity of Illness, and Volume of Care: A Systematic Review and Meta-Analysis." *PLOS One* 9(10): e109975.
Peterson, L. A., D. W. LeChauncey, T. Urech, C. Daw, and S. Sookanan. 2006. "Does Pay-For-Performance Improve the Quality of Care?" *Annals of Internal Medicine* 145(4): 265–72.
Prada, G., and T. Brown. 2012. *The Canadian Health Care Debate: A Survey and Assessment of Key Studies.* Ottawa, ON: The Conference Board of Canada.
Premier's Advisory Council on Health for Alberta (Mazankowski Report for Alberta). 2001. "A Framework for Reform." *Report of the Premier's Advisory Council on Health.* December.
Robson, W. B. P. 2001. *Will the Baby Boomers Bust the Health Budget? Demographic Change and Health Care Financing and Reform.* Ottawa: CD Howe Institute.
Royal College of Physicians and Surgeons of Canada. 2010. "Bridging the Gap. Building Collaborative Foundations for an Effective and Efficient Health Care System." Brief to the House of Commons Standing Committee on Finance, August 13. http://www.royalcollege.ca/portal/page/portal/rc/common/documents/advocacy/bridging_the_gap_e.pdf
Simpson, J. 2015. "Why a Health-Care Report was Dead on Arrival in Ottawa." *The Globe and Mail,* July 22. http://www.theglobeandmail.com/ opinion/why-a-key-health-care-report-was-dead-on-arrival-in-ottawa/article25608277/
Stahl, T., M. Wismar, E. Ollila, E. Lahtinen, and K. Leppo (editors). 2006. *Health in All Policies: Prospects and Potentials.* Helsinki: Finnish Ministry of Social Affairs and Health.
Standing Senate Committee on Social Affairs, Science and Technology (Kirby Report). *The Health of Canadians—The Federal Role.* 2002. www.parl. gc.ca/Content/SEN/Committee/372/SOCI/rep/repoct02vol6-e.htm
Sutherland, J. 2011. "Hospital Payment Mechanisms: An Overview and Options for Canada." *CHSRF* series on cost drivers and health system efficiency: Paper 4. Ottawa ON: Canadian Health Services Research Foundation.
Taber, Jane. 2012. "Provinces to Bulk-Buy Generic Drugs in Bid to Cut Health

Costs." *Globe and Mail*. 26 July. http://www.theglobeandmail.com/news/
politics/provinces-to-bulk-buy-generic-drugs-in-bid-to-cut-health-costs/article4442541/

Taylor, M. G. 1978. *Health Insurance and Canadian Public Policy: The Seven Decisions that Created the Canadian Health Insurance System*. Montreal: McGill-Queen's University Press.

Tuohy, C. H. 1999. *Accidental Logics: The Dynamics of Change in the Health Care Arena in the United States, Britain, and Canada*. Oxford: Oxford University Press.

Van Notten, P. W. F., J. Rotmans, M. B. A. van Asselt, and D. S. Rothman. 2003. "An Updated Scenario Typology." *Futures* 35: 423–443.

Vollmar, H. C., T. Ostermann, and M. Redaelli. 2015. "Using the Scenario Method in the Context of Health and Health Care—a Scoping Review." *BMC Medical Research Methodology* 15(89): doi:10.1186/s12874-015-0083-1

Wilkinson, A, and R. Kupers. 2013. "Living in the Futures." *Harvard Business Review*.

Wranik, D., and A. Katz. 2015. "A Typology of Pay-For-Performance Programs in Publicly Funded Primary Health Care Systems." *Health Systems and Policy Research* 2: 1.

Chapter 10

AN ACTION PLAN FOR REFORMING HEALTHCARE IN CANADA

DON DRUMMOND AND TALITHA CALDER

The purpose of this chapter is to set out a strategy for government action to reform healthcare in Canada. It picks up from earlier work (Drummond 2015), which argued that there is enough consensus on the substance of meaningful healthcare reform in Canada, but a lack of political will to deliver. Furthermore, it suggested that the conditions could be put in place to bolster that political will and create an environment in which governments would deliver meaningful reform over the next few years.

A number of recent studies and events have done a great deal to create the conditions needed for political will. In particular, they have illuminated the present problems with healthcare and offered good suggestions for improvement. Perhaps most importantly, they have conditioned the public to expect—and even want to see—healthcare reform. The absence of a sharp rebound in government revenues since the 2009–10 recession has kept the fiscal imperative of containing healthcare cost growth top of mind. The time has come for governments to broaden and deepen the piecemeal reforms underway. But they must do so strategically in this, perhaps the most politically sensitive of all policy fields.

Drummond's 2015 paper suggested that the healthcare reform debate should look at the conditions that supported bold policy reforms in other areas, including deficit reduction, free trade, value-added sales taxes, public pensions, and

Managing a Canadian Healthcare Strategy, edited by A. Scott Carson and Kim Richard Nossal. Montreal and Kingston: McGill-Queen's University Press, Queen's Policy Studies Series. © 2016 The School of Policy Studies, Queen's University at Kingston. All rights reserved.

others. In each of those cases, governments acted boldly despite considerable opposition from the public and legislatures. Certain common conditions can be found, or in many cases were created, with each of these major reforms. They are

- identification of a clear, significant problem with negative externalities beyond the community directly affected;
- a critical mass of analysis and research suggesting a course for policy reform;
- a clear sense of the objectives of reform;
- models upon which to base policy reform, often drawing upon international experience;
- alignment of at least some key stakeholders with the intended direction of reform and vocal supporters; and
- options to phase in reforms.

In the strategy for healthcare reform set out here, we will be addressing how to complete the creation of favourable conditions for reform, and then how to move forward in the political space opened.

The chapter is structured in accordance with a sensible sequence for reform in any policy area, outlined below in Figure 10.1:

Figure 10.1
Sequence for Policy Reform

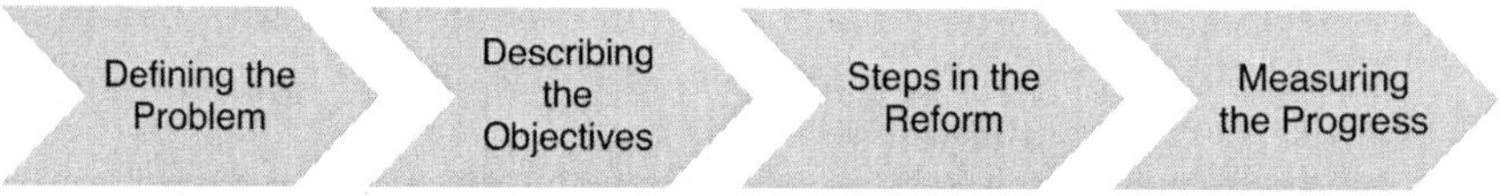

| Defining the Problem | Describing the Objectives | Steps in the Reform | Measuring the Progress |

Before this, however, it is first necessary to situate proposals in the context of reforms undertaken, to identify the governments that constitute the target audience, and to address how to engage stakeholders in reform processes.

RECOGNIZING REFORMS UNDERWAY

No jurisdiction in Canada is starting healthcare reform from scratch. Most provinces and territories would argue, with considerable justification, that they are already in the midst of health policy reform; some would even argue that reform is a continuum. So it is necessary to define what changes in strategy are in order.

The most basic distinction between what we are calling for in this chapter and existing processes is the need to emphasize system-wide strategies. Healthcare consists of many parts, but these too often operate as silos. A central tenet of most reform proposals is to make the parts work better together to improve health outcomes at the same or at lower costs. System-wide strategies change the nature of the reform process considerably, most notably by involving stakeholders, including the public, more directly. We argue that this requires governments to be clearer and more transparent in their reform intentions, and to work more closely with stakeholders than would be required under piecemeal change.

WHAT GOVERNMENT IS BEING ADDRESSED?

A national focus on health policy reform has some attractive features, such as supporting portability of care across provinces and territories, lowering costs through economies, and creating comparable standards for all Canadians. During its nine years in office, the Harper Conservative government showed little interest in playing a large role in healthcare, and provinces to date have only dealt collectively with healthcare in selective areas. The lack of federal involvement over almost 10 years may have been, in part, a reflection on previous federal-provincial accords, where the federal government provided funding, but the provinces did not give a detailed account of improvements in return for the money. This speaks to a classic challenge in federal systems where one level of government provides funding for policies and programs, which are properly in the jurisdiction of another level of government. The resulting muddled lines of accountability can compromise the transparency and efficiency of how the funds are used. The Liberal federal government elected in October 2015 may be more involved in healthcare than their predecessors. However, it seems as if much of the health policy reform that will be implemented over the next few years will be driven by provinces and territories acting without federal leadership—or the federal government may play a supporting or co-ordinating role. Such an approach may still yield common factors across the country over time as success in one jurisdiction is modelled in others.

In general, the strategy for health policy reform set out in this chapter is targeted at a specific province or territory. However, there are at least four aspects of reform where a broader, and pan-Canadian or national, perspective might be particularly applicable. First, some have argued that a national pharmacare program should be a top priority, even though this has been debated in Canada for decades with no progress. However, provincial governments have recently been working together on obtaining better pharmaceutical prices than could be accessed by provinces acting individually. As well, the federal minister of health recently asked Ontario to lead discussions about national pharmacare. At a minimum, a pan-Canadian approach could be strengthened to obtain better pharmaceutical prices.

Second, better care for the rapidly growing number of elderly Canadians is a high priority for reform. This, too, could have national elements. For example, governments in Canada could set out common standards of care for the elderly that each jurisdiction could work toward, with a number of provinces working together to achieve those standards.

Third, the federal government could play a lead role in healthcare innovation. This could be shaped by the July 2015 report of the Advisory Panel on Healthcare Innovation chaired by Dr. David Naylor. Federal action could lead to pan-Canadian improvements, particularly if the federal government established an innovation fund, and if the ideas were supported by all provinces.

Finally, there is a need for better health information. There would be economic and portability advantages to developing this on a national, pan-Canadian basis. For our purposes here, efforts to establish national pharmacare and eldercare programs will be encouraged, but will not be assumed. Instead, the focus in these and other areas will be on individual provinces and territories. In contrast, much of the focus on improved information will be at the national level, building upon institutions already in place.

National or pan-Canadian elements of healthcare could result from two opposing strategies. One could be a top-down approach, where the federal or provincial and territorial governments act together to set standards to be adopted within their respective jurisdictions. This seems unlikely over the next few years, other than in selected areas such as pharmaceutical pricing.

A second approach would be a bottom-up approach, in which best practices from one province or territory are emulated by others. Given contemporary conditions, this seems a more likely possibility. The strength of such a bottom-up approach would be bolstered by improved capacity of health information, and in particular the capacity to compare health outcomes and the efficiency of healthcare across provinces and territories. This would help identify best practices that could be adopted by others. It would also highlight jurisdictions that lag in the quality and efficiency of healthcare delivery. Individual provinces could and should look for such best practices, but an enhanced pan-Canadian capacity is also advised.

ENGAGING STAKEHOLDERS AND THE PUBLIC

We need to recognize that some aspects of healthcare reform are likely to be of limited interest to large numbers of Canadians. In those cases, governments can and should proceed with as little fanfare as possible. However, almost anything that involves system-wide reform will come to the attention of stakeholders, and that attention is likely to generate concerns. If not managed properly, those concerns may lead to governments backing down on reforms. The better course is to involve stakeholders, including the public, from the outset.

Healthcare reforms over the next 10 years will likely take place in an environment of ongoing fiscal constraint. Most jurisdictions will not try to lower healthcare costs, but most will be striving to slow down cost growth relative to revenues. This fiscal environment will preclude governments from injecting new funding that might "buy" support from those working in the health sector. Instead, workers in the sector may perceive that they could potentially lose something. So in addition to public wariness over change in healthcare, internal stakeholders may feel defensive and hence resist change. This is another reason to work closely with the healthcare workforce in the reform process and to ensure that to the greatest extent possible cost constraint results from efficiency gains rather than austerity measures.

We believe health policy reform in any Canadian jurisdiction should be anchored by a public document that accurately sets out the problem, the objectives, the steps to be taken, and the way that progress will be measured. Such policy statements proved crucial in the case of other major Canadian public policy initiatives. For example, the Conservative government of Brian Mulroney telegraphed much of its economic agenda in 1984 with the release of *A New Direction for Canada: An Agenda for Economic Renewal*. Similarly, 10 years later, the Liberal government of Jean Chrétien laid out its economic and fiscal plans in the so-called Purple and Grey Books. These documents conditioned the public to upcoming changes, drew stakeholders into reform processes, and provided a common script to bureaucrats and politicians in discussing change.

Despite the reforms underway in various provinces, no jurisdiction has yet communicated such a grand vision for health to the public and the healthcare sector's stakeholders. Presenting the larger picture for reform permits everyone to see how the pieces of change are to fit together to achieve a better outcome. Challenges in particular areas of reform should then become more manageable.

Stakeholders should be involved in a consultation exercise leading up to and following a public report on healthcare reform. This has been facilitated by the involvement of many stakeholder groups in recent years in publishing position papers on aspects of healthcare reform. Table 10.1 and Appendix A set out a selection of recent policy position papers by major healthcare stakeholder groups. It must be noted that the majority of stakeholder reports by national organizations are aimed at national reforms. So here we are disjointed. The policy capacity of stakeholder groups tends to be at the national association level, whereas the thrust of policy change of late—and, we suggest, for the foreseeable future—will be at the provincial level. This has created an unfortunate disconnect between healthcare stakeholders and policy development. Various stakeholder groups will need to make more of an effort to address their policy recommendations to the provinces.

Interactions with stakeholders during a reform process need not be acrimonious. Recent policy papers from organizations such as the Canadian Medical Association (CMA) and the Canadian Nurses Association (CNA) have been very much in line with the recommendations heard during the Queen's Health Policy Change Conference Series and are reflected in this chapter. This is not to say all would be smooth sailing, however. Attempts to address scope of practice, for example, could be highly contentious. It is noteworthy that the CMA and CNA have purposely chosen to leave this controversial area aside in their collaborative efforts. But all the major stakeholder groups support the general thrust of a high-quality, efficient, integrated, accessible, and equitable health system focused on individuals and families. Further, there are examples of collaborative input from stakeholders in previous reform exercises, including 10 health professional organizations working together under the Primary Health Care Transition Fund (PHCTF) in the early 2000s to enhance interdisciplinary collaboration in primary healthcare.

It would be advantageous for each jurisdiction to have a fairly independent

TABLE 10.1
Policy Position Papers by Canadian Healthcare Stakeholders

	Canadian Medical Association (CMA)	Canadian Nurses Association (CNA)	CMA & CNA	British Columbia Medical Association	New Brunswick Medical Society	Health Action Lobby	Health Council of Canada	Council of the Federation	Canadian Physiotherapy Association	Canadian Academy of Health Sciences	Canadian Health Services Research Foundation
Access	✓	✓	✓	✓	✓	✓					
Choice	✓				✓	✓		✓	✓	✓	✓
Clinical Autonomy	✓				✓						
Accountability			✓					✓	✓	✓	✓
Patient-Centred Care	✓	✓	✓	✓	✓		✓			✓	✓
Continuum of Care	✓	✓					✓			✓	
Quality	✓	✓	✓	✓	✓						
Sustainability	✓	✓	✓	✓	✓		✓				
Efficiency	✓			✓	✓						
Effectiveness	✓			✓							
Equity	✓	✓	✓								
National Leadership		✓				✓	✓	✓	✓	✓	
Triple Aim[1]	✓	✓	✓			✓	✓	✓	✓	✓	

[1] Better health, better care, better value

review of its healthcare as part of the process leading to such a public document. That provides the government with a reading of stakeholder perspectives and allows various reform ideas to be floated without the government having to take ownership and becoming defensive if there is controversy. Such reviews also condition the public and stakeholders to the notion of reform. Table 10.2 and Appendix B set out which provinces have had such reviews completed during the past four years. Many provinces have had recent external reviews of important segments of healthcare in recent years, but only Ontario and New Brunswick have had system-wide reviews. The other provinces should contemplate doing likewise.

TABLE 10.2
Independent Reviews of Provinces' Healthcare

	BC	AB	SK	MB	ON	QC	NB	NS	NL	PEI
Healthcare System			2008		2012	2001	2012/ 2013	2007		2008
Healthcare Governance		2013		2008						
Healthcare Funding						2013				
Hospital Care	2011									
Emergency Care	2014			2013				2010		
Ambulatory Care									2013	
Cancer Care	2013									
Long-Term Care					2012					
Rural Healthcare		2015								

We now return to the elements of a public document needed to launch broader healthcare reforms: defining the problem, describing the objectives, determining steps in the reform process, and then outlining how to monitor and measure progress.

THE STARTING POINT: DEFINING THE PROBLEM

Communication with the public should start with a better definition of the problem, in that the fiscal element is broadened by references to mediocre health outcomes and care and inefficiency. To the degree that the Canadian public is aware of problems with healthcare in the country, attention is likely on just two facets: rising costs and long wait times, especially for specialists. For those who contemplate efficiency, they are likely struck by the frequent necessity of going to hospitals when other sites of care (e.g., community health centres) have lower costs and higher client satisfaction.

When governments incurred large deficits in the late 2000s, they put enormous emphasis on how healthcare costs were rising faster than revenues. By now, numerous studies have pointed out how healthcare will continue to consume larger portions of revenues and hence threaten the sustainability of other programs or require ever-rising tax rates, which have likely caught the public's attention. So the "fiscal problem" has some traction. However, we argue that policy reform based solely on fiscal matters will not be successful; indeed, we believe that they will likely be met with public suspicion. There will be no support for reforms interpreted to solely drive down costs and save money, as Canadians will interpret cost cutting to healthcare as putting their health at risk.

In contrast to the fiscal dimension, there is little public awareness of the quality of Canadian healthcare and the efficiency with which it is delivered. These data are not available to make strong, sweeping statements about the quality of Canadians' health and how their healthcare compares to that of other countries, in part because the results vary widely by particular ailments. However, as documented in Carson (2015a) and Carson et al. (2015), the health of Canadians, and the quality of their overall healthcare, are about average in comparison to other developed economies. Yet in terms of dollars spent per capita, or as a ratio of Gross Domestic Product, international comparisons (e.g., OECD 2010), show that Canada, with some provincial variation, is part of a small group of countries that have one of the most expensive healthcare systems; indeed, it comes after the United States, which truly is in a universe of its own and thus should not even be used as a comparator (though Canadians always tend to compare their healthcare system with the US). Putting the two sides of the equation, outcomes and costs, together, means that Canada has inefficient healthcare. As Srivastava (2014) has noted, Canada spends 30 percent more public funding on health than would be required under an "efficient system" (based upon a hybrid of the best features across OECD countries).

Affordability of healthcare will be a third facet of concern to a portion of the Canadian public. Most Canadians are conditioned to believe we have a public healthcare system so affordability is not an issue. But that is only true of primary care. Overall, according to a report by the Canadian Institute for Health Information (CIHI), *National Expenditure Trends, 1975 to 2014*, private spending accounts for 30 percent of health-related costs in Canada. This is considerably higher than the average of developed countries. Private spending accounts for more than half of drug costs and more than 90 percent of non-primary, non-pharmaceutical costs, and that includes many aspects of mental health, one of the fastest growing areas of healthcare spending (CIHI 2014). Private insurance, both commercial and not-for-profit, is maturing to address private health costs. In 2012, a bit more than 40 percent of private healthcare costs were covered by private insurance, up from just over 29 percent in 1988 (CIHI 2014). Private insurance covers 60 percent of private drug costs and a similar coverage ratio applies in dental. In vision care, private insurance coverage is only 26 percent of private costs (CIHI 2014). Given the extensive public coverage in primary care and the availability to some people of private insurance for pharmaceuticals and other aspects of non-primary care, the affordability issue is not generalized for the whole population but rather acute for certain demographics, mainly for those who do not have access to employer-sponsored insurance plans.

Public acceptance of—and even support for—healthcare reforms will be more likely once the public is aware that Canada delivers mediocre healthcare at a high and rapidly rising cost, and that a significant number of Canadians face affordability barriers to accessing appropriate care.

DESCRIBING THE OBJECTIVES OF HEALTHCARE REFORM

A public document setting out a reform process must address the necessity of containing healthcare cost growth. But it should not unduly dwell on this problem, since that would frame the issue in a negative fashion for the public. So an accurate description of the problems should transition into clear objectives to demonstrate that with a more efficient approach better health outcomes are feasible.

The objectives of healthcare reform should be a high level of health, superior results from healthcare interventions in terms of measured health improvement, and patient and family satisfaction, delivered in an efficient manner that is accessible and affordable for all Canadians. In a public discussion paper these objectives can be described in an absolute sense and relative to other jurisdictions (where better outcomes that are realistic can be cited).

THE STEPS IN HEALTHCARE REFORM

All of the major steps in healthcare reform should be set out in a public document from the particular province or territory. But all are not equal in importance or in approach. Some steps will involve the public directly and these must be communicated and proceeded with carefully with extensive public consultation. Other steps will be contentious with particular healthcare stakeholders. Yet others are more internal matters that will be less visible to the public.

Enhancing the Role of External Agencies

The first major decision that must be made in the reform process is the division of roles between government and an independent body appointed by the government. We have argued that governments should use an independent body to provide an assessment of the provision of healthcare along with recommendations, informed by extensive consultations with stakeholders. There is an option to go further and have some of the reforms implemented by an external body similar to the Ontario Health Services Restructuring Commission chaired by Dr. Duncan Sinclair from 1996 to 2000. This option could relieve some of the political pressure, although ultimately all stakeholders will hold the relevant government accountable.

A second major decision must focus on how to organize the management of healthcare. Some have argued that responsibility must be moved away from the political realm (Carson 2015b). Since 2005, all provinces have devolved important parts of healthcare administration to arm's-length agencies. The agencies typically have their own boards, but provincial governments tend to appoint, or at least nominate, board members. The structure is there for the agencies to have a fair degree of independence, but the length of the arm, be it short or long, is influenced by practice as much as by design. There has been a great deal of change in the structure of these agencies, particularly over the number of entities in a province. In recent years there has been a trend toward consolidation into fewer regional agencies. However, on 18 March 2015, the Government of Alberta announced its intent to introduce eight to 10 "operational districts" within the highly centralized Alberta Health Authority (Alberta 2015a). Table 10.3 and Appendix C provide a summary of the diverse management structures of healthcare across the provinces.

Table 10.3
Administrative Management Structure of Healthcare in the Provinces

	BC	AB	SK	MB	ON	QC	NB	NS	NL	PEI
Provincial Health Authority	✔									
Local Health Integration Networks					✔					
Health Networks						✔				
Regional Health Authorities	✔		✔	✔					✔	
Single Health Authority		✔						✔		✔
Health and Social Service Agencies						✔				
First Nations Health Authority	✔									

Big Decisions Required: Pharmacare and Seniors' Care

The two steps in healthcare reform that would have the greatest impact on the public are a new pharmaceutical program and a different approach to seniors' care.

A national pharmacare program that would extend coverage to all Canadians and replace the current piecemeal provincial plans and the bits and pieces of private insurance that exist would inevitably create inefficiencies because most of the levers for controlling the use of pharmaceuticals are in the hands of the provinces and their agents. It would also raise tricky issues of federal-provincial transfers. A federally funded program would not only transfer money from people paying private insurers to paying the public insurer, but it would save billions of dollars to the provinces as well. Would the federal government then want a transfer of tax points back to them in return? ·

Given the division of responsibilities and budgeting for healthcare, it is inevitable that the provinces would need to be intimately involved in any national pharmacare program. That would clearly require a great deal of discussion at all levels of government, all the more so because there are important distinctions across existing provincial pharmaceutical policies, which could create challenges and even opposition to adopting a new, common scheme across the country. This necessary dialogue can be made easier by moving beyond the current mindset that a pharmacare program has to be either federally or provincially driven. It can, and should, be both. A pharmacare program in Canada could be modelled after the Canadian Pension Plan where the federal and provincial governments are joint custodians. Employees and employers make contributions to the Canada Pension Plan, and to a large extent this would likely be the structure of a pharmacare program as well. So that is another potential parallel. At any rate, the latest dialogue on a national program has just begun. Keeping in mind that such a scheme has been discussed in Canada for decades, no one should hold their breath waiting for it to happen. Yet the case for major reform in pharmaceuticals in Canada is compelling.

Relative to other countries, pharmaceuticals are expensive in Canada, and until recently the costs kept rising rapidly. In 2011, Canadians spent an average of $701 on pharmaceuticals, the second highest within the OECD, and well above the OECD average of $483 (U.S. dollar at PPP; OECD 2013). From the early 1990s until 2010, pharmaceuticals were one of the fastest growing cost components of healthcare in Canada. According to CIHI (2012, vii), drug costs increased slightly less than 0.1 percent in 2012. However, this may be due in part to temporary factors, such as fewer new drugs coming to market, some major ones coming off patent protection, and recent provincial moves to lower generic drug prices. In other words, these recent developments should not necessarily be taken as a sign that the cost curve has been permanently dampened. On the cost side, pharmaceuticals are consistent with overall healthcare in that Canada has a more expensive system compared to almost all other developed countries, except the United States.

In the case of primary care, Canadians can at least console themselves that the relatively high cost comes with comprehensive public coverage of costs, albeit with waiting times that are much longer than in most other developed countries. High public coverage of costs cannot be said for pharmaceuticals. Statistics Canada's Canadian Community Health Survey of 2007 indicated that almost 10 percent of Canadians do not take pharmaceuticals as directed due to cost considerations. Common factors for those unable to afford prescribed medication include poor health, low income, and lack of access to a private insurance plan. Of Canadian families without insurance, 26.5 percent were not able to afford the drugs as prescribed (Statistics Canada 2007). As some provinces cover drug costs for people on social assistance, the affordability issue is particularly acute for the low-income and working poor who do not have access to an employer-sponsored insurance plan. Indeed, in absolute level terms, the highest spending on prescription drugs occurs with the second lowest income quintile (CMA 2014a). There can still be affordability issues in families with some form of insurance as co-payments can be high.

There is great variation in provincial pharmaceutical plans (Dixon 2015). At the aggregate level, provincial plans pay 41.6 percent of drug costs, but this varies from a low of 23.9 percent in New Brunswick to 47.6 percent in Saskatchewan (CIHI 2012). Some provinces base coverage largely on income while others use age (as with seniors). Low-income residents on social assistance are typically covered, but in several provinces there is weak coverage, or relatively high co-payments for the working poor. Quebec has a unique model in that people who do not have private insurance are obliged, at a cost, to take public coverage.

A 2013 Commonwealth Fund General Public Survey found 8 percent of Canadians did not fill a prescription or skipped a dose in the last 10 months because of cost. This compares to only 2 percent in the United Kingdom. There was considerable variation across provinces, although at around 5 percent even the best Canadian performers, namely Saskatchewan and Quebec, are still not close to the UK. The affordability challenge was particularly acute in New Brunswick and Ontario with avoidance rates above 10 percent (Busby and Peddle 2014).

The overall approach to pharmaceuticals in Canada gets low marks for efficiency. At the aggregate level this is obvious from the high cost relative to other countries, which co-exists with poor access and affordability for low-income people. The fragmentation of the system has compromised purchasing power in getting better prices for brand and generic drugs, although recent initiatives are helping somewhat on that front. The multiple payers in the system raise administrative costs. And evidence exists that co-payments reduce optimal use of pharmaceuticals (see, for example, Tang, Ghali, and Manns 2014).

A fairly standard rationale for the lack of government drive to establish national pharmacare is the public cost. But a number of studies question whether there would be a significant net cost compared to the status quo. A public pharmacare system would lower costs through more efficient administration, greater ability to direct lower-cost pharmaceutical use, and lower prices through the benefits of greater bargaining power. To be netted against these gains are the costs the public sector would have to pick up from current private sector spending.

First, it should be clear that this is largely an issue of perception. Some form of taxpayer contribution might need to rise to cover this transfer of expenditure, but from the individual's perspective this is simply a transfer of a payment from a private insurer to the public sector. Second, the net increase in public spending may not be that large once the economies are considered. Marc-André Gagnon (2010) has argued that total costs would be reduced $10.7 billion per year under a public system. Morgan et al. (2015) calculate that total spending on pharmaceuticals would be $7.3 billion per year lower under a public program and this would break out as $8.2 billion in savings to the private sector and a net incremental public sector cost of around $1 billion per year— all figures from the central tendency estimates. To be sure, the Canadian Life and Health Insurance Association (CLHIA) disputes the very large estimates of cost savings from converting to a public pharmaceutical plan (Swedlove 2014). They argue that the estimates rely upon CIHI data on existing (partial) public administration that are not fully inclusive. Therefore, the CLHIA believes that the extrapolation to a cost estimate under a fully public system is substantially underestimated.

In light of a pan-Canadian dialogue on a national pharmacare program, it is troubling that there are such disparate views on the likely financial consequences. As support for that dialogue, a credible, independent body should be charged with examining the existing cost estimates and rendering a view on the differences and likely cost implications of a public system. In the absence of this, it is very difficult to assess the pros and cons of going in this direction. A round of talks with the provinces and the federal government is being launched on a national pharmacare program. Such an objective is worthy of support, but provinces may not wish to count on a positive outcome given Canada's long-suffering efforts aimed at such a national program.

In the meantime, there are many steps that can be taken, some nationally and some within provinces. From a financial perspective, the claimed benefits of sweeping pharmaceuticals into public coverage, as with primary health, are lower drug prices, greater facility to control costs through what drugs are used and how, and lower administration costs. Some gains can certainly be made on the first two fronts without going all the way to a public pharmacare program.

First, the Patented Medicine Prices Review Board could be strengthened. At present, the Board compares prices in Canada with seven countries that have comparatively high drug prices. It could shift the countries in the base, and it could extend its purview to generic drugs. This may be particularly important with the enactment of the Comprehensive Economic and Trade Agreement between Canada and the European Union. A great deal of attention has been paid to the prospect of higher brand drug prices in Canada due to the imposition of Europe's longer patent protection period. Less attention has been paid to the lower generic drug prices in much of Europe.

Second, the provinces could continue strengthening their efforts under the pan-Canadian Pharmaceutical Alliance (pCPA) to establish an opt-in system to "bulk buy" pharmaceuticals, meaning that lower base prices for both brand name and generic drugs would be established. If prices negotiated by the pCPA are not disclosed, it may be difficult for private insurers to benefit from the strides made by the public bodies. However, there should be a way to allow private insurers to benefit from price discounts negotiated by governments.

Third, the effectiveness and efficiency of pharmaceutical use could be improved in several ways. Better data and analysis on the effectiveness of medication would help if the findings were shared with physicians and pharmacists.

Provinces could tighten systems to monitor prescription use by individuals. As people can get prescriptions through different doctors and pharmacies they often end up with too many medications, some of which may essentially just be countering the effects of others. As in the case of British Columbia, greater latitude on therapeutic substitutes could also improve cost and efficiency.

Steps could also be taken within current structures to improve affordability. Some provinces are already addressing this. To be sure, Alberta, Ontario, Nova Scotia, and Prince Edward Island all have plans that are age-based rather than income-based other than to cover recipients of social welfare, or in some cases where drug costs exceed a certain percentage of family income. A minimalist reform in this area could be for these provinces to shift to an income-based plan, as already exists in the other provinces. This would require some political maneuvering as some seniors may lose the automatic subsidies they now enjoy, but low-income seniors would still be covered, as would the working poor who are now left to shoulder the full burden if they do not have a private plan. Going one step forward would be to consider the Quebec model with mandatory public coverage, at a cost, for those not in a private insurance plan. Premiums could be based on income, with care taken not to create steep marginal effective tax rates as income rises. In provinces with co-payments that may be creating affordability issues, a tighter link could be made to income and/or the medical value of the pharmaceutical. In general, the most likely reform model for improved affordability will be public coverage based on income with a deductible and co-payments that do not unduly impinge upon prescribed drug use. But lest it be thought that adopting a Quebec-style program is a simple answer for some other provinces, it must be pointed out that in March 2015 Quebec's Health and Welfare Commissioner reported that the prescription rate is too high in Quebec, drugs covered by the plan are not reviewed sufficiently often, insufficient efforts are made to use less expensive drugs, and too much is paid for pharmaceuticals in Quebec relative to the rest of Canada and other countries. The report is a sobering reminder that pharmaceutical policy needs to move on many fronts if it is to be fiscally sustainable and equitable to access.

As with healthcare in general, seniors' care features widespread problems of cost, inefficiency, access, and poor satisfaction of the elderly and their caregivers. Under the current system, the cost of long-term care services will roughly triple in constant dollars over the next 40 years. Public costs are estimated to rise from $24 billion to $71 billion (inflation-adjusted dollars) while private costs are expected to rise even faster from $44 billion to $116 billion (Blomqvist and Busby 2014). A survey commissioned by the Canadian Medical Association (2014b), *National Report on Health Care: Seniors Health Issues and the Impact of an Ageing Population*, revealed that only half of the respondents agree they can afford, or will be able to afford, to pay for the extra healthcare services that are not covered by medicare or their health insurance. In response to a slightly different question, 70 percent expressed concern about having enough money for uninsured services. The stress involved in seniors' care also comes through in the CMA survey, where 60 percent of respondents who participate in providing care report experiencing a high level of stress because of this.

There are a number of parallels between pharmacare and seniors' care. Neither is close to being fully covered by public sector plans. Private sector plans, usually through an employer, have filled part of the vacuum. But gaps remain for some people, typically those in the low to middle income range without access to a comprehensive employer-sponsored insurance plan. In the 2014 CMA survey on seniors' healthcare, 40 percent of respondents said they were very concerned about having enough money for a long stay in a long-term care facility or a long period of nursing care at home, and another 34 percent indicated they were somewhat concerned. Greatest concern is found among those close to retirement. So access and affordability of seniors' care are serious issues for a substantial portion of Canada's population.

Governments, whether federal or provincial, could move to sweep seniors' care more fully into the public sphere so that it is paid for through general tax revenues. Alternatively, the financing could be done through a more comprehensive system of co-payments. Alternatively, a new program could be introduced to encourage and facilitate individual savings accounts targeted at care in the later years of life. The latter two seem more likely given the significant tax increases that would be required under the first possibility and the widespread existence of private insurance plans. However, before delving more intensively into funding, it is advisable to address the uncertainty of costs people will face in their later years and the inefficiency of current seniors' care.

The most likely scenario for funding seniors' care would be for governments to cover some basic level of care, with individuals and their families responsible for anything above that. This could be a purely provincial scheme, or a federal-provincial program. A major problem with such a scenario is that there is tremendous uncertainty over what individuals and their families would be responsible for. In a perfect world, people would have a good idea of how much of a nest egg they need to accumulate before they reach the older, frailer years. But few have such insight because the present system is not transparent on cost and future directions are uncertain. It is not surprising, then, that the cost of home care or long-term care is not explicitly factored into people's lifetime savings plan. A high priority should be to change this approach. Most likely, the realistic amounts people will need to accumulate by age 65 or so are much higher than most are now contemplating. In the absence of such clarity, it is hard to imagine that any new savings vehicle tied to seniors' care could be successful.

We should also first ensure that the money for seniors' care is being used efficiently before settling on a path to raise more funding. Present systems are certainly not efficient. Dr. Chris Simpson, past-president of the CMA, refers to the system as "warehousing our seniors in hospitals" (2015). He points to the 15 percent of acute care hospital beds in Canada occupied by patients who do not need and are not receiving acute care and observes almost all of them are seniors. The hospitals are not equipped to deal with their chronic care needs and in the meantime these patients are "deconditioned, they fall, and they suffer hospital-acquired infections." In a study for the Ontario government in 2011,

Caring for Our Aging Population and Addressing Alternate Level of Care, Dr. David Walker (2011) describes how the situation begins with emergency rooms far too often being the point of entry for an elderly person into healthcare. Once in the hospital the elderly often languish without receiving the treatment and rehabilitation they need. Discharge procedures are often inefficient in that the elderly are not directed to the care that would maximize their prospects of returning to an independent life. Long-term care facilities do not tend to include a capacity to, in the words of Dr. Walker, "assess and restore." Simpson estimates the cost of a hospital bed at $1,000 per day compared to $130 for long-term care and $55 for home care. The potential savings from shifting from hospitals to long-term care and home care are estimated by the CMA at $2.3 billion a year.

One objective of a better seniors' care system is, of course, a more sustainable financial situation. That would involve extracting a dividend from making care more efficient. And it would require identifying and securing a source of funds for the increase in costs due to the sharply rising number of elderly. There are many options to consider for how to cover the inevitable rise in the cost of seniors' care. Private savings could play a larger role. That could happen through greater promotion of existing vehicles such as RRSPs, TFSAs, and reverse mortgages, or it could occur through the creation of a new savings vehicle, such as Medical Savings Accounts, modelled after the TFSA, but for the explicit use of funding long-term care.

Alternatively, there could be more formal reliance on private insurance, such as through a system where individuals contribute to a risk pool and draw from that pool on the basis of the evaluation of their needs by a multidisciplinary assessment team. Another option that combines private insurance with public support is a voucher system whereby governments provide means-tested subsidies (vouchers) and individuals are left to cover the rest of the costs. Or the public sector could take on most or all of the cost, funded either through general revenues or a new contribution plan along the lines of Employment Insurance and the Canada Pension Plan.

While the discussion on future funding should begin in earnest, we must recognize that there are many other aspects of seniors' care that need immediate attention. We must start by looking at seniors' care from the perspective of elders themselves. Dr. Duncan Sinclair (2015), former vice principal (Health Sciences) and dean of Queen's Faculty of Medicine, spoke from a personal perspective in remarks to the Tech Value Net Conference on Improving Care for the Frail Elderly in February 2015. Dr. Sinclair acted as an eloquent spokesperson for many Canadians when he said that when he becomes frail, dependent, and in need of on-going care, his wants and needs would include continued dignity, remaining in his home, avoiding pain and suffering, and not being a burden to others. Current arrangements are not suitable to deliver on these fronts for many seniors.

An instinctive reaction to projections of sharply rising numbers of elderly people is to build more long-term care facilities. But that goes against the grain of care efficiency and the aspirations enunciated by Dr. Sinclair and likely felt by the majority of people. The Danish model, which prohibited building more long-term care facilities and instead focused on improving home-based care, is a better course for Canada. Not only is this a lower-cost option, but it also results in higher satisfaction of the elderly and their families. Provinces would need to increase their resources for home care and the attendant co-ordination required in order to move in this direction. In part, this funding could and should come from money now being given to hospitals, as the number of seniors in hospitals should be reduced. In most provinces, other steps required would include increasing programs to provide house-calls by nurse practitioners, enhancing integration of community care and service providers and hospitals, promoting renovation tax credits for homes, and establishing standards for personal care workers.

Many changes would be required to provide better quality and more efficient care for the elderly. The starting point would be to move the focal point from the emergency wards of hospitals to community care settings. There, a better capacity could be built to assess the needs of the elderly and design appropriate care strategies, with an emphasis on supporting people in their homes. Primary care providers would need to be much more involved in the diagnosis and rehabilitation plans. And long-term care facilities would need to devote a good portion of their resources to these providers in order to ensure that a number of their clientele do not become permanent residents.

It is critical to ask who should take the lead. The CMA calls for a "national seniors' healthcare strategy" and this was backed up by 95 percent of the respondents in their 2014 survey. Of those respondents, 91 percent agreed that the strategy should find ways to "keep elderly patients living at home for as long as possible and not in hospitals or long-term care facilities." It is encouraging that there is an alignment of the aspirations of people with the analysis of efficiency of care. The CMA has been less clear on why the strategy needs to be national and what exactly that means. However, it is clear they mean for the federal government to take a prominent role. A natural reason for a broad initiative is that similar situations appear across the country, so common approaches would be sensible. But that does not mean the drive must necessarily be from the federal government or even "national" as opposed to "pan-Canadian." As with other aspects of healthcare, a national approach has the advantage of providing consistent standards of care across the country. Some political cover would be offered to individual jurisdictions if all or at least many moved in a similar fashion at the same time. Any new savings vehicle would be facilitated if operated through the national tax system. As with most other aspects of healthcare, reform of seniors' care could at least start at the provincial level, whether by an individual province or more than one operating together. Progress need not be stymied if a national approach is not forthcoming over the next few years.

One strategy for moving toward what might ultimately be a national seniors' care system is for governments across Canada to begin discussing standards of care to which each of them could aspire. Even if the standards were common, they might get there in different ways and at different paces. As often happens in Canada, a study for a particular province has applicability across the country. In this regard, all provinces should look at the study done for Ontario in 2012 by Dr. Samir Sinha, "Living Longer, Living Well." The report revolves around five principles for seniors' care: equity, access, choice, value, and quality. These principles would likely be agreed to by all jurisdictions. Dr. Sinha went on to make specific recommendations that are, on occasion, somewhat specific to Ontario, but that for the most part apply, perhaps with a few tweaks, to other provinces. For example, he addressed the promotion of health and wellness, improved funding for house calls to reduce the incidence of seniors going to and staying in hospitals, enhanced home and community care services, and improved flows to and from long and short stay care facilities, among many other areas (Sinha 2012, 11–15).

Steps to Increase Efficiency

Several provinces are already implementing steps to drive up efficiency of healthcare and this effort should be continued. Examples include moving away from cost-plus budgeting of hospitals to basing financing on performance; shifting some portion of physician compensation away from a per service fee to a salary model; greater differentiation across institutions that reflects their relative efficiency in particular areas; and more and better use of health information and records. The structural changes need to be complemented by clearer objectives and measurement against those objectives. For example, Ontario and other provinces have moved more care to healthcare clinics. In theory this makes sense as it moves care aware from higher-cost hospitals while still allowing economies across caregivers. But expected outcomes were not clearly set for the clinics and outcomes have been only weakly recorded, so it has been difficult to measure their efficiency.

A second priority would be better integrated care across the sectors—hospital, community, primary care, specialty, home care, social welfare, and so on. In general, less emphasis should be placed on hospitals as the epicentre of care. They have high costs, increased risk of infection, and generally result in lower patient satisfaction. Several provinces have expanded the use of healthcare clinics. In Ontario, there has been an expansion of nurse-led clinics and these have recorded lower costs and higher levels of patient satisfaction.

Considerable savings would likely be realized in every province and territory through paying more attention, and better coordinating the care of the small portion of the population accounting for a very large share of the costs. For example, in Ontario, about 1 percent of the population accounts for 49 percent of hospital and home care costs, and 10 percent of the population accounts for 95 percent of such costs (Drummond 2012, Ch. 5). The costs will always be sharply skewed because some people are very sick and require expensive care while the majority enjoys good health. But a good portion of the high cost of the minority results from weak co-ordination of their care. Indeed, until recently, little was known about this group. Patients with congestive heart failure might be dismissed from hospital without notice to their physician or community nurse. A timely visit by that nurse, which is often not feasible due to lack of notice, might prevent an expensive and dissatisfying return to hospital.

Stronger standards for medical approaches and conducts of practice would improve the quality and efficiency of care. In some areas these are strong now, such as in certain areas of cancer, but in general there is little guidance provided to physicians and other caregivers.

Scope of Practice

The Ontario Nurses' Association has argued that 70 percent of what physicians do can be completed by nurses. This finding has also been supported by an extensive body of research, which has found that nurses and physician assistants can handle up to 70 to 80 percent of the care that primary care physicians typically provide (Scheffler 2008). To a degree, the efficiency gains associated with this are being garnered by nurse-led clinics. One could argue that a more efficient allocation of care across stakeholders would involve more than shifting roles between physicians and nurses. This would obviously be a contentious area of reform within stakeholder groups who may perceive change as a threat to their incomes. Thus, close consultation with stakeholders would be required. An option to be explored is the extent to which responsibility for scope of practice could be shifted to the local or hospital level. Informal discussions among hospital administrators during the second Queen's Health Policy Change conference led to suggestions that very large reductions in budget, with no loss and possible improvements to quality, could result if there were greater local autonomy in human resource management.

Human Resources Planning

Human resources planning in healthcare is largely the responsibility of the provinces and territories, either directly or through their faculties of medicine. The shortages of some specialists, and hence the long wait times, can be laid at the doorstep of this planning process and interaction with other elements of public policy such as compensation. For example, the shortage of gerontologists has long been known and will get worse with the ageing of the population. This is not likely unrelated to gerontology being one of the lowest paid fields within medicine. Closer attention needs to be paid to demographic and technological changes (for example, fewer physicians in certain areas such as cataract surgery, radiology, cardiac surgery, and so on are now required), and this insight must be used to change the inflows into medical schools and alter compensation schemes to provide the required incentives.

Blomqvist, Busby, Jacobs, and Falk (2015) add another human resources reason to consider in terms of giving more authority to hospitals for budgeting. They argue that hospitals should pay for specialists' services and that this should include negotiating pay and access to hospitals' facilities. The case is made that this would better match available specialists with hospital capacity.

Full Circle to The Ultimate Goal: Promoting and Maintaining Good Health

In the long run, improving health outcomes at a sustainable, affordable cost to society will require the promotion and maintenance of good health, and not just efficiency gains in biomedical care. Most provinces are active in public education campaigns on the negative health effects of smoking and alcohol abuse, there have been some provincial and federal participACTION initiatives, and some jurisdictions dabble in student nutrition program initiatives. But, in general, Canada's healthcare system is inadequate to tackle public health challenges and must be improved. This should extend to long-run perspectives on who is most likely to get sick and under what conditions. In doing so, greater attention would be paid to the conditions that lead to such poor health outcomes for the most vulnerable and marginalized Canadians, including indigenous and racialized people, immigrants and newcomers, women, children, and the low-income and working poor. A more holistic approach may well determine that the best way of lowering future healthcare costs is to invest in the education of high-risk youth, or in more affordable housing for low-income families.

More specific changes could be instituted in the area of health promotion. For example, it is probably not a coincidence that Canada has one of the highest rates in the developed world of hospitalization of adults with Type II diabetes, and one of the lowest incidences of people with diabetes or at risk of diabetes taking the recommended, regular blood tests. If there were a tighter link between health promotion and healthcare, these rates would be reversed. (It is both ironic and perverse that our cars tell us how many kilometres until the next oil change but we have no equivalent for our bodies.)

Much of the problem with promoting and maintaining good health comes down to the objectives and compensation models for healthcare providers. As the objectives are largely around healthcare interventions rather than promoting good health and as much of the compensation is based on fees for these interventions, it is not surprising that the focus is largely on addressing health problems after they have struck rather than promoting good health in the first place.

A good part of the thrust on health promotion could include an important role for the federal government. One fairly easy step would be to coordinate the work being done in this area by the provincial health research councils or institutes in British Columbia, Alberta, Saskatchewan, Manitoba, Ontario, Quebec, New Brunswick, Nova Scotia, and Newfoundland and Labrador.

MEASURING OUTCOMES

Public policy often sets out lofty objectives but does not track their realization. This must not be the case with healthcare. Currently, health data focuses on outputs and especially inputs, but not on the outcomes of general health and healthcare interventions. If outcomes are more effectively tracked, this could result in better evaluations of the value-added aspect of healthcare interventions. Moreover, the measurement of outcomes should reflect the perspective of patients and their families, not just as to their medical outcome, but also their satisfaction with treatment and associated processes.

One fairly easy step would be to help coordinate, or at least compile, the work being done. Better data would facilitate analysis of quality and efficiency of care and enable identification of best (and worst) practices. One of the most powerful ways to improve the quality of healthcare across Canada will be a facility to compare and contrast results across provinces and territories, other countries, and even across institutions. Several institutions already exist in Canada to do this. So the thrust for better measurement should begin at the national (but not necessarily federal) level, as opposed to many of the other steps in this report that are targeted more at provinces and territories. It would be desirable to have a few degrees of freedom from political input for the data collectors, disseminators, and analyzers.

At the aggregate or more "macro" level, the Canadian Institute of Health Information has ventured more into cross-jurisdictional comparisons, and this should be encouraged. Infoway's work should be continued on a national electronic health record system and there should be a comprehensive evaluation to ensure that there is value added and, if not, how practices should be amended. Further, the Canadian Foundation for Healthcare Improvement (CFHI) highlights best practices across the country. Through continuation of the CFHI's work or through another agency, this analytical capacity should be strengthened and expanded.

In recent years, massive electronic health records have been created across Canada, at great expense. However, the level of health information exchanges across organizations and care settings remains astonishingly low. For example, only 12 percent of primary care physicians are "notified electronically of patients' interactions with hospitals or send [or] receive electronic referrals for specialist appointments" (Protti 2015, 1). Moreover, "fewer than three in 10 primary care physicians have electronic access to clinical data about a patient who has been seen by a different health organization" (Protti 2015, 1). This all adds up to one of the poorest levels of health information exchange across organizations and care settings among developed countries. To the degree that the inefficiency and mediocre quality of healthcare in Canada relates to the difficulty in bringing the various silos of care together, electronic health records have so far failed to deliver on their promise. A new era must be launched to ensure connectivity of records, and as with all public policy challenges, this should start with an analysis of what is going wrong.

With a focus on healthcare interventions as opposed to health outcomes more generally, and with most physicians still being compensated on a fee-for-service basis, it is not surprising there has been so little progress in connecting electronic health records across organizations and care settings. Too few of the players involved have an incentive to devote the necessary time, as connectivity is neither explicitly in their objectives nor reflected in their compensation. As with other challenges in health, then, success in connectivity with electronic health records will require a shift toward targeting the health of people rather than just the results of health interventions, and as part of that shift in objective, the relevant stakeholders should be incentivized to spend the time required in building these information bases to best serve people's overall health.

ALL TOGETHER NOW

There are many strands to needed healthcare reform, but they can and should be held together through a public document that accurately sets out the problems, objectives, and steps to reform, and then determines how to regularly measure and report progress. Nothing in what is recommended above seems heroic relative to the kinds of reform that have been implemented in other areas—or indeed even compared to what has already been done in healthcare in Canada. It just takes a few more steps to create the winning conditions to get the public and stakeholders onside and then a comprehensive strategic plan. At the moment, it seems change will most likely occur at the provincial or territorial level, but these individual jurisdictions will likely quickly emulate success observed elsewhere. A national approach is wise in some areas, in particular for building upon some of the information infrastructure already in place. There should be an effort to create national standards for seniors' care and pharmaceuticals. Provinces could work toward the standards in their own ways and at their own pace. In time there might be greater comparability of healthcare across the country. Further, there might even be programs like a national pharmaceutical plan or national seniors' care. But these can be gradual evolutions and do not need to be starting points because they could also be stumbling points.

Many of the conditions needed for successful provincial healthcare reform have been established within the last few years, with the Queen's Health Policy Change Conference Series playing a crucial role. Moving forward, provinces, either acting alone or together, can put the remaining pieces in place and act now to create positive change for our healthcare system.

REFERENCES

Alberta. 2013. *Working Together to Build a High Performance Health Review System*. Edmonton, AB: Ministry of Health. http://www.health.alberta.ca/documents/High-Performance-Health-System-2013.pdf

———. 2015a. *Action Underway to Improve Rural Health Care*. Edmonton, Alberta: Ministry of Health. Press release, 18 March. http://alberta.ca/release.cfm?xID=37883C5BA8FE0-EA79-D893-B8A2F0F535B9A063

———. 2015b. *Rural Health Review Final Report*. Edmonton, AB: Ministry of Health. http://www.health.alberta.ca/documents/Rural-Health-Services-Review-2015.pdf

Black, Charlyn, Dawn Mooney, and Sandra Peterson. 2014. *Patient Experiences with Outpatient Cancer Care in British Columbia, 2012/13*. Vancouver, BC: UBC Centre for Health Services and Policy Research. http://www.health.gov.bc.ca/library/publications/year/2014/patient-experiences-outpatientcancer-care.pdf

Blomqvist, Ake, and Colin Busby. 2014. *Paying for the Boomers: Long-Term Care and Intergenerational Equity*. Toronto, ON: C.D. Howe Institute. September. http://www.cdhowe.org/pdf/Commentary_415.pdf

Blomqvist, Ake, Colin Busby, Aaron Jacobs, and William Falk. 2015. *Doctors without Hospitals: What to do about Specialists Who Can't Find Work*. Toronto, ON: C.D. Howe Institute. 5 February. http://www.cdhowe.org/pdf/ Ebrief_204.pdf

Busby, Colin, and Jonathan Peddle. 2014. *Should Drug Plans be based on Age or Income?* Toronto, ON: C.D. Howe Institute. December. http://www.cdhowe.org/pdf/Commentary_417.pdf

Campbell, Bradley J. 2007. *Changing Nova Scotia's Health Care System: Creating Sustainability Through Transformation*. Halifax, NS: Department of Health and Wellness. https://novascotia.ca/health/reports/pubs/Provincial_ Health_Services_Operational_Review_Report.pdf

Canadian Health Services Research Foundation (CHSRF). 2011. *Assessing Initiatives to Transform Healthcare Systems: Lessons for the Canadian Healthcare System*. CHSRF series on healthcare transformation: Paper. Ottawa, ON: Canadian Health Services Research Foundation. http://www.cfhi-fcass. ca/sf-docs/default-source/commissioned-research-reports/JLD_REPORT. pdf?sfvrsn=0

Canadian Institute for Health Information (CIHI). 2012. *Prescribed Drug Spending in Canada 2012: A Focus on Public Drug Programs*. Ottawa, ON: CIHI. https://secure.cihi.ca/free_products/Prescribed_Drug_Spending_in_ Canada_EN.pdf

———. 2014. *National Health Expenditure Trends, 1975 to 2014*. Ottawa, ON: CIHI. http://www.cihi.ca/web/resource/en/nhex_2014_report_en.pdf

Canadian Medical Association. 2010. *Healthcare Transformation in Canada— Change that Works, Care that Leads*. Ottawa, ON: Canadian Medical Association. http://policybase.cma.ca/dbtw-wpd/PolicyPDF/PD10-05.PDF

———. 2014a. *Access to Prescription Drugs in Canada: Costing the Gap*. Report on the 2012 Statistics Canada Family Expenditure Survey. February.

———. 2014b. *National Report on Seniors Healthcare: Seniors Health Issues and the Impact of an Ageing Population*, 18 August. Ottawa, ON: Canadian Medical Association. https://www.cma.ca/En/Lists/Medias/2014_Report_ Card-e.pdf

Canadian Medical Association, and Canadian Nurses Association. 2011. *Principles to Guide Health Care Transformation in Canada*. Ottawa, ON: Canadian Medical Association and Canadian Nurses Association. https://www. cnaaiic.ca/~/media/cna/files/en/guiding_principles_hc_e.pdf

Canadian Nurses Association. 2012. *A Nursing Call to Action: The Health of Our Nation, the Future of Our Health System*. Ottawa, ON: Canadian Nurses Association. https://www.cna-aiic.ca/~/media/cna/files/en/nec_report_e.pdf

Canadian Physiotherapy Association. 2014. *Submission to the Advisory Panel on Health Care Innovation*. Ottawa, ON: Canadian Physiotherapy Association. http://www.physiotherapy.ca/getmedia/b954618b-3c9e-4eb7-a42e-

32d7223e5499/2014-12-08_Federal_Advisory_Panel_on_Healthcare_Innovation.pdf.aspx

Carson, A. S., 2015a, "Why Canadians Need a System-Wide Healthcare Strategy." In *Toward a Healthcare Strategy for Canadians,* edited by A. S. Carson, J. Dixon, and K. R. Nossal, 11–37. Montreal and Kingston: McGill-Queen's University Press.

Carson, A. S. 2105b. "If Canada Had a Healthcare Strategy, What Form Could it Take?" In *Toward a Healthcare Strategy for Canadians,* edited by A. S. Carson, J. Dixon, and K. R. Nossal, 255–276. Montreal and Kingston: McGill-Queen's University Press.

Carson, A. S., Dixon, J., and Nossal, K. R. 2015. *Toward a Healthcare Strategy for Canadians.* Montreal and Kingston: McGill-Queen's University Press.

Chodos, Howard. 2001. *Quebec's Health Review* (The Clair Commission). Ottawa, ON: Government of Canada. http://publications.gc.ca/Collection-R/LoPBdP/BP/prb0037-e.htm

Council of the Federation. 2012. *From Innovation to Action: The First Report of the Health Care Innovation Working Group.* Ottawa, ON: Council of the Federation. http://www.pmprovincesterritoires.ca/phocadownload/publications/health_innovation_report-e-web.pdf

Dagnone, Tony. 2009. *For Patients' Sake: Patient First Review Commissioner's Report to the Saskatchewan Minister of Health.* Regina, SK: Ministry of Health. http://www.health.gov.sk.ca/patient-first-commissioners-report

Dixon, J. 2015. "No Undue Hardship: A Way Forward for Canadian Pharmacare." In *Toward a Healthcare Strategy for Canadians,* edited by A. S. Carson, J. Dixon, and K. R. Nossal. Montreal and Kingston: McGill-Queen's University Press.

Doctors of B.C. 2012. *Charting the Course: Designing British Columbia's Health Care System for the Next 25 Years.* Vancouver, BC: Doctors of B.C. https://www.doctorsofbc.ca/sites/default/files/charting_the_course_final.pdf

Drummond, Don. 2012. *Commission on the Reform of Ontario's Public Services.* Toronto, ON: Government of Ontario. http://www.fin.gov.on.ca/en/reformcommission/chapters/report.pdf

———. 2015. "Health Policy Reform in Canada: Bridging Policy and Politics." In *Toward a Healthcare Strategy for Canadians*, edited by A. Scott Carson, Jeffrey Dixon, and Kim Richard Nossal, 237–54. Montreal and Kingston: McGill-Queen's University Press.

Gagnon, Marc-Andre. 2010. *Why Canadians Need Universal Pharmacare.* Ottawa, ON: Canadian Centre for Policy Alternatives. 16 September. https://www.policyalternatives.ca/publications/commentary/why-canadians-needuniversal-pharmacare

Health Action Lobby (HEAL). 2014. *The Canadian Way: Accelerating Innovation and Improving Health Performance.* Ottawa, ON: Health Action Lobby. http://www.healthactionlobby.ca/images/stories/publications/2014/HEAL_TheCanadianWay_EN_NoEmbargo.pdf

Health Council of Canada. 2013. *Better Health, Better Care, Better Value for All: Refocusing Health Care Reform.* Toronto, ON: Health Council of Canada. https://www.cahspr.ca/web/uploads/conference/2014-02-14_Better_Health_Better_Care_Better_Value_For_All.pdf

IPAC. 2013. *Health Care Governance Models in Canada: A Provincial Perspective.* Ottawa, ON: IPAC. http://www.ipac.ca/documents/ALL-COMBINED.pdf

Manitoba. 2008. *Report of the Manitoba Regional Health Authority External Review Committee.* Winnipeg, MB: Department of Health and Healthy Living and Seniors. http://digitalcollection.gov.mb.ca/awweb/pdfopener?smd=1&did=16959&md=1

Morgan, Steven G., Michael Law, Jamie Daw, Liza Abraham, and Danielle Martin. 2015. "Estimated Cost of Universal Public Coverage of Prescription Drugs in Canada." *Canadian Medical Association Journal,* 16 March. doi:10.1503/cmaj.141564

Murray, Michael A. 2012. *Patient Experiences with Acute Inpatient Hospital Care in British Columbia, 2011/12.* Victora, BC: Ministry of Health. http://www.health.gov.bc.ca/library/publications/year/2012/patient-experience-sacute-in patient.pdf

Nelson S., J. Turnbull, L. Bainbridge, T. Caulfield, G. Hudon, D. Kendel, D. Mowat, L. Nasmith, B. Postl, J. Shamian, and I. Sketris. 2014. *Optimizing Scopes of Practice: New Models of Care for a New Health System.* Ottawa, ON: Canadian Academy of Health Sciences. http://www.cahs-acss.ca/wp-content/uploads/2014/05/Optimizing-Scopes-of-Practice_-Executive-Summary_E.pdf

New Brunswick. 2013. *Benchmarking and Performance Improvement Process.* Fredericton, NB: Department of Health and Wellness. http://www.gnb.ca/0212/values/pdf/OHSR%20Phase%201%20Final%20Report%2025-04-2013.pdf

New Brunswick Medical Society. 2013. *Fixing New Brunswick's Health Care System.* Fredericton, NB: New Brunswick Medical Society. http://www.nbms.nb.ca/assets/Care-First/NBMSPolicyENG.pdf

Newfoundland and Labrador. 2013. *Newfoundland and Labrador Ambulance Program Review.* St. John's, NL: Department of Health and Community Services. http://www.health.gov.nl.ca/health/publications/nl_ambulance_review.pdf

Nova Scotia. 2014. *Emergency Care Standards Update.* Halifax, NS: Department of Health and Wellness. http://novascotia.ca/dhw/publications/Emergency-Care-Standards-Update-2014.pdf

OECD (Organisation for Economic Co-operation and Development). 2010. *Health Data 2010: Statistics and Indicators for 32 Countries.* Paris, France: OECD.

————.2013. *Health at a Glance.* Paris, France: OECD.

Prince Edward Island (PEI). 2008. "An Integrated Health System Review in PEI." *A Call to Action: A Plan for Change.* Charlottetown, PE: Department of Health and Wellness. http://www.gov.pe.ca/photos/original/doh_csi_report.pdf

Protti, Denis. 2015. *Missed Connections: The Adoption of Information Technology in Canadian Healthcare*. Commentary 422. March. Toronto, ON: C.D. Howe Institute. http://www.cdhowe.org/pdf/commentary_422.pdf

Quebec. 2014. Pour que l'argent suive le patient: l'implantation du financement axé sur les patients dans le secteur de la santé. Quebec City, QC: Ministry of Health and Social Services. http://www.groupes.finances.gouv.qc.ca/santefinancementactivite/wp-content/uploads/2014/02/Rapport-Financ-axe-patients-19fev14.pdf

Ross, John. 2010. *The Patient Journey through Emergency Care in Nova Scotia: A Prescription for New Medicine*. Halifax, NS: Department of Health and Wellness. http://novascotia.ca/dhw/publications/Dr-Ross-The-Patient-Journey-Through-Emergency-Care-in-Nova-Scotia.pdf

Scheffler, Robert. 2008. *Is there a Doctor in the House? Market Signals and Tomorrow's Supply of Doctors*. Stanford University Press.

Simpson, Christopher. 2015. "Code Gridlock: Why Canada needs a National Seniors Strategy." *Inside Policy—The Magazine of The Macdonald-Laurier Institute*. February. Ottawa, ON: Macdonald-Laurier Institute. https://www.cma.ca/En/Lists/Medias/Code_Gridlock_final.pdf

Sinclair, Duncan. 2015. "Remarks." Tech Value Net (TVN) Conference on Improving Care for the Frail Elderly. February.

Sinha, Samir K. 2012. *Living Longer, Living Well*. Toronto, ON: Ministry of Health and Long-Term Care. http://www.health.gov.on.ca/en/common/ministry/publications/reports/seniors_strategy/docs/seniors_strategy.pdf

Srivastava, Divya. 2014. "Creating Strategic Change in Canadian Healthcare." Presentation at Queen's Health Policy Change Conference, 15–16 May 2014.

Statistics Canada. 2007. Canadian Community Health Survey (Rapid Response on Prescription Drug Expenses). http://www23.statcan.gc.ca/imdb/p2SV.pl?Function=getSurvey&Id=29539

Swedlove, F. 2014. Correspondence to Ms. Linda Silas, 2 September.

Tang, Karen L., William A. Ghali, and Braden J. Manns. 2014. "Addressing Cost-Related Barriers to Prescription Drug Use." *Canadian Medical Association Journal* 186 (4) (March 4): 276–80.

Toews, Reg. 2013. *Manitoba EMS System Review*. March. Winnipeg, MB: Department of Health and Healthy Living and Seniors. http://www.gov.mb.ca/health/documents/ems.pdf

University Health Network (UHN). 2015. *Laboratory Medicine Program Review of Eastern Health Laboratory Medicine Program*. 6 March. http://www.easternhealth.ca/publicreports.aspx

Walker, David. 2011. *Caring for Our Aging Population and Addressing Alternate Level of Care*. 30 June. Toronto, ON: Ministry of Health and Long-Term Care. http://www.health.gov.on.ca/en/common/ministry/publications/reports/walker_2011/walker_2011.pdf

Appendices

Managing a Canadian Healthcare Strategy, edited by A. Scott Carson and Kim Richard Nossal. Montreal and Kingston: McGill-Queen's University Press, Queen's Policy Studies Series. © 2016 The School of Policy Studies, Queen's University at Kingston. All rights reserved.

Appendix A
Summary of Recommendations

General Strategy	
R1.	The piecemeal reforms of healthcare across the country should broaden to system-wide change.
R2.	National leadership and design in healthcare reform are welcome, but provinces can choose to act together.
R3.	Each province should commission an external review of its healthcare system that closely involves stakeholders, including the public.
R4.	Each province should anchor its healthcare strategy in a public document that accurately explains the problems, the objective(s), the steps in reform, and how progress will be monitored and measured.
R5.	Key stakeholder groups should engage more directly with provinces on healthcare reform.

Steps in Healthcare Reform	
R6.	Provinces should consider a greater role for an arm's length agency, both in healthcare administration and in implementing reforms.
R7.	While discussions are being launched on a national pharmaceutical program, provinces should focus (individually and, where feasible, together) on more affordable drug prices (with a federal role here as well), better access/affordability through reforms of public support systems, and tighter protocols and monitoring of the use and effectiveness of pharmaceuticals.
R8.	To better inform the dialogue on a national pharmacare program, a credible, independent body should be charged with examining the differing views of the cost implications of public administration.
R9.	Governments should facilitate discussions on national standards of seniors' care, with an aim to improve efficiency and quality of seniors' care through reducing hospital use, expanding home care, and ensuring flow into and out of long-term care.
R10.	Recent efforts to improve the efficiency of healthcare delivery should be continued, including moving further away from cost-plus budgeting for hospitals and fee-for-service for doctors and making greater and better use of electronic health records.
R11.	Provinces should focus on better coordination of care across the various sites of care and pay greater attention to coordinating the care of the small portion of the population that accounts for much of total healthcare spending.
R12.	Provinces should examine potential efficiency gains and cost savings through scope-of-practice changes, including giving hospitals a greater voice in the delineation of duties.
R13.	Provinces and medical schools should put more emphasis on human resources planning in light of demographic and technological changes, and strive for a better match of the supply of healthcare providers with patient demand.

...continued

Appendix A, continued
Summary of Recommendations

R14.   The emphasis should shift from healthcare to health promotion, along with appropriate shifts in the incentives to healthcare providers.

Measuring Outcomes

R15.   Existing pan-Canadian institutions such as CIHI, CFHI, and Canada Health Infoway can lead in generating better data and analysis on health outcomes and the results of healthcare interventions, including comparisons across institutions and provinces.

R16.   Incentive systems need to be further changed to give healthcare providers the motivation to focus on health outcomes and to better use electronic health records in that pursuit.

Appendix B
Policy Position Papers by Healthcare Stakeholders

Year	Stakeholder Group & Report	Reference
2010	Canadian Medical Association: Health Care Transformation in Canada—Change that Works, Care that Leads	(Canadian Medical Association 2010) http://policybase.cma.ca/dbtw-wpd/PolicyPDF/PD10-05.PDF

The CMA has created an extensive framework for healthcare transformation, listing the actions needed for change under five main pillars. A copy of this transformation framework is included below:

1. Building a culture of patient-centred care;
   a. Key action: Create a Charter for Patient-Centred Care
2. Incentives for enhancing access and improving quality of care;
   a. Key action: Change incentives to enhance timely access
   b. Key action: Change incentives to support quality care
3. Enhancing patient access along the continuum of care;
   a. Key action: Universal access to prescription drugs
   b. Key action: Continuing care outside acute care facilities
4. Helping providers help patients;
   a. Key action: Ensure Canada has an adequate supply of health human resources
   b. Key action: Improve adoption of health information technologies
5. Building accountability/responsibility at all levels;
   a. Key action: Build system accountability
   b. Key action: Build system stewardship.

The CMA has made 14 recommendations to achieve these objectives:

1. Gain government and public support for the CMA's Charter for Patient-Centred Care.
2. Improve timely access to facility-based care by implementing partial activity-based funding for hospitals.
3. Implement appropriate pay-for-performance systems to encourage quality of care at both the clinician and facility levels.
4. Establish an approach to comprehensive prescription drug coverage to ensure that all Canadians have access to medically necessary drug therapies.
5. Begin construction immediately on additional long-term care facilities.
6. Create national standards for continuing care provision in terms of eligibility criteria, care delivery, and accommodation expenses.
7. Develop options to facilitate pre-funding long-term care needs.
8. Initiate a national dialogue on the Canada Health Act in relation to the continuum of care.
9. Explore ways to support informal caregivers and long-term care patients.
10. Develop a long-term health human resources plan through a national body.
11. Accelerate the adoption of Health Information Technology (HIT) in Canada.

...continued

Appendix B, continued
Policy Position Papers by Healthcare Stakeholders

12. Accelerate the introduction of e-prescribing in Canada.
13. Require public reporting on the performance of the system, including outcomes.
14. Establish an arm's-length mechanism to monitor the financing of healthcare programs at the federal and provincial/territorial levels and assess comparability of coverage.

Year	Stakeholder Group & Report	Reference
2012	Canadian Nurses Association: A Nursing Call to Action: The Health of Our Nation, the Future of Our Health System	(Canadian Nurses Association 2012) https://www.cna-aiic. ca/~/media/cna/files/en/ nec_report_e.pdf

In May 2011, the Canadian Nursing Association established an independent National Expert Commission to evaluate the most efficient, effective, and sustainable ways to meet the changing and pressing health needs of Canadians in the 21st century.

The Commission made a number of recommendations, including:

- Addressing the social determinants of health.
- Improving access to primary healthcare for vulnerable populations (immigrant and refugees, Aboriginal, low-income populations).
- Reinforcing the shift to team-based medical care and changing the way healthcare professionals are educated.
- Bringing pharmacare under medicare.
- Enhancing federal funding to develop a national home care and palliative care program.
- Integration across the continuum of care, and increasing public financing across the continuum of care.
- Improving the selection of indicators and data that more effectively measures progress of healthcare systems.
- Utilizing technology to improve access to care (e.g., Skype, telemedicine, email).
- Safer, higher quality of care.

The Commission found that nurses are underemployed and underutilized outside of acute and long-term care settings. In 2010, public sector healthcare nurses worked a total of 20,627,800 hours of overtime. Hospital over capacity is a key contributor to over utilization of the existing nursing workforce and it is having a negative impact on patients, families, and health outcomes.

...continued

Appendix B, continued
Policy Position Papers by Healthcare Stakeholders

Year	Stakeholder Group & Report	Reference
2011	Canadian Medical Association & Canadian Nurses Association: Principles to Guide Health Care Transformation in Canada	(Canadian Medical Association, and Canadian Nurses Association 2011) https://www.cna-aiic.ca/~/media/cna/files/en/guiding_principles_hc_e.pdf

This brief report outlines the principles that the CMA and CNA came up with together to guide healthcare transformation in Canada. The goal of this report is to have these principles guide discussions at the provincial/territorial and federal levels, leading to the signing of a new healthcare accord among the governments. The principles are summarized as follows:

- Patient-centred: Patient must be at the centre of healthcare, with seamless access to a continuum of care; services must be based on need, not ability to pay; and health professionals must treat patients with respect and dignity.
- Quality: Canadians deserve quality services that are appropriate for patient needs, respect individual choice, and are delivered in a manner that is timely, safe, effective, and according to the most currently available scientific knowledge.
- Health promotion and illness prevention: The health system must support Canadians in the prevention of illness and the enhancement of their well-being, with attention paid to the social determinants of health.
- Equitable: The healthcare system has a duty to Canadians to provide and advocate for equitable access to quality care and commonly adopted policies to address the social determinants of health.
- Sustainable: Sustainable healthcare requires universal access to quality health services that are adequately resourced and delivered across the board in a timely and cost-effective manner.

Accountable: The public, patients, families, providers, and funders all have a responsibility for ensuring the system is effective and accountable.

In addition to the principles developed by the CMA and the CNA, the action plan should continuously build on the five principles of the Canada Health Act to guide the transformation of Canada's healthcare system toward one that is publicly funded, sustainable, and adequately resourced, and provides universal access to quality care.

Year	Stakeholder Group & Report	Reference
2013	British Columbia Medical Association: Charting the Course: Designing British Columbia's Health Care System for the Next 25 Years	(Doctors of B.C. 2012) https://www.doctorsofbc.ca/sites/default/files/charting_the_course_final.pdf

In a written submission to the standing committee on health in 2013, the British

...continued

Appendix B, continued
Policy Position Papers by Healthcare Stakeholders

Columbia Medical Association (BCMA) authoured a report entitled Charting the Course: Designing British Columbia's Health Care System for the Next 25 Years, which examined the policy measures the province must pursue to build a healthcare system that will serve the aging population and address the rising incidence of chronic diseases.

This report made six recommendations to the Ministry of Health in British Columbia:

1. Continue to implement and expand patient-centred funding.
2. Pursue and implement public health strategies, which address chronic illnesses such as obesity, mental health, and chronic diseases of the circulatory system.
3. Invest in health capital infrastructure and community-based programs.
4. Coordinate physician workforce planning, both federally and with other provincial governments.
5. Pursue better efficiencies in terms of cost and supply of medications.
6. Introduce evidence-based wait time benchmarks for the timely delivery of healthcare services.

Year	Stakeholder Group & Report	Reference
2014	New Brunswick Medical Society: Fixing New Brunswick's Healthcare System	(New Brunswick Medical Society 2013) http://www.nbms.nb.ca/assets/Care-First/NBMSPolicyENG.pdf

The New Brunswick Medical Society has published a submission to government, entitled Fixing New Brunswick's Health Care System. This review focused on the following areas of reform in New Brunswick's healthcare system: primary care, electronic medical records, better care for seniors, aligning people and processes more effectively, and creating inter-professional healthcare teams.

Year	Stakeholder Group & Report	Reference
2014	Health Action Lobby (HEAL): The Canadian Way: Accelerating Innovation and Improving Health Performance	(HEAL 2014) http://www.healthactionlobby.ca/images/stories/publications/2014/HEAL_The-CanadianWay_EN_No-Embargo.pdf

The Health Action Lobby represents more than 650,000 healthcare providers and consumers of healthcare. This consensus statement was created to identify the various ways the federal government can play a role in improving the health and healthcare of Canadians.

The statement focuses on six main issues:

...continued

Appendix B, continued
Policy Position Papers by Healthcare Stakeholders

- Improved collaboration between the federal government and the provinces and territories.
- A performance framework that is consistent with the Triple Aim approach to guide improvements and innovation in health systems and healthcare delivery.
- A commitment to stable and reliable transfer payments to go towards healthcare in the provinces and territories.
- Collaboration with healthcare providers to ensure the delivery of health promotion and illness prevention initiatives are evidence-based and cost effective.
- Strategic federal investments related to Canada's aging population, access to prescription drugs, and the spread of on-the-ground health innovations.
- The development of a common set of national health system performance indicators.

The statement calls on the federal government to participate in the Council of the Federation's Health Innovation Working group, and for combined, time-limited strategic funds to spur system improvements, including a "National Health Innovation Fund focused on primary care, health human resources and mental health and addictions, as well as a Community-Based Health Infrastructure Fund" to help the provinces and territories accelerate the building of much needed long-term care facilities.

As part of the statement, HEAL advocates for the federal government to contribute 25 percent annually to healthcare funding in Canada. The present federal share of health system funding is estimated to be 23 percent this year and will drop to 13.3 percent by 2037 if no changes are made.

Finally, the statement proposes a new vision statement for healthcare: "to advance the health and health care of Canadians, working collaboratively with the provinces and territories, health-care providers and the public to ensure the promotion and delivery of appropriate, integrated, cost-effective, and accessible health services and supports."

Year	Stakeholder Group & Report	Reference
2013	Health Council of Canada: Better Health, Better Care, Better Value for All: Refocusing Health Care Reform	(Health Council of Canada 2013) https://www.cahspr.ca/ web/uploads/confer- ence/2014-02-14_Bet- ter_Health_Better_Care_ Better_Value_For_All.pdf

This report looks back on the last decade of healthcare reform, and finds that changes made to healthcare have not kept pace with the evolving needs of Canadians:

...continued

Appendix B, continued
Policy Position Papers by Healthcare Stakeholders

- Progress on wait times for key procedures cited in the Health Accords have stalled.
- Primary healthcare services lag behind other countries.
- Home care services do not address long-term needs.
- Prescription drug costs remain beyond the means of many Canadians.
- Health disparities and inequities continue to persist across the country.

The Health Council builds off the Triple Aim framework and proposes that better health, better care, and better value for all can be achieved through sustained support of five key enablers: (i) leadership at both the policy and delivery level; (ii) linking health system change to policies and legislation; (iii) capacity building through increasing resources and the effectiveness and efficiency of existing resources; (iv) innovation and spread; and (v) measurement and reporting.

The report concludes that enablers were not aligned to support the above system goals of better health, better care, and better value for all. The healthcare system can be improved in the following ways:

- patient engagement (e.g., active participation in their care);
- individual contributions of health care providers (e.g., nursing care);
- management processes at the organizational level (e.g., operationalizing a hospital surgical checklist); and
- strategic planning and policy decisions at the regional health authority level (e.g., implementing integrated service plans) and health ministry levels (e.g., implementing a provincial disease strategy).

Year	Stakeholder Group & Report	Reference
2012	Council of the Federation: From Innovation to Action: The First Report of the Health Care Innovation Working Group	(Council of the Federation 2012) http://www.pmprovinces-territoires.ca/phocadownload/publications/health_innovation_report-e-web.pdf

In July 2012, the HCIWG released its report: From Innovation to Action. As discussed in the report, the HCIWG's work is guided by the premiers' view that innovation needs to be the cornerstone of improved healthcare for Canadians. This report focuses on three priority areas: clinical practice guidelines that are consistent across provinces, team-based healthcare delivery, and health human resources. Additionally, the report considers how to create opportunities for the provinces and territories to work together to improve health outcomes.

The report lists 12 recommendations for improvement across the three focus areas identified above:

- Clinical practices:
  - Adopt clinical guidelines on heart disease and foot ulcers.

...continued

Appendix B, continued
Policy Position Papers by Healthcare Stakeholders

- −Work with clinical communities and health offices with the objective of developing, within six months, provincial and territorial-specific deployment strategies.
- −Report back within 24 months with an update on implementation.
- −Encourage national health providers to promote the adoption of clinical practice guidelines.
- −Identify other leading practices in clinical practice guidelines that could be shared among provinces and territories.
- Team based models of care:
  - −Working group identified best practices of team-based care in provinces and territories across Canada (for example collaborative emergency centres in Nova Scotia).
  - −Define options for a platform for ensuring the ongoing identification and dissemination of information on innovative models.
- Health human resources:
  - −Adopt guiding principles for health human resources management.
  - −Work with ministers to create a health human resources website to better facilitate communication of information about health human resources labour markets across provinces and territories.
- Generic drugs:
  - −Identify three to five generic drugs to include in a provincial/territorial competitive value price initiative.
  - −Initiate a national competitive bidding process that would result in lower prices by April 1, 2013.
- Advancing the work:
  - −Monitor the progress made on the initiatives contained in this report.

Year	Stakeholder Group & Report	Reference
2014	Canadian Physiotherapy Association: Submission to the Advisory Panel on Health Care Innovation	(Canadian Physiotherapy Association 2014) http://www.physiotherapy.ca/getmedia/b954618b -3c9e-4eb7-a42e- 32d7223e5499/2014- 12-08_Federal _Advisory_Panel_on_ Healthcare_Innovation .pdf.aspx

This policy position paper focuses on innovative models that feature the role of physiotherapy in improving patient flow and maximizing system resources for better health outcomes.

CPA calls on the federal government to lead in three specific ways:

1. Support direct access to healthcare providers in the public and private systems through mechanisms that prohibit third party payer requirements for physician referral. This may be achieved through changes within federal

...continued

Appendix B, continued
Policy Position Papers by Healthcare Stakeholders

departments responsible for health services.

2. Invest in health services research and design to bridge the gap between demonstrated success in pilot projects to system-wide implementation and reform.

3. Dedicated funding for community-based well-being and injury prevention initiatives to target aging populations appropriately. The new federal funding model does not account for the fiscal disparities of provinces with older populations. A targeted investment program would allow provincial health savings from prevention-based care to be reinvested into continuing innovation and health services improvement that meets the needs of an older population.

Year	Stakeholder Group & Report	Reference
2014	Canadian Academy of Health Sciences: Optimizing Scopes of Practice: New Models of Care for a New Health System	http://www.cahs-acss.ca/wp-content/uploads/2014/05/Optimizing-Scopes-of-Practice_-Executive-Summary_E.pdf

This report acknowledges that Canada's health system has been difficult to change because of enshrined legislative, regulatory, and financial schemes.

The assessment directly addresses the optimal scope of practice of healthcare providers through an examination of these barriers to change, and calls for a system-wide transformation that builds upon ongoing quality improvement initiatives to better meet patient, community, and population needs.

This report identifies the misalignment of health human resources (HHR) capacities with the need to provide healthcare services relevant to population demands as the current problem with Canada's healthcare system. In response to the challenge of providing high-quality and accessible care, the scopes of practice of some healthcare professionals, such as pharmacists and nurse practitioners, have been extended and new professions and roles, such as pharmacy technicians and health navigators, have been developed in several jurisdictions across Canada. In some cases, however, these roles have been introduced without full articulation of how they will be integrated into existing service delivery models or how they will impact the scopes of practice of existing health professions.

A new healthcare strategy for Canada must focus on the patient, be flexible and accountable, and will ensure that the right provider gives the best care in the most appropriate location. Further recommendations:

-   The federal government to provide national leadership to support collaborative care models and the evolution of this scope of practice
-   An infrastructure that provides arm's-length evidence and evaluation of the

...continued

Appendix B, continued
Policy Position Papers by Healthcare Stakeholders

health workforce with both HHR planning and deployment through optimal scopes of practice as its mandate
- Research funds earmarked to address gaps in the literature on HHR planning
- Provincial governments should take the lead on funding, financing, and remuneration that would enable collaborative models of care that align with patient outcomes

Year	Stakeholder Group & Report	Reference
2011	Canadian Health Services Research Foundation: Assessing Initiatives to Transform Healthcare Systems: Lessons for the Canadian Health Care System	(CHSRF 2011) http://www.cfhi-fcass.ca/ sf-docs/default-source/ commissioned-research- reports/JLD_REPORT. pdf?sfvrsn=0

This report recognizes that a clear vision and strategy is required to better align between the care offered and the care the population needs in Canada. The report looks at different healthcare systems and comes up with six different themes to address strategic areas in healthcare.

An analysis of the current health system in Canada shows that there are six areas in need of reform:
- Strategic alignment: The healthcare system must be realigned to meet patients' needs and demands. Large reforms at the system level and implementing more effective chronic disease management and population health interventions can help to achieve this objective.
- Organizations as the engine for delivery and change: Through encouraging more inter-professional teams to deliver healthcare, this can transform organizational behaviour to meet evolving and shifting demands in the population. However, organizational change can be challenging and it is essential for reforms to be closely and deliberately managed during the change process.
- Professional cultures: Transformation of the healthcare system also requires new professional roles and the engagement of the medical profession. The report recommends that more attention be paid to nurse practitioners, patient navigators, and health assistants in delivering healthcare. Other suggestions include the development of new professional roles that link clinical and managerial functions.
- Creating an enabling environment: Achieving improvements also requires effective governance, well-defined and appropriate goals and targets, effective reporting mechanisms, and well-designed financial (for example, hospital funding, pay for performance) and non-financial incentives.
- Patient engagement: Patient care takes place not only between physician and patient, but also as a function of organizational context and system policies; therefore, patients must be included in policy decisions and the design of health services.
- Evidence-informed policy and decision making: Strategies must enhance healthcare organizational capacity to integrate evidence into practice, as well

Appendix B, continued
Policy Position Papers by Healthcare Stakeholders

---

as better coordination among research-based evidence, policy making, and politics. Structural changes to healthcare systems are constantly being implemented without improved patient outcomes. There is a need for innovations and experiments that will increase communications between the research community, policymakers, and the political sphere. Professionals should take on a more significant role in transforming Canada's health system.

Appendix C
Independent Review of Provinces' Healthcare

British Columbia
A comprehensive external review of British Columbia's healthcare system has not been conducted; however, there have been several external reviews of different healthcare sectors.

UBC Health Services and Policy Research has conducted external reviews of patient experiences in different sectors of BC's healthcare system. In 2011/12, they focused on acute inpatient hospital care in British Columbia (Murray 2012), and in the most recent 2012/13 report, they examined patient experiences with outpatient cancer care (Black, Mooney, and Peterson 2014).

Alberta
In April 2013, the Government of Alberta organized a task force that was responsible for interviewing individuals in leadership positions about how to improve the healthcare governance system. The main finding of this research was to make Alberta Health work more effectively by clarifying roles and responsibilities, developing a partnering culture, and building the capacity of all individuals to deal with the challenges the system will face in the future. The task force made 10 recommendations that focused on three key themes:

1. All parties must be clear about their roles and responsibilities and be committed to achieving excellence in their execution, including having the minister and the Alberta Health Services Board adopt a procedure for the recruitment and selection of new board members that is competency-based, nonpartisan, and transparent.

2. Alberta Health works with the Alberta Health Services to achieve targets set out in the health plan.

3. Albertans require the full engagement of physicians in order to benefit from the effectiveness and quality outcomes that the health system should deliver (Alberta 2013).

The Ministry of Health in Alberta recently conducted a comprehensive review of rural health in the province to better understand the concerns and challenges of Albertans living in rural and remote communities. The final report was released in March 2015. Fifty-six recommendations were made which focused on six main themes: greater community engagement; team-based primary healthcare services; addressing EMS dispatch issues; retention of healthcare professionals; enhancing utilization of existing healthcare facilities; and acknowledging the role of healthcare facilities and services in the economic viability of rural communities (Alberta 2015b).

Saskatchewan
In November 2008, the minister of health launched the independent patient-first review of the Saskatchewan health system, entitled For Patients' Sake (Dagnone 2009).

The review comprised two distinct streams of research: an examination of the patient experience across the full continuum of healthcare services and the administration of healthcare in regional health authorities (health regions), the Saskatchewan Cancer Agency, and the Saskatchewan Association of Health Organizations

...continued

Appendix C, continued
Independent Review of Provinces' Healthcare

(SAHO).
Similar to the Alberta report, Saskatchewan's external health review recommended that no major changes be made to the existing regional healthcare governance model. The report made 16 recommendations which fell under three broad themes:

1. "Patient first" must be embedded as a core value in healthcare: The best interests of patients and families must be the primary driver of policy decisions, collective agreements, priority setting and resource allocation decisions, and the operation of workplaces.

2. Healthcare in Saskatchewan needs to function as a cohesive system: There is a lack of coordination and standardization within the health system's administrative and leadership structures.

3. Frontline providers must be empowered to deliver patient- and family-centred care: Effective leadership and improved system performance are critical to supporting a family- and patient-centred care model.

Manitoba
The province of Manitoba has not had a comprehensive external health review. However, in 2008 an independent task force was convened to conduct a governance review of regional health authorities across the province (Manitoba 2008).

In March 2013, a large-scale review of Manitoba's emergency medical services system was completed. This report recommended closing 18 low-volume EMS stations and upgrading others, as well as setting a province-wide standard for ambulance wait times (Toews 2013).

Ontario
The 2012 Commission on the Reform of Ontario's Public Services made over 100 recommendations on improving the efficiency of the healthcare system in Ontario. Some of the key recommendations include:

• Giving local health integration networks (LHINs) more responsibility over funding and integration.

• Diverting patients who do not need acute care in hospitals to family doctors, clinics, and nursing homes.

• Increasing university nursing programs and using nurse practitioners more effectively.

• Expanding the role of pharmacists to permit them to give routine injections, inhalations, and immunization.

• Creating an online system for prescription refills, test results, and appointment scheduling.

• Linking the Ontario Drug Benefit program, currently for seniors and social assistance recipients, directly to income (Drummond 2012).

In the 2011 report Caring for our Aging Population and Addressing Alternate Levels of Care, Dr. Walker made 32 recommendations to the Ontario government for improving the care for alternate level-of-care patients in the province,

...continued

Appendix C, continued
Independent Review of Provinces' Healthcare

---

including:

- Primary Care: Primary care providers identify seniors for early risk of frailty and help seniors manage other health challenges.
- Community Care Continuum: Additional and sustained resources are provided to integrate, coordinate, and enhance community care.
- Access Centres (CCACs), Community Support Service (CSS) agencies, and assisted living arrangements.
- Cross-System Responsiveness to Special Needs Populations: Integrated care for populations with special needs across the care continuum.
- Assess and Restore: Enhance "Assess and Restore" programs, which are interventions for short-term rehabilitative and restorative care treatments for seniors and other people who have experienced a reversible loss of their functional ability and who risk losing their independence.
- Role of Acute Care Hospitals in Seniors' Care: Hospitals must become more effective in optimizing this capacity, while applying best practices as related to discharge planning.
- Specialized and Differentiated Long-Term Care Capacity: Increase capacity for cyclical, restorative, transitional, and respite care programs for seniors, while maintaining permanent placement programs for seniors with more complex needs.
- System Enablers: Strengthen governance and accountability of LHINs. LHINs must be responsible for meeting targets and objectives and aligning incentives with desired outcomes. Additionally, a comprehensive needs-based service planning and forecasting model is necessary to inform decision making on the type and number of beds and services to be funded in each community.

In 2012, Dr. Samir Sinha released the Living Longer, Living Well report to the minister of health and long-term care and the minister responsible for seniors on recommendations to inform a seniors strategy for Ontario. The report outlined five principles for a seniors' strategy (equity, access, choice, value, and quality) and proposed a number of key recommendations to improve seniors' care in Ontario, including:

- Promoting Health and Wellness: Increase the availability of accessible exercise, falls prevention, and health promotion classes across the province.
- Strengthen Primary Care for Older Ontarians: Ensure that its development of Quality Improvement Plans in Primary Care and Health Links supports a core focus around the care of older Ontarians, and maintain and improve funding to support the number of house calls made by physicians.
- Enhance the Provision of Home and Community Care Services: Increase home and community service funding by 4 percent, support LHINs, CCACs, and CSSs to formalize a Standardized Collaborative Care Model, and encourage the development of more assisted living and supportive housing units as alternatives to long-term care homes.
- Improve Acute Care for Elders: Promote the development of senior-friendly hospitals, explore the development of community paramedicine programs,

...continued

Appendix C, continued
Independent Review of Provinces' Healthcare

---

and support the development and launch of the successful Hospital at Home model in Ontario.

- Enhancing Ontario's Long-Term Care Home Environments: Develop new LTC home-based service models, and improve flow to and from LTC home long-stay and short-stay services by reviewing the existing application and transfer processes and policies.

- Addressing the Specialized Care Needs of Older Ontarians: Leverage the success of the Behavioural Supports Ontario (BSO) Initiative and support the LHINs in broadening palliative care.

- Medications and Older Ontarians: Conduct full review of the MedsCheck Program, reform the Ontario Drug Benefit Program, and develop best practice guidelines and knowledge transfer mechanisms to improve prescribing practices.

- Caring for Caregivers: Improve the awareness of services and supports available to unpaid caregivers with improved single points of access, promote the awareness of tax credits for unpaid caregiving, and encourage the standardization of services and supports offered through the Alzheimer Society's First Link program and fully support the implementation of this program in every LHIN across Ontario.

- Addressing Ageism and Elder Abuse: Raise public awareness about the abuse and neglect of older adults, provide training for front-line staff, and co-ordinate community services to better assist victims of elder abuse in communities across the province.

- Addressing Needs of Older Aboriginal Peoples in Ontario: Aboriginal peoples start to deal with chronic illnesses and geriatric issues at younger ages than other populations and have more challenges finding culturally appropriate care; a separate seniors strategy must be designed for Aboriginal peoples to accommodate their unique needs and circumstances.

- Supporting the Development of Elder Friendly Communities: Enable older Ontarians to adapt their homes to meet their needs. Further enhance the development and availability of non-profit, safe, dignified, and consumer-oriented transportation systems for older Ontarians.

- System Enablers: Provide more financial support to PSWs, finalize the Alternate Funding Plan to support geriatricians, and require that health, social, and community service providers streamline their assessment and referral processes.

Quebec
In 2001, the Clair Commission proposed 36 recommendations to improve Quebec's healthcare services. Included among those recommendations are a number of innovative suggestions, such as:

- the reorganization of the delivery of primary healthcare services by encouraging the formation of group family practices made up of six to 10 physicians who would provide care to a roster of patients 24 hours a day, 7 days a week; and

- the creation of a dedicated "loss of autonomy" insurance fund financed by

...continued

Appendix C, continued
Independent Review of Provinces' Healthcare

---

taxpayers that would be used to pay for an expansion of home care and institutional services to the growing number of elderly persons (Chodos 2001). In 2013, an advisory committee was convened to look at how to implement patient-focused funding in Quebec. At the end of its work, the panel submitted its report to the government on the implementation of patient-focused funding in the health sector. This report reflects the unanimous conclusions of the members of the expert group (Quebec 2014).

New Brunswick
In the spring of 2012, the Government of New Brunswick created the Office of Health System Renewal (OHSR), with a two-year mandate to encourage and assist health system partners and the NB health system to improve its performance.

The OHSR found that the NB healthcare system was not aligned, integrated, citizen-centred, innovative, affordable, or sustainable. Based on this analysis, the OHSR recommended that the goal should be to achieve a per capita public healthcare cost equal to the Canadian average by the 2016 fiscal year; according to the OHSR, this represents a total annual reduction in healthcare spending of approximately $250M by 2017.

In order to achieve this, the OHSR developed an eight-point action plan that includes benchmarking NB healthcare expenditures against Canadian provinces and identifying and implementing best practices.

The OHSR also focused on the following priorities:
- An organizational review, leading to management efficiencies within the healthcare system.
- Monitoring the regional health authorities' progress in implementing the cost per weighted case initiative.
- A review of shared services, including participation in a feasibility study of integrating FacilicorpNB operations with the new Department of Government Services.
- Identification and implementation of health innovations and best practices most promising to health renewal in New Brunswick.
- Monitoring and accountability of health renewal results (New Brunswick 2013).

Nova Scotia
The last comprehensive external review of the health system took place in 2007. The report provides over 100 recommendations, under the following themes:
- Renew emphasis on primary and continuing care, including shifting everything other than acute care out of acute care hospitals.
- Improve access to alternate levels of care and create care options in private homes, and dedicate facilities geared to long-term and chronic healthcare conditions.
- Review the scope of practice of nursing and other non-physician professionals to find innovative means to provide services.

...continued

Appendix C, continued
Independent Review of Provinces' Healthcare

• Review and assess technology-oriented services (e.g., computerized patient records; Campbell 2007).

In September 2009, the Nova Scotia government appointed Dr. John Ross as its provincial adviser on emergency care. Dr. Ross's report, The Patient Journey Through Emergency Care in Nova Scotia, contained 26 recommendations to improve emergency care in the province. As a follow-up to his report, Dr. Ross also developed minimum care standards for emergency care in November 2010. In response to his recommendations, Better Care Sooner: The Plan to Improve Emergency Care was released in December 2010 by the Department of Health and Wellness. Adoption and implementation of the Emergency Care (EC) Standards is one of the action items in the plan. The purpose of the provincial EC Standards is to provide consistency and high quality care in the emergency care system in Nova Scotia (Nova Scotia 2014).

Prince Edward Island
The last comprehensive external health review in PEI took place in 2008. An Integrated Health System Review in PEI—A Call to Action: A Plan for Change made recommendations for all sectors of PEI's healthcare system, but found that the most serious gaps observed in the health system were in primary care. The recommendations included changes to governance and management, and the operating framework.

Newfoundland and Labrador
A comprehensive external review of Newfoundland and Labrador's regional healthcare system has not been conducted.

On 12 March 2015, Newfoundland and Labrador's largest health authority released the results of an external review that gave several recommendations to improve its pathology laboratory. The review was conducted by the Ontario-based University Health Network (UHN), and recommends hiring a medical director, establishing a training program for pathology assistants, setting up a new reporting procedure, and conducting a workload analysis (UHN 2015).

A program review in 2013 was conducted on the ambulance program in Newfoundland and Labrador. The report made 10 recommendations to improve the ambulance care system in Newfoundland and Labrador, including improving accountability, building a medical dispatch centre, and enacting EMS legislation to govern ambulance services in the province.

Appendix D
Administrative Management Structure of Healthcare in the Provinces

British Columbia	http://www.health.gov.bc.ca/socsec/roles.html

In 2002, the BC government reduced the network of regional authorities to create the current system of five regional health authorities and one provincial authority. British Columbia's regional health authorities are responsible for governing, planning, and delivering healthcare services within their geographical regions. More specifically, the RHAs are responsible for identifying population health needs, planning appropriate programs and services, ensuring programs and services are properly funded and managed, and collecting data and tracking performance objectives. The Provincial Health Services Authority (PHS) oversees the work of the RHAs and governs and manages their performance. Additionally, the PHS works with the five RHAs to coordinate and deliver highly specialized services, including cardiac care and transplants. British Columbia has a separate health authority for First Nations peoples, which is responsible for planning and delivering First Nations health services and programs.

Alberta	http://www.albertahealthservices.ca/204.asp

In 2008, 10 RHAs and three health agencies in Alberta were amalgamated into one authority called Alberta Health Services (AHS). Currently, the AHS is the largest single health authority in Canada and delivers medical care through 400 facilities throughout the province. The AHS was established to improve access, quality, and sustainability of healthcare services. Since its inception, the AHS has been organized so as to separate acute hospital facilities from small hospitals and community services, which are organized into five separate zones. The AHS reports to a board of directors, appointed by the minister of health and wellness. Under the AHS, there are 12 health advisory councils who are charged with fostering community engagement.

On 18 March 2015, it was announced that Alberta Health Services would establish eight to 10 "operational districts" within the AHS. The new AHS operational districts, to be implemented by 1 July, will be responsible for delivering local health services and meeting performance objectives. Under the new model, each operational district will have more authority on how money is spent on services, facility repairs, and staff recruitment. They will receive advice from new 10–15 member local advisory committees.

Saskatchewan	http://www.health.gov.sk.ca/health-system

Since 2002, Saskatchewan's 12 regional health authorities (RHAs) and cancer agencies have provided health services either directly or through healthcare organizations. The RHAs' scope of responsibilities include hospitals, health centres, wellness centres, social centres, emergency response services, supportive care, home care, community health services, mental health service, and rehabilitation services. Boards and chairs of the RHAs are appointed by order-in-council. Saskatchewan is the first jurisdiction in Canada to apply a lean approach to patient care; more than 700 lean projects have been launched across Saskatchewan, with the goal of improving patient outcomes.

...continued

Appendix D, continued
Administrative Management Structure of Healthcare in the Provinces

Manitoba	http://www.gov.mb.ca/health/rha/

The Regional Health Authorities of Manitoba (RHAs) are mandated to promote and provide patient-centred, integrated, province-wide, sustainable solutions to healthcare services and programs. Manitoba's five RHAs are composed of healthcare providers who coordinate, manage, deliver funds to, and evaluate healthcare and health promotion in their region. All RHAs receive funding from the provincial government and are governed by a board of directors. In the spring of 2012, the provincial government reduced the number of RHAs in Manitoba from 11 to five. Through the merger process, 81 board member positions were eliminated. The amalgamation is intended to realize $10 million in savings over three years.

Ontario	http://www.lhins.on.ca/

Ontario was the last province in Canada to devolve healthcare to regional decision making. In 2005, Local Health Integration Networks (LHINs) were created as the health system designer and manager in Ontario. LHINs are charged with building and funding regional systems of integrated care and aligning health systems with the Ministry of Health's priorities and local needs. Responsibilities of the LHINs do not include the delivery of healthcare services. The LHINs delegate the delivery of healthcare services to Health Services Provider Boards. Currently, there are 14 LHINs across Ontario, with an average of 900,000 persons per LHIN.

Quebec	http://www.msss.gouv.qc.ca/en/reseau/services.php

Quebec's healthcare system is divided into three levels: provincial, regional, and local. At the provincial level, the Ministry of Health and Social Services manages the health and social services system. It is responsible for overall organization and allocates budgetary resources. At the regional level, 18 health and social services agencies (ASSS) are charged with regional planning, resource management, and budget allocation to institutions in each region of the province. Below the ASSS are local health and social services networks (there are 94), certain hospitals, children and youth protection centres, long-term care centres, and rehab centres. Health and social services networks (CSSS) provide services directly to citizens and follow up on the care they receive.

...continued

Appendix D, continued
Administrative Management Structure of Healthcare in the Provinces

Nova Scotia	http://novascotia.ca/dhw/about/DHA.asp

Currently, Nova Scotia's healthcare services are delivered by nine district health authorities (DHA) and the IWK Health Centre. These health authorities are responsible for all hospitals, community health services, mental health services, and public health programs in their districts. However, on 1 April 2015, the Province of Nova Scotia will amalgamate these nine DHAs into a unified provincial authority. The purpose of amalgamation is to enhance patient care and safety, streamline administration, and provide more timely and consistent access to care. Under this new structure, nine vice presidents will report to the president/CEO, with one position shared with the IWK. In addition, there will be two executive directors in each zone, one for medical leadership and one for operational leadership.

New Brunswick	http://www2.gnb.ca/content/gnb/en/departments/health.html

In 2008, New Brunswick reformed its healthcare system from eight regional health authorities (RHAs) to two health networks, in order to improve integration, consistency, and the effectiveness of the healthcare system. Since then, the New Brunswick Health Council has been responsible for oversight and accountability of the two health networks in the province (Horizon Health Network and Vitalite Health Network). Similar to RHAs across Canada, New Brunswick's health networks are responsible for delivering heathcare services and programs. The health networks are governed by a 17-member board of governors, appointed by the lieutenant governor, on the recommendation of the minister of health. The health networks receive support services, including supply chain, clinical engineering, information technology and telecommunications, and laundry and linen services, from FacilicorpNB, a public sector agency created by the New Brunswick government in 2008.

Newfoundland and Labrador	http://www.health.gov.nl.ca/health/

Currently, healthcare services and programs in Newfoundland and Labrador are delivered through four regional health authorities (RHAs). The RHAs are charged with the delivery, administration, and assessment of health and community services in a specified area. Each RHA delivers similar services across Newfoundland and Labrador, but are structured differently, using different divisions for lines of business. The programs and services delivered through RHAs cover the full spectrum of hospital and community services, including acute care hospital services, long-term care services, and community-based services. The RHAs are governed by a CEO and a voluntary board of trustees, who are appointed by the minister of health.

...continued

Appendix D, continued
Administrative Management Structure of Healthcare in the Provinces

Prince Edward Island	http://www.healthpei.ca/

In 1993, PEI created the first five regional health authorities in Canada. However, the RHA model was not effective for PEI because it required a large administrative structure for a small population. These boards were dissolved in 2005, with responsibility transferred to the Department of Health. The system changed once again in July 2010, with the government transferring power from the Department of Health and Wellness (renamed) to Health PEI, an arm's-length crown corporation. Currently, Health PEI is governed by a board of directors, which ensures that the approved programs are delivered in accordance with the Ministry of Health's priorities. Health PEI's organizational structure is arranged in seven divisions that cover the full spectrum of healthcare services. Each year, the Quality and Safety Council evaluates Health PEI's programs and services on the basis of a balanced scorecard system that measures achievement against numerous key performance indicators.

Queen's Policy Studies
Recent Publications

The Queen's Policy Studies Series is dedicated to the exploration of major public policy issues that confront governments and society in Canada and other nations.

Manuscript submission. We are pleased to consider new book proposals and manuscripts. Preliminary inquiries are welcome. A subvention is normally required for the publication of an academic book. Please direct questions or proposals to the Publications Unit by email at spspress@ queensu.ca, or visit our website at: www.queensu.ca/sps/books, or contact us by phone at (613) 533-2192.

Our books are available from good bookstores everywhere, including the Queen's University bookstore (http://www.campusbookstore.com/). McGill-Queen's University Press is the exclusive world representative and distributor of books in the series. A full catalogue and ordering information may be found on their website (**http://mqup.mcgill.ca/**).

For more information about new and backlist titles from Queen's Policy Studies, visit http://www.queensu.ca/sps/books.

School of Policy Studies

Handbook of Canadian Higher Education Laew, Theresa Shanahan, Michelle Nilson, and Li-Jeen Broshko (eds.) 2015. ISBN 978-1-55339-442-6

The Politics of Canadian Foreign Policy, 4th edition, Kim Richard Nossal, Stéphane Roussel, and Stéphane Paquin (eds.) 2015. ISBN 978-1-55339-443-3

Thinking Outside the Box: Innovation in Policy Ideas, Essays in Honour of Thomas J. Courchene, Keith G. Banting, Richard P. Chaykowski, and Steven F. Lehrer (eds.) 2015. ISBN 978-1-55339-429-7

Toward a Healthcare Strategy for Canadians, A. Scott Carson, Jeffrey Dixon, and Kim Richard Nossal (eds.) 2015. ISBN 978-1-55339-439-6

Work in a Warming World, Carla Lipsig-Mummé and Stephen McBride (eds.) 2015. ISBN 978-1-55339-432-7

Lord Beaconsfield and Sir John A. Macdonald: A Political and Personal Parallel, Michel W. Pharand (ed.) 2015. ISBN 978-1-55339-438-9

Canadian Public-Sector Financial Management, Second Edition, Andrew Graham 2014. ISBN 978-1-55339-426-6

The Multiculturalism Question: Debating Identity in 21st-Century Canada, Jack Jedwab (ed.) 2014. ISBN 978-1-55339-422-8

Government-Nonprofit Relations in Times of Recession, Rachel Laforest (ed.) 2013. ISBN 978-1-55339-327-6

Intellectual Disabilities and *Dual Diagnosis: An Interprofessional Clinical Guide for Healthcare Providers,* Bruce D. McCreary and Jessica Jones (eds.) 2013. ISBN 978-1-55339-331-3

Rethinking Higher Education: Participation, Research, and Differentiation, George Fallis 2013. ISBN 978-1-55339-333-7

Making Policy in Turbulent Times: Challenges and Prospects for Higher Education, Paul Axelrod, Roopa Desai Trilokekar, Theresa Shanahan, and Richard Wellen (eds.) 2013. ISBN 978-1-55339-332-0

Building More Effective Labour-Management Relationships, Richard P. Chaykowski and Robert S. Hickey (eds.) 2013. ISBN 978-1-55339-306-1

Navigationg on the Titanic: Economic Growth, Energy, and the Failure of Governance, Bryne Purchase 2013. ISBN 978-1-55339-330-6

Measuring the Value of a Postsecondary Education, Ken Norrie and Mary Catharine Lennon (eds.) 2013. ISBN 978-1-55339-325-2

Immigration, Integration, and Inclusion in Ontario Cities, Caroline Andrew, John Biles, Meyer Burstein, Victoria M. Esses, and Erin Tolley (eds.) 2012. ISBN 978-1-55339-292-7

Diverse Nations, Diverse Responses: Approaches to Social Cohesion in Immigrant Societies, Paul Spoonley and Erin Tolley (eds.) 2012. ISBN 978-1-55339-309-2

Making EI Work: Research from the Mowat Centre Employment Insurance Task Force, Keith Banting and Jon Medow (eds.) 2012. ISBN 978-1-55339-323-8

Managing Immigration and Diversity in Canada: A Transatlantic Dialogue in the New Age of Migration, Dan Rodríguez-García (ed.) 2012. ISBN 978-1-55339-289-7

International Perspectives: Integration and Inclusion, James Frideres and John Biles (eds.) 2012. ISBN 978-1-55339-317-7

Dynamic Negotiations: Teacher Labour Relations in Canadian Elementary and Secondary Education, Sara Slinn and Arthur Sweetman (eds.) 2012. ISBN 978-1-55339-304-7

Where to from Here? Keeping Medicare Sustainable, Stephen Duckett 2012. ISBN 978-1-55339-318-4

International Migration in Uncertain Times, John Nieuwenhuysen, Howard Duncan, and Stine Neerup (eds.) 2012. ISBN 978-1-55339-308-5

Centre for International and Defence Policy

Afghanistan in the Balance: Counterinsurgency, Comprehensive Approach, and Political Order, Hans-Georg Ehrhart, Sven Bernhard Gareis, and Charles Pentland (eds.), 2012. ISBN 978-1-55339-353-5

Institute of Intergovernmental Relations

Canada: The State of the Federation 2012, Loleen Berdahl, André Juneau, and Carolyn Hughes Tuohy (eds.), 2015. ISBN 978-1-55339-210-1

Canada: The State of the Federation 2011, Nadia Verrelli (ed.), 2014. ISBN 978-1-55339-207-1

Canada and the Crown: Essays on Constitutional Monarchy, D. Michael Jackson and Philippe Lagassé (eds.), 2013. ISBN 978-1-55339-204-0

Paradigm Freeze: Why It Is So Hard to Reform Health-Care Policy in Canada, Harvey Lazar, John N. Lavis, Pierre-Gerlier Forest, and John Church (eds.), 2013. ISBN 978-1-55339-324-5

Canada: The State of the Federation 2010, Matthew Mendelsohn, Joshua Hjartarson, and James Pearce (eds.), 2013. ISBN 978-1-55339-200-2

The Democratic Dilemma: Reforming Canada's Supreme Court, Nadia Verrelli (ed.), 2013. ISBN 978-1-55339-203-3